NEW DEVELOPMENTS IN MEDICAL RESEARCH

MEDICAL AND BIOLOGICAL FRONTIERS RESEARCH COMPENDIUM

New Developments in Medical Research

Additional books in this series can be found on Nova's website under the Series tab.

Additional e-books in this series can be found on Nova's website under the E-book tab.

NEW DEVELOPMENTS IN MEDICAL RESEARCH

MEDICAL AND BIOLOGICAL FRONTIERS RESEARCH COMPENDIUM

TSISANA SHARTAVA
EDITOR

NOVA BIOMEDICAL

New York

For permission to use material from this book please contact us:
Telephone 631-231-7269; Fax 631-231-8175
Web Site: http://www.novapublishers.com

Library of Congress Cataloging-in-Publication Data

ISBN: 978-1-62417-022-5

Library of Congress Control Number: 2012949635

Published by Nova Science Publishers, Inc. † New York

Contents

Preface

This book compiles articles from the International Journal of Medical and Biological Frontiers which publishes original research on the leading edge of research in biology and medicine. Some of the topics discussed include current advances in nucleic acid-based antiviral therapy; the role of platelet rich plasma injections in Achilles Tendonoses; advances in tissue engineering application for ligament repair; advances in ceramic bearings for total hip replacement and liver metastases of colorectal carcinoma.

Chapter 1 – In recent years, the emergence and reemergence of infectious viral diseases has promoted intense research to explore new approaches for drug development. Targeting of a specific viral gene(s) to inhibit viral replication is one of the newly developing strategies of experimental research. In this regard, nucleic acid (NA)-based antiviral agents, such as ribozymes, antisense oligonucleotides, aptamers, short interfering RNA, MicroRNAs (miRNAs), and artificial miRNAs (AmiRNAs), represent a new collection of potential gene targeting tools. These therapeutic sequences can be designed to target the viral genome or messenger RNAs (mRNAs), leading to down regulation of a specific viral gene. Cellular miRNAs and DNA virus-encoded miRNAs play important roles in viral replication and pathogenesis. Thus, silencing of these miRNAs using specific inhibitors, such as antagomirs or miRNA sponges, is another promising strategy for inhibition of viral replication. AmiRNAs are mimics of endogenous miRNAs, which can be designed to target viral mRNAs and inhibit viral infection with mutational tolerance. The NA-based antiviral strategy has been applied experimentally to inhibit many RNA and DNA viruses, such as the highly pathogenic avian influenza (H5N1), SARSCoV, Hepatitis C virus (HCV), and Hepatitis B virus (HBV).

This strategy has many advantages, particularly the drug specificity and high affinity to the viral gene targets. Here, the authors highlight current research progress in the field of viral gene targeting in regards to several viral diseases of both human and animal origin. Additionally, the authors discussed the limitations and pitfalls that pertain to this new class of antiviral therapies.

Chapter 2 – Tendon disorders include Achilles tendonoses and are common. Achilles tendonosis has poor results with conservative surgery and many patients eventually require surgical management. There has been an increasing interest in the use of platelet rich plasma for Achilles tendonosis supported by the fact that it is a less invasive treatment option with a good safety profile, and the availability of new devices for outpatient preparation and delivery. It is thought that platelet rich plasma injection for Achilles tendonosis is effective because of the high concentration of platelets it delivers. Although recent reviews report promising results of the use of platelet rich plasma in tendonosis, a recent systematic review of randomised controlled trials showed that platelet rich plasma was not more efficacious than placebo for Achilles tendonosis. There is only limited evidence in the literature supporting the use of platelet rich plasma in Achilles tendonosis, and it is based on animal studies and clinical studies with limitations. There is only one high quality randomised control study that compared platelet rich plasma with control saline injection in Achilles tendonosis, and showed no significant difference between both groups. Control subjects may have responded to saline injections as active therapy as these produce some local trauma and bleeding, and this has shown to have a stimulatory effect on the tendon. Injection of any fluid invariably changes the pressure-volume relationship within a given anatomical space and can potentially destroy pathological vascular and neural growth. The authors conclude that platelet rich plasma injection in Achilles tendonosis is effective not because of the high concentration of platelets it delivers, but due to the local injection effects of percutaneous tenotomy, local bleeding and changes in pressure-volume relationship.

Chapter 3 – Ligament injuries form a significant proportion of musculoskeletal injuries with resulting disability and mobidity to patients worldwide. Current treatment regimens may not result in the ligament achieving its pre-injury characteristics or function. The use of mesenchymal stem cells to repair injured ligament tissue is an emerging novel technique, that holds great promise due to its unique characteristics. This review highlights these characteristics, and what makes mesenchymal stem cells so amenable to use in tissue engineering in the arena of ligament regeneration. It discusses the current research evidence and clinical trials in the application of mesenchymal stem cells in ligament injury and the future challenges and potential of this exciting and expanding area of functional tissue engineering.

Chapter 4 – The search for the perfect bearing in hip arthroplasty remains elusive with all combinations proving over time to have their own idiosyncrasies, benefits and problems. It has become increasingly clear that it is the bearing couple which presents the major obstacle to increasing the longevity of hip arthroplasties. Over the years the femoral stem has evolved and most available prostheses in wide usage can boast survival data far in excess of what may have been expected a few deacades ago. Similarly although the debate over fixation methods of the acetabular component persists, expected survival of the shell is unlikely to be limited by wear. The use of ceramics as either ceramic on ceramic (COC) or ceramic on polyethylene (COP) has been a popular choice of surgeons worldwide during a period which has seen significant improvements in materials manufacture and machining tolerances. At the time of writing Ceramic on Metal is also undergoing trial.

Using COC or COP can be an attractive option; particularly in younger and more active patients with the likelihood of much improved longevity. Over recent years there has been increased focus on Metal-on-metal (MOM) articulations and metal ion levels due to wear and corrosion. Any factor resulting in high metal ion levels appears to be associated with an increased failure rate. Young females are one risk factor for failure, possibly due to their small size, and are therefore more likely to receive COC or COP bearings as a primary hip arthroplasty [2] COC or COP have the potential advantage of excellent wear characteristics from high wettablilty, scratch resistance and hardness – only diamond being harder. Zirconia rates 8.5 on Mohs scale of mineral hardness with diamond rating 10. Ceramics are inorganic, crystalline materials whose popularity in hip arthroplasty is growing - ceramic femoral heads are likely to overtake metallic heads in the National Joint Registry of England and Wales in numbers used.

Chapter 5 – The early detection of (especially malignant) focal liver lesions is of utmost importance. For example, the resection of liver metastases of some malignancies (including colorectal cancer) has been shown to improve the survival of the patients. Exact knowledge of the number, size, and regional distribution of colorectal liver metastases is essential to determine their resectability. Almost all colorectal liver metastases larger than 10mm are demonstrated with current imaging techniques but the detection of smaller colorectal liver metastases is still relatively poor.

One of the advantages of Magnetic Resonance Imaging (MRI) of the liver is the better soft tissue contrast (compared to other radiologic modalities), which reveals better detection and characterization of the colorectal liver metastases in question. Developments in MRI hardware and software and the availability of novel MRI contrast agents have further improved the diagnostic yield of MRI in lesion detection and characterization. Although the primary modalities for liver imaging are ultrasound and Computed Tomography, recent studies have suggested that MRI is the most sensitive method for detecting small colorectal liver metastases and MRI is now considered the pre-operative standard.

Two recent developments in MRI sequences for the upper abdomen comprise (unenhanced) diffusion-weighted imaging (DWI) and T1-weighted keyhole-based dynamic contrast-enhanced MRI (T1w DCE MRI).

DWI using low b-values, allows improved detection ($b=10s/mm^2$) of (especially) small (<10mm) colorectal liver metastases because of the black-blood effect and thus is useful as a road map sequence. The black-blood effect facilitates detection of colorectal liver metastases by better differentiation between vascular branches, colorectal liver metastases and surrounding liver parenchyma. Using higher b-values, the calculation of Apparent Diffusion Coefficient (ADC) value, true diffusion coefficient (D) and the perfusion fraction f has been used for the characterization of focal liver lesions. The true diffusion coefficient D is a parameter for the (patho)physiologic molecular diffusion of focal liver lesions. It therefore permits characterization of tissues and pathologic conditions. The perfusion fraction f is a parameter for the (patho)physiologic microperfusion of focal liver lesions.

T1w keyhole-based DCE MRI enables perfusion imaging of the liver with high temporal and spatial resolution with full liver coverage. T1w keyhole-based DCE MRI (4D THRIVE sequence) improves the evaluation of focal liver lesions by providing multiple arterial and venous phases and allows the calculation of parametric maps displaying different perfusion parameters using pharmacokinetic models. The use of 4D THRIVE with parametric mapping enables spatially matching tumour vascular characteristics such as blood volume, blood flow, permeability and leakage space. Parametric maps therefore have the advantage that they can be used in clinical practice and might also be useful for follow-up purposes (e.g. during therapy in an oncological setting).

Chapter 6 – Cheese is a versatile, nutrient-dense dairy food, i.e. a good source of protein, vitamins and minerals particularly calcium and phosphorus, which is an important component in highly consumed convenience foods. However, cheese is perceived as being high in saturated fat, which might contribute to risks of atherosclerosis, and sodium. There is considerable evidence that excess or high sodium intake, which is the case in Western countries, is associated with hypertension and strokes, hence, dietary guidelines recommend that sodium intake be reduced.

This review covers the scientific and technological aspects of the role of sodium in cheese manufacture and functional properties and highlights various strategies for reducing the sodium. The focus is on natural cheese, made from milk by acid and/or rennet-coagulation, and process cheese. This cheese differs from natural cheese in that it is made from natural cheese or casein, which is blended with the necessary emulsifying salts and in the presence of heat, leading to the formation of a homogeneous product with extended shelf-life. Process cheese has numerous end-use applications in processed foods, which counts for ~75% of the dietary sodium in industrialized diets.

The source of sodium in cheese is mainly the added salt (sodium chloride). Salt acts primarily as food preservative and flavor enhancer and also interacts with major components in the cheese and thereby affecting the functionality, e.g. salt increases the protein hydration during manufacture which affects the stability and textural properties. Process cheese contains much higher sodium content, compared to natural cheese, due to the necessity of using emulsifying salts, such as sodium citrate and phosphate. These salts are crucial for the hydration of the protein, emulsification of fat and the stability of the final product.

Strategies for reducing sodium in cheese are mainly outlined in the reduction of the salt and/or emulsifying salts used and their substitution by the potassium equivalents salts. However, these strategies present many challenges, such as adverse effects on flavor and microbiological stability. In process cheese, a high reduction of emulsifying salts does not allow for the formation of a homogeneous end product. Recent approaches of reducing emulsifying salts used are also discussed, such as utilizing of emulsifiers or protein hydrolyzates in the manufacture of cheese.

A final section in this review is about the future of low sodium cheese manufacture, including suggestions for reducing sodium that has not been systematically investigated in research on various cheese types.

Chapter 7 – Alterations in Angiotensin II (Ang II) and Peroxisome Proliferator-Activated Receptor-γ (PPAR-γ) affect cardiovascular diseases, diabetes and metabolic disorders, suggesting that these two systems intersect at some common biochemical pathways. Elucidating common cellular signaling factors between these two systems are important for better design of combinatorial drugs for treating patients with these disorders. Inhibitors of Ang II and agonists of PPAR-γ appear to have similar and beneficial effects. Ang II, a pro-fibrotic factor, enhances collagen synthesis and contributes to adverse remodeling in case of hypertensive heart diseases that damage tissue structure and alter cardiac function. In contrast, increased PPAR-γ activity inhibits collagen synthesis, reduces fibrosis and adverse remodeling of the cardiac tissue. Treatments with Ang II blockers or with PPAR-γ agonists improve cardiac function. These effects are evident in cardiac myofibroblasts, which appear at the site of myocardial infarction. Cardiac myofibroblasts are the major cell types involved in tissue repair and remodeling. In this article, the authors review Ang II and PPAR-γ pathways operative in cardiac myofibroblasts and provide evidence for interactions between these two systems.

Chapter 8 – The essential feature of sex common to both bacteria and eukaryotes is information exchange (recombination) between two genomic DNA molecules derived from different individuals. In bacteria a naturally occurring sexual process termed transformation is characterized by transfer of DNA from one bacterium to another, followed by recombination between the resident DNA and the incoming DNA. In eukaryotes, the sexual cycle involves recombination between paired DNA molecules (chromosomes) in which the two DNA molecules are derived from two different parents. This process occurs in diploid cells during meiosis, and is followed by formation of haploid gametes. The fusion of gametes from different individuals to generate diploid progeny completes the eukaryotic sexual cycle.

DNA damage appears to be a fundamental problem for life. Here, the authors present evidence for the view that the enzymatic machinery for carrying out recombination, during transformation in bacteria and meiosis in eukaryotes, is an adaptation for DNA repair. Both bacterial and eukaryotic cells, generally, contain repair enzymes that are adept at removing DNA damages. However there are limits to the capability of cells during ordinary cell divisions to repair their DNA. Damages causing loss of information in both DNA strands (double-strand damages) are particularly difficult to handle since they require information from a second homologous chromosome. A repair process referred to as homologous recombinational repair (HRR) appears designed to carry out repair of such double-strand damages.

Evidence is presented for the hypothesis that sexual processes (i.e. transformation in bacteria and meiosis in eukaryotes) are maintained as evolutionary adaptations to facilitate HRR. In bacteria and microbial eukaryotes the problem of DNA damages is particularly acute during periods of stress, especially oxidative stress. It is during such stressful conditions that sex (which facilitates HRR) tends to occur in these facultatively sexual organisms. In multicellular eukaryotes, meiosis facilitates HRR and appears to be designed to protect against damages to the DNA of gametes, thus minimizing infertility and defective progeny.

Another consequence of recombination during sex is increased genetic variation among progeny. Increased variation appears to have significant consequences at the population level over the long-term and is sometimes considered the primary adaptive function of sex. However, the authors present evidence that the machinery for sexual recombination is maintained primarily by the strong short-term advantage of passing relatively undamaged DNA from one generation to the next. The genetic variation that is generated appears to be a byproduct of HRR.

Chapter 9 – Amyotrophic lateral sclerosis (ALS) is a progressive neurodegenerative disease affecting brain, brainstem and spinal cord motor neurons.

Muscle weakness is a hallmark sign in ALS, occurring in approximately 60% of patients. Early symptoms vary with each individual, but usually include tripping, dropping things, abnormal fatigue of the arms and/or legs, slurred speech, muscle cramps and twitches and/or uncontrollable periods of laughing or crying. There are spinal-onset or bulbar-onset disease forms, according to the first involvement of limbs or speech/swallowing muscles, respectively. With voluntary muscles progressively affected, patients in the later stages of the disease may become totally paralyzed.

In this paper, ALS diagnostic issues, and methods and techniques for assessing severity of motor deficits are discussed. Various treatment options for limb and bulbar palsies are reviewed: in addition to drugs, assistive rehabilitation approaches are presented, from physiotherapy to occupational therapy, from respiratory exercises to swallowing manoeuvres and postures.

Chapter 10 – Serum concentration of chromium and oxidative stress (malondialdehyde) were measured in Types I and II diabetic patients. The nature of the relationship between serum chromium and oxidative stress was also assessed in Types I and II diabetic patients. Results showed that both Types I and II diabetes were associated with a significantly elevated serum chromium levels. Serum chromium increased by 22.6% in Type I diabetic patients and 25.3% in their Type II counterparts, $p < 0.05$. Oxidative stress level as indicated by serum malondialdehyde (MDA) was also elevated in both Type I and Type II diabetes. Malondialdehyde concentration was 7.44 ± 0.53 µmol and 9.88 ± 0.91 µmol in Types I and II diabetic patients respectively, values that are higher than the control serum malondialdehyde concentration of 5.51 ± 0.52 µmol, $p < 0.05$.

The correlation between serum chromium and oxidative stress in both controls and Types I and II diabetic patients shows a weak relationship between these parameters. This indicates the difference in the pattern of the influence played by this metal in the phenomenon of oxidative stress induced by diabetes mellitus and the differences in the pathogenesis, etiology and severity of types I and II diabetes. The elevated levels of serum chromium can potentiate further production of reactive oxygen species, and hence contribute to an increase in the oxidative stress phenomenon already found to be associated with both Types I and II diabetes.

Chapter 11 – The "Biomaterial Consensus Conference" in 1983, reached an agreement on the definition of biomaterial: the substance (or combination of substances), natural or synthetic, that can be used alone or in combination, and for a variable period of time, that can treat, increase or replace a function of the body. It can therefore be defined as all materials reachable as metals and alloys, ceramics, carbon derivatives, polymers and biological tissues, which have been used and are still used in surgical treatments. Only some of these are components of the prostheses used today in surgery for inguinal hernia.

Amid's classification proposed in 1997, provides three sets of synthetic prostheses in response to the diameter of the pores, but basically marking guidelines application of different prosthetic materials has now been relegated due to the emergence of next-generation prosthesis.

They seek to achieve the best possible integration into the tissues, improve their performance on all interfaces and avoid complications.

Chapter 12 – Human melanin is synthesized in melanosomes located in melanocytes of the skin, hair, eyes, ears, and leptomeninges. Melanin not only determines skin color, but also protects the skin from UV damage by absorbing UV light. Congenital pigmentary disorders that result in skin and hair depigmentation, such as Hermenksky Pudluk Syndrome, Chediak Higashi Syndrome, and Griscelli Syndrome are due to various gene mutations that cause defects in melanin synthesis. Excessive production of melanin, which occurs in response to UV-induced DNA damage, inflammation, or other skin injuries, however, can result in skin hyperpigmentation including freckles, melasma, solar lentigo, age spots, and post-inflammatory hyperpigmentation. In this chapter the authors review the synthesis of melanin, the signaling pathways related to the regulation of melanogenesis, the factors influencing melanogenesis and various pigmentation disorders, as well as the effectiveness of various natural products at reducing hyperpigmentation.

In: Medical and Biological Frontiers Research Compendium ISBN: 978-1-62417-022-5
Editor: Tsisana Shartava

Chapter 1

Current Advances in Nucleic Acid Based Antiviral Therapy

Maged Gomaa Hemida, Xin Ye, Mary Zhang, Paul J. Hanson, Bruce McManus and Decheng Yang*

Department of Pathology and Laboratory Medicine, University of British Columbia, James Hogg Research Centre, Institute for Heart + Lung Health, Vancouver, Canada

Abstract

In recent years, the emergence and reemergence of infectious viral diseases has promoted intense research to explore new approaches for drug development. Targeting of a specific viral gene(s) to inhibit viral replication is one of the newly developing strategies of experimental research. In this regard, nucleic acid (NA)-based antiviral agents, such as ribozymes, antisense oligonucleotides, aptamers, short interfering RNA, MicroRNAs (miRNAs), and artificial miRNAs (AmiRNAs), represent a new collection of potential gene targeting tools. These therapeutic sequences can be designed to target the viral genome or messenger RNAs (mRNAs), leading to down regulation of a specific viral gene. Cellular miRNAs and DNA virus-encoded miRNAs play important roles in viral replication and pathogenesis. Thus, silencing of these miRNAs using specific inhibitors, such as antagomirs or miRNA sponges, is another promising strategy for inhibition of viral replication. AmiRNAs are mimics of endogenous miRNAs, which can be designed to target viral mRNAs and inhibit viral infection with mutational tolerance. The NA-based antiviral strategy has been applied experimentally to inhibit many RNA and DNA viruses, such as the highly pathogenic avian influenza (H5N1), SARSCoV, Hepatitis C virus (HCV), and Hepatitis B virus (HBV).

This strategy has many advantages, particularly the drug specificity and high affinity to the viral gene targets. Here, we highlight current research progress in the field of viral gene targeting in regards to several viral diseases of both human and animal origin.

* Corresponding Author: Dr. Decheng Yang, 166-1081 Burrard Street, The Heart + Lung Institute, St. Paul's Hospital, Vancouver, B. C., V6Z 1Y6, Canada. Tel (604) 682-2344 Ext. 62872,Fax (604) 806-9274. E-mail: *decheng.yang@hli.ubc.ca.*

Additionally, we discussed the limitations and pitfalls that pertain to this new class of antiviral therapies.

1. Introduction

Viruses are a unique group of pathogens characterized by many criteria making their treatment or even prophylaxis very difficult. They are obligate intracellular parasites. In addition, high rates of mutation and even the viral genome itself being infectious are especially apparent among several types of RNA viruses. Another concern is the emergence of new viruses, such as the severe acute respiratory syndrome coronavirus (SARSCoV) outbreak in 2002 in China, Tawian and Canada [1]. Several approaches have been used for either treatment and/or prevention such as; virusides, immunomodulators, and antiviral drugs with minimal success [2].

New approaches in the field of antiviral therapy and prophylaxes are in urgent need. Currently, there are three major gene silencing approaches that can be implemented to selectively target and cleave mRNAs which include, single stranded antisense oligonucleotides, ribozymes, and RNA interference (RNAi) molecules, as well as other approaches that may target proteins such as aptamers [3]. These approaches are aimed at inhibition of a specific protein at the level of translation by targeting the associated mRNA rather than binding directly to the protein to modify its function, as conventional drugs did [3]. Zamenick and Stephanson used nucleic acid (NA)-based agents such as oligonucleotides for the first time to inhibit the replication of Rous sarcoma virus *in vitro* [4, 5]. Since then, several studies focused on targeting essential viral genes and proteins (6) however, high viral mutation rates limit the success of this antiviral strategy [6]. Using NA-based therapeutic molecules is a new trend in antiviral research.

This strategy is based on targeting of specific viral genes essential to viral replication, resulting in the inhibition of virus replication [7]. The NA-based antiviral strategies include aptamers, antisense oligonucleotides, ribozymes and the RNA interference [7]. Our goal is to summarize the recent progress in the development of each of these new antiviral agents, which includes discussion of their mechanisms of action, advantages and the major concerns associated with this antiviral approach.

2. NA-Based Antiviral Agents and Their Mechanism of Actions

The ultimate goal of using the nucleic acid molecules as antiviral agents is to ensure the specific and effective targeting of viral genes and/or proteins (for aptamers) without any deleterious effects on the host cells. In this portion, we will mainly focus on the mechanism of action for each category of antiviral agent such as ribozymes, antisense oligonucleotides, and the RNAi molecules in addition to aptamers, which are designed to target certain viral proteins.

2.1. Ribozymes and Deoxyribozymes

Ribozymes are short nucleic acid molecules with enzymatic activity. They have the ability to recognize and cleave a specific target sites in a certain messenger RNA (mRNA) (Figure 1) [8]. Ribozymes are currently considered to be one of the most promising antiviral agents due to their ability to downregulate the expression of several viral genes [8].

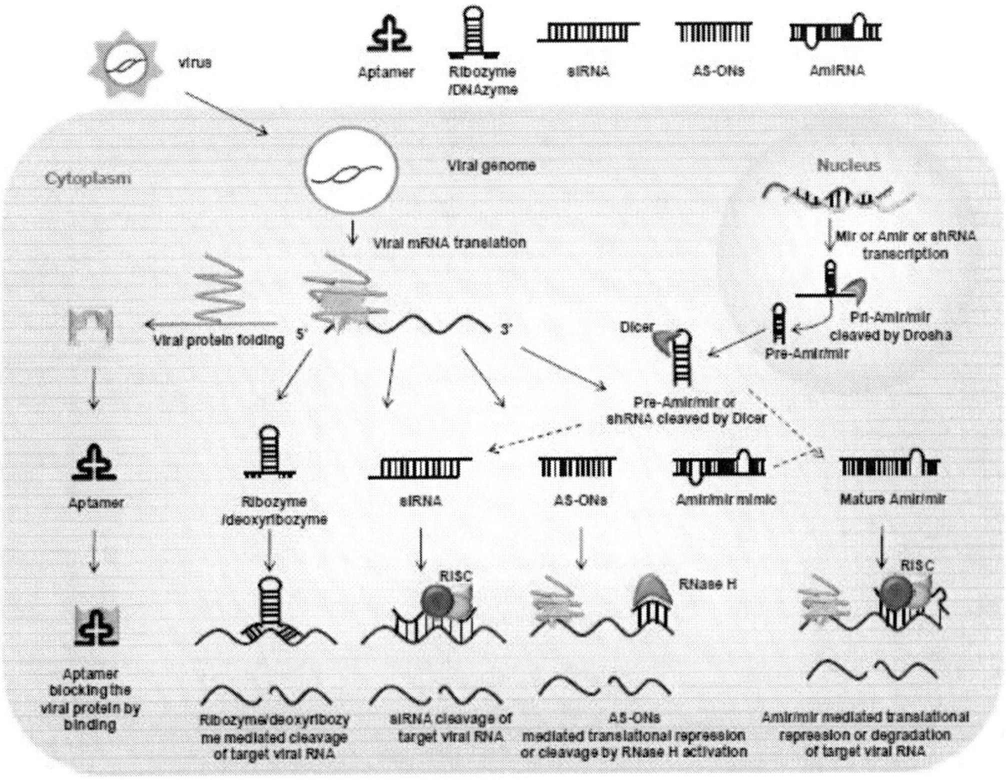

Figure 1. Mechanisms of action of the NA-based antiviral agents. Nucleic acid-based antiviral agents can be delivered by either transfection into the cells (aptamers, ribozymes/DNAzymes, siRNA, AS-ONs or AmiR/miRNA mimics) or vector expression of the transcripts in the cells (AmiR/miRNA or shRNA). Selected Aptamers are capable of binding to certain viral proteins and block their activity leading to the inhibition of viral replication. Ribozymes/DNAzymes with their enzymatic activity can recognize and cleave the target viral RNA in a sequence specific manner. AS-ONs, often optimized by chemical modification, have high affinities to their targets and are able to induce blockage of the viral protein translation by hindering the ribosome or cleavage of the target RNA by recruiting RNase H. siRNA and shRNA are designed perfectly matching with the target sequence of viral RNA. They hybridize with the viral RNA and trigger the RISC-mediated cleavage of the targets. AmiR/miRNA are similar to siRNA but harboring mismatches with their target sequences. They can bind to their targets, causing the degradation of the target viral RNA or inhibition of gene translation of the virus.

Presently, they are only used in catalyzing the cleavage of RNA molecules. However, new modifications have been made, which allow ribozymes to catalyze the enzymatic degradation of DNA molecules. This new modification is termed DNA enzymes, DNAzymes or deoxyribozymes [8].

Ribozymes are generally classified according to their size, mechanism of action and structure, which includes the distinction of hammerhead, hairpin, hepatitis delta and the varkud satellite ribozymes [8]. Ribozymes may be designed in a way to target several potential sites in any mRNA. This multisite potential makes them promising antiviral agents (Table 1) [9]. In theory, ribozymes may be designed to degrade and destruct any RNA molecule regardless its origin [10]. Both the hammerhead and the hairpin ribozymes were used to combat HIV and showed promising results (Table 2) [11-13].

Table 1. NA-based antiviral agents

NA agent	Mechanism of Action	Advantages	Disadvantages	Ref.
Ribozymes.	Enzymatic cleavage of target mRNA.	-Target specificity for host or viral factors. -induce little or no immune response.	-Point mutations results in loss of their function. -Degree of efficacy depends on the target.	[10]
Aptamers.	- Recognize their targets based on the complementation in shape. - Targeting protein directly and bind to them resulting in alteration of their function.	-Can block the function of one domain of protein without affecting its three-dimensional structure. -Can disrupt the interaction between different proteins. -High affinity binding and specificity. -Trigger negligible immune response. -Can be designed and target various molecules such as proteins, carbohydrates, nucleic acids and even organisms.	-Only designed for extracellular targets. -Carry lots of electric charges. -High cost of production especially at the beginning of their discovery.	[202]
AS-ODs.	- AS-ODs induce translation arrest by - block ribosome reading -RNase H mediated cleavage of mRNA -Compete with ribosome for the binding to mRNA-5'UTR	-Specific targeting. -Easy to design. -Can be designed to target several regions of one mRNA.	-Easy to degrade in biological environment. - relatively their large molecular weight make them difficult to be uptake by cells. -Potential toxicity.	[69, 171]
siRNA/ shRNA.	-Enzymatic cleavage of target mRNA -Degradation of target mRNA	-Highly specific. - Can target several stages of virus replication. -Can be designed to target virus and/or host genes. -Trigger little immune response.	-Efficacy is dependent on the target gene. -Point mutation result in loss of function. - delivery limitations. - often result in viral escape mutants - off-target effect.	[25, 43]
miRNA/ amiRNA.	-Inhibits mRNA translation by destabilization of mRNA and block translation initiation and elongation	- Easily to synthesis. -Can target many genes at the same time. -mutation tolerance.	delivery limitations. -instability. - off-target effect.	[48, 109]

2.2. Aptamers

Most NA-based antiviral agents act by targeting a certain RNA or DNA sequence; however, aptamers are a class of nucleic acid ligands with high affinity binding to their target molecules because they can bind only to certain viral and/or host protein targets. Unlike the other NA-based molecules, aptamers act on the protein level rather the mRNA level (Figure 1). This specific binding to their targets is very similar to the binding of the monoclonal antibodies to certain epitopes (Figure 1). This affinity biding is very specific and mainly depends on the complementation between the aptamer and its target protein [14]. This binding usually affects the function of the target protein [15]. They are produced by process called systematic evolution of ligands by exponential enrichment (SELEX) [16]. Simply, aptamers could be prepared from a random pool of nucleic acid sequences and can be selected and separated by repeated cycles of separation and amplification. This is mainly based on their affinity binding to their target sequence [17]. Some RNA aptamers such as Pegaptanib have been approved for treatment of some ocular vascular diseases [18]. Aptamers have been used as antiviral agents for several viruses such as Human immunodeficiency virus (HIV), Hepatitis B Virus (HBV), Hepatitis C virus (HCV), influenza avian viruses myeloblastosis virus and human cytomegalovirus (Table 2) [19-24]. Aptamers may be used to inhibit the viral replication or for target based inhibition as in case of some DNA aptamers designed to block the receptor binding for influenza A virus [20].

Table 2. NA-based molecules targeting different virus genes

Virus	Family	Genome	NA agent	Viral target	Reference
				HA	
				PB1	[20, 202, 203]
Influenza	*Orthomyxoviridae*	ss RNA (-)	Aptamers	PB1, PB2, PA, and NP	[67]
			Ribozymes	NP, PA	[204]
			AS-ONs	M2 splice junction	[205]
			siRNA	PB1	[206]
			shRNA	NS3, helicase, RdRp, and	[207]
			miRNA	IRES	[23, 208-211]
HCV	*Flavivirdae*	ss RNA (+)	Aptamers	IRES	[212]
			Ribozymes	5'UTR	[213]
			AS-ONs	NS5B	[84, 85, 214]
			siRNA	La, PTB, hVAP-33	[215]
			shRNA	N, helicase,	[216, 217]
SARS-CoV	*Coronaviridae*	ss RNA (+)	Aptamers	NTPase/Helicase	[218]
			Ribozymes	Viral RNA	[219]
			AS-ONs	E, M, S, N	[94, 220]
			siRNA	Rep 1 A, and Leader	[221]
			shRNAs-	N	[222]
RSV	*Paramyxoviridae*	ss RNA (-)	AS-ONs	L and M2	[118, 223]
			siRNA	N, P, E, F, and SH	[224]
			shRNA	N, and L	[225-228]
HIV	*Retroviridae*	RNA (+)	Aptamers	Tat, TAR, Rev, gp120	[9, 229]
			Ribozymes	Gag, LTR,	[230-232]
			AS-ONs	Rev, TAR, LTR, and Tat	[104, 105]
			siRNA	Rev, Gag, Tat, TAR, LTR,	[104, 105, 233,
			shRNA	and Nef	234]
CVB3	*Picornaviridae*	RNA (+)	AS-ONs	Rev, Gag, Tat, and Nef	[135, 235]
			siRNA	5'UTR, IRES, 3'UTR	[125, 126, 129,
			shRNA	2A, IRES, 3C, 3D, VP1,	173]
	Rhabdoviridae	ss RNA (-)	siRNA	2C	[130, 131, 216]
				VP1, and 3D, 5' and	[236]
				3'UTR	

Table 2. (Continued)

Virus	Family	Genome	NA agent	Viral target	Reference
Rabies HBV HSV HCMV HPV	*Hepadnaviridae* *Herpesviridae* *Herpesviridae* *Herpesviridae*	ds DNA ds DNA ds DNA ds DNA	amiRNA Ribozymes Aptamers AS-ONs siRNA shRNA Ribozymes Aptamers AS-ONs siRNA shRNA Aptamers AS-ONs siRNA shRNA Ribozymes Aptamers AS-ONs siRNA shRNA	N N S P Core , N HBsAg, C C, S, P, and X UL20 US11 IE4, IE5 UL27, UL29, E gD, gE UL84 IE2 UL54, UL122 UL54, IE86 E6, E7and and E6/E7 E6, E7 E6, E7 E6, E7 E6, E7	[61] [237] [22] [238] [239, 240] [240-242] [243] [244] [245] [246, 247] [243, 246] [248] [171] [142, 143] [249, 250] [153, 251] [252] [157] [165, 253, 254] [249]

2.3. Antisense Oligonucleotides

Antisense oligonucleotides (AS-ONs) are single stranded DNA fragments (15-20 nucleotides) [3] that can bind to their complementary sequence in any mRNA. They form a DNA-RNA complex that can inhibit the translation of protein encoded by this mRNA.

Antisense may work at different stages of protein synthesis. On the level of transcription they may bind to certain target DNA in the nucleus leading to inhibition of its transcription. AS-ONs may also target specific nuclear localization signals of certain proteins, which results in the inhibition of the transport of these transcripts to the cytoplasm [25]. AS-ONs may exert their actions by several mechanisms (Figure 1 and Table 1). The first one is the induction of the RNase H cleavage of target mRNA by AS-ONs, resulting in the inhibition on the translation.

The other mechanism is targeting of the 5' end of the mRNA, resulting in the prevention of binding and the assembly of the translation machineries [3]. These AS-ONs undergo rapid degradation by the host cells nucleases. To date, three generations of chemically modified AS-ONs have been developed to overcome this rapid nuclease degradation [26].

In the first generation, one oxygen atom in the phosphodiester bond is replaced with sulfur atom. This approach has been used for example to inhibit HIV replication [27]. This modification resulted in increasing the nuclease resistance and consequently increasing their serum half life time up to 9-10 h compared to the non-modified AS-ON molecules [3].

The second generation is the AS-ON molecules containing nucleotides with alkyl modification at the 2' position in the ribose, termed 2'-O-methy RNA. This approach cannot trigger the RNAse H activity and their action depends on the steric blockage of the ribosome [28]. The third generation comprises a wide range of modifications; the most important one is the locked nucleic acid (LNA). In this modification, there is a methylene bridge which connects the 2'-oxygen of the ribose group [29]. This approach has been used to inhibit the replication of many viruses, such as HIV-1 Tat gene [30]. The AS-ONs have been used successfully to either inhibit or decrease the expression levels of key genes involved in several viral diseases such as HCV, H5N1 influenza virus, West Nile virus, and HIV [31-36], which will be discussed below.

2.4. siRNA and shRNA

The small interfering RNA (siRNA) was discovered in 1998 [37]. Elbashir and his colleagues in 2001 started to use them for the first time as NA-based therapeutic molecules. They reported the silencing of some genes in the mammalian cells [38, 39]. Since that time, people have been exploring the possibility of using siRNAs as antiviral agents, in fact, several siRNAs are in clinical trials now [40]. The strategy is to use siRNAs on a large scale to silence important viral genes on the mRNA level, leading to the subsequent inhibition of viral replication [41]. One of the advantages of siRNA technology is the relatively small size (about 21 nucleotides) of the molecule, which can bypass the interferon response in the mammalian cells [42]. There are two common ways to use the siRNA technology; the first is the use of chemically synthesized double stranded siRNA (Figure 1). The second is the use of the vector-based short hairpin RNA (shRNA) [43]. The phenomenon of RNA interference (RNAi) is a natural process through which knocking down of certain gene is achieved using host cell machinery. Simply, the presence of dsRNA molecules in the host cell initiates several processes, leading to their cleavage into small RNA molecules (about 21 nucleotides in length) by the RNAse III enzyme (Dicer). These siRNA molecules are then loaded onto the RNA induced silencing complex (RISC), resulting in degradation of the target RNA [44]. In the light of the mechanism of this process, several studies implemented this technology for limiting the expression levels of certain genes. In these studies, they used chemically synthesized siRNA molecules. This technology has shown a promising trend across different fields which includes inhibiting several viral genes which resulted in downregulation of the viruses replication [45]. Respiratory syncytial virus (RSV) was one of the first viruses in which RNAi technology was used to inhibit its replication by targeting some of its genes [117].

2.5. miRNAs and Artificial miRNAs

miRNAs are a group of endogenous small non coding RNAs ranging from 18- 23 nucleotides (nt) in length [46]. They are involved in the regulation of gene expression in a wide range of biological processes, as well as in the regulation of different viral infections [47]. Meanwhile, several viruses, especially the DNA viruses, may encode their own miRNAs, which are involved in their pathogenesis and infection. Therefore silencing these miRNAs may represent a novel antiviral therapeutic approach [48]. The biogenesis of miRNAs is well understood now [49-52]. Briefly, the miRNAs encoded genes are transcribed in the nucleus by the RNA polymerase II enzyme into pri-miRNAs. These pri-miRNAs are subjected to another cleavage modification in the nucleus, giving rise to pre-miRNAs (hairpin like structures) using another enzyme that resides in the nucleus, called Drosha. This is generally accomplished with the help of some cellular factors, such as the DGCR8/Pasha. The pre-miRNAs are transported to the cytoplasm using special fairy called the Exportein-5 in a RAN GTP dependant manner. In the cytoplasm, the pre-miRNAs are further modified through cleavage by another enzyme called Dicer, to produce short miRNA duplex. One of the two strands is usually undergoes degradation by cellular nucleases, while the other remains as a mature miRNA (Figure 1). Detailed description of the miRNA biogenesis can be found also elsewhere [50-53]. The seeding region of miRNA (the 2-7 nt in relation to the 5' end of the mRNA) was found to play an important role in the mechanism of action of each miRNA. For example, if the miRNA displays high degree of complementation between its seeding region and the target mRNA sequence, the result may be the cleavage of this target mRNA however, if there is a low degree of complementation between the previously mentioned sequences, this will result in translational repression of the target gene [54, 55]. Using miRNAs as antiviral therapy has been approached from several different aspects, for example; silencing of virus encoded miRNAs may result in the inhibition of its replication, as in case of SV40, EBV, and HIV [56-58]. On the other hand, manipulating certain host cell miRNAs involved in the viral replication may represent one of the promising antiviral strategies as in case of silencing of miR-122, which resulted in the inhibition of HCV replication [59]. Artificial microRNAs (AmiRs) are synthetic miRNAs designed to specifically target and downregulate certain genes. AmiRs represent the next logical step for the use of miRNAs as antiviral therapy. They act in the same manner as endogenous miRNAs (Figure 1) and they have been recently used as antiviral agents by targeting some viral genes involved in the viral pathogenesis and replication (Table 2) [60]. Several studies have designed and used the AmiRs to inhibit the replication of HIV and Rabies viruses [60, 61].

3. Uses of NA-Based Approaches for Inhibiting Different Viruses

Several NA-based antiviral agents have been designed to target and inhibit key genes and proteins involved in the replication of many RNA and DNA viruses. This approach resulted in the inhibition of those viruses replication. In the following section we will highlight the progress of this novel antiviral therapeutic approach for many viruses.

3.A. RNA Viruses

NA-based antiviral agents used for many RNA viruses with different genome (single stranded, segmented and double stranded) and different sense of genome (ssRNA (+), and ssRNA (-)).

3.A.1. Influenza Virus

Influenza viruses are group of single stranded RNA viruses having segmented genome (7-8 segments). They belong to the family *Orthomyxoviridaes* and there are three types of influenza viruses (A, B, and C) based on their antigenic and genetic properties [62]. Currently, there are two common approaches for either the treatment or prophylaxis of influenza viral infection including the antiviral drugs and the influenza virus vaccines, respectively. Those two approaches have been used for some time now, however, their roles in either treatment or prophylaxes of influenza viruses is still questionable [63]. Due to the high mutation frequency of influenza viruses, a new approach targeting the highly conserved regions of the viral genome could be the most realistic antiviral approach for these kinds of viruses. Several NA-based approaches targeting different genes of influenza virus have been explored. These antiviral agents adopt several strategies to combat influenza virus at different levels such as; induction of wide spectrum of antiviral immunity, inhibiting virus replication and suppression of viral gene expression by cleavage and degradation of the viral mRNAs [64, 65]. These approaches resulted in a significant reduction of the influenza virus particle formation [16, 66-69]. AS-ODs have been designed to target influenza A virus polymerase *PB1* gene. This approach was successful in the inhibition of the virus replication in cell culture and achieved a reduction in the number of virus plaques up to 10^6 [68]. Another study designed different antisense phosphothioate molecules targeting the starting codon of *PB2* and PA genes respectively. These AS-ODs delivered to the Clone 76 cells in liposome encapsulated form and. resulted in the significant inhibition of virus replication [70]. Another approach to inhibit influenza virus replication in cell culture is the use of specific aptamers to target the *PB1* gene. This approach achieved 93.5 % reduction of viral replication [66, 67]. The segmented nature of the genome makes it an ideal target for several siRNA molecules at the same time. Most viral genes play essential roles during virus replication. This approach enables us to use a combination of different siRNA molecules targeting different genes at the same time. This will minimize the chance of developing viral resistance or escape mutants due to the use of single siRNA molecule as well [66]. According to the same study they designed 20 siRNAs molecules targeting different influenza virus genes such as (NP, PB1, PB2, M and NSP) but not the HA and NA. They assessed the inhibitory effects of those siRNAs on the virus replication and found that some siRNAs were able to inhibit the virus replication in both cell culture and embryonated eggs. The siRNAs designed to target the NP and PA genes led to the inhibition of the mRNA of not only the corresponding genes but also the vRNA and the complementary RNA strand (cRNA). Theses potent inhibitory effects were also observed in Vero cells lacking the interferon genes. This confirmed the independent effect of those siRNA molecules from the action of different types of interferons, which may lead to the global shutdown of transcription of the host cell genes during some viral infection [66]. Although this NA-based approach as antiviral therapy against influenza virus showed promising results, many challenges facing this new approach still exist and will be discussed in Section 5.

3.A.2. Hepatitis C Virus (HCV)

According to the most recent epidemiological studies, more than 3% of the human populations are affected by the HCV. This virus cause liver cirrhosis, hepatocellular carcinoma and death [71]. There is no available vaccine so far and the only available treatment is the use of combination between the interferon alpha and the ribavirin. These treatments usually result in different side effects such as depression, hemolytic anemia and fever [72]. Thus, targeting the HCV genome using different NA-based molecules could be one of the most promising options at present. The HCV genome is a single stranded positive sense RNA and the single open reading frame is flanked at the 5' and 3' untranslated regions (UTRs). The 5'UTR is about 324-341 nucleotides in length and harbors an internal ribosome entry site (IRES) which plays important roles in translation of the viral RNA in a cap-independent manner [73]. The translated single polyprotein is further processed into four structural (Core, E1, E2/p7) and six nonstructural proteins (NS2, NS3, NA4a, NS5a and NS5B) [74, 75], which are potential targets for drug design. Antisense oligonucleotides have been designed to inhibit HCV replication in several studies [76-79]. The most promising approach was the design of 20-mer phosphorothioate (PO-ON AS-ON) targeting specific sequence around the initiation codon near the 5'UTR. This siRNA, called ISIS 14803 (Hepa Sense ^{TM}), showed marked inhibition of HCV replication *in vitro*. The application of ribozymes represents another approach used to target HCV genome and inhibit its replication. Several ribozymes have been designed to target the 5'UTR and showed great reduction in the virus replication up to 50 % [80]. One of the most promising targets for ribozymes is the nucleotide 195 in the IIIb loop of the 5'UTR. Chemical modification of this ribozyme-195 was done by introducing PO linkage at the 5' end. This modification makes it more stable against the ribonuclease cleavage. In addition, the chemically modified ribozyme 195 triggered antiviral effect of IFN-α in a response to the HCV-poliovirus chimera. Ribozyme-195, later called Heptazyme, was evaluated in clinical trial; however, the study was aborted mainly due to its toxic effect [80]. Many siRNA molecules have been designed and used to control HCV infection. Some siRNAs target the coding region of core, NS3, NS4B and NS5B. This resulted in up to 80% reduction in the virus replication. Other siRNAs targeted the NS3 and NS5B inhibited the virus replication without triggering the interferon response [81-85]. As mentioned earlier, the IRES of HCV plays important roles during virus replication. Targeting this particular conserved sequence using some siRNAs molecules resulted in inhibition of HCV replication up to 80% (86). In a similar manner targeting the same sequence with some shRNAs molecules resulted in marked reduction in the HCV replication in cell culture [87]. According to the most recent literatures most of the HCV genome regions showed a potential to be targeted by different siRNAs molecules [71]. Another interesting novel approach in the HCV therapy is the silencing of miRNA-122, which is one of the most abundant miRNAs expressed in the liver. There are two target sites of this particular miRNA in the 5' UTR of the HCV. Usually, miRNA-122 binds to their recognition sites and resulted in the upregulation of the HCV infection. The most logical way is to inhibit the miR-122 using different chemicals, such as antagomir, in order to control the HCV replication. This approach had been designed and used to control the HCV in mammals by injecting the anti-miRNA-122 antagomir by intravenous route. This approach led to the sustained inhibition of the HCV loads in the infected animals. This approach is currently under clinical trials in chimpanzees [88-90].

3.A.3. Severe Acute Respiratory Syndrome Virus (SARS-CVv)

SARS-CoV is one of the most recently identified contagious human diseases. It was characterized for the first time in 2002-2003 as almost 8000 people were affected by this virus from 30 countries on 5 continents in a very short time [91]. This virus had been classified and placed in the family *Coronavirdae*. It is an enveloped, single stranded RNA virus with positive polarity flanked with the 5' and 3'UTRs. The viral genome encodes 23 proteins. The genome organization is; 5'UTR-replicase-spike(S)-envelope (E)-, membrane (M)-nucleocapsid (N) and 3'UTR [92]. Because the sudden onset and rapid spread of this virus, there was an urgent needs for the development of immediate effective antiviral therapy. Several antiviral approaches were tested in many laboratories including the use of AS-ON, siRNA, shRNA, locked nucleic acids, etc [91, 93-95]. Targeting the nonstructural replicase gene of SARS-CoV (especially the most conserved region among all coronaviruses) using specific shRNA plasmid resulted in the inhibition of the virus replication in 293T cells and HeLa cells. Meanwhile, it also resulted in the reduction in the number of plaques produced by SARS-CoV in Vero cell line [91]. On the other hand, targeting the SARS-CoV structural genes (S, E, M, and N) using 26 different siRNA molecules also resulted in reduction of the expression of the targeted genes by 80% in Vero E6 cells [95]. The S protein plays important roles during viral infection and pathogenesis because it carries an ectodomain that is exposed on the surface of the virus and responsible for the interaction with the cellular receptors. Previous studies using specific monoclonal antibodies against S glycoprotein resulted in the inhibition of coronavirus infection [96, 97]. Taking this in consideration, one study designed specific siRNA molecules targeting different regions in the S glycoprotein of SARS-CoV. This study showed a great reduction in the S gene mRNA level in 293T cells [98]. Another study designed 48 siRNAs for screening the entire SARS-CoV genome and evaluated their effects on the virus replication in vitro. Two of the 48 siRNAs showed downregulation of the spike gene and the NSP12. Those two siRNAs were also validated *in vivo* using the Rhesus Macaque model by inoculation of a combination of those siRNAs intranasally. The obtained results showed great inhibition of virus replication and minimized the virus spread in the lung. This is in addition to inhibition in the development of the classical SARS-CoV clinical signs such as marked reduction in the body temperature of the treated group of animals as well as less lung damage in the necropsy findings [99].

3.A.4. Human Immunodeficiency Virus (HIV)

HIV is the etiological agent of the acquired immune deficiency syndrome (AIDS). According to the most recent studies done by the Joint United Nations Program, more than 42 million people are affected by HIV. Almost 21.8 millions of them died. HIV belongs to the family *Retroviridae* and its genome encodes nine open reading frames which produce 15 proteins [100]. The HIV genome is composed of two identical copies of single stranded RNA molecules about 9.6 kb in length. This viral genome must be converted to DNA using the reverse transcriptase enzyme, and then integrated into the host cell genome before the expression of the viral genes. Three genes encode the Gag, Pol, and Env polyproteins. They undergo further cleavage to produce the 9 genes. Both Gag and Env genes produce structural proteins. The Gag gene produce 4 protein (matrix, capsid, nucelocapsid and p6) while the Env produce two protein (surface or gp120 and trans-membrane or gp41). The Pol gene produces three proteins mainly having enzymatic functions (protease, reverse transcriptase, and integrase) [100]. (During HIV replication, the reverse transcriptase enzyme used to convert the ssRNA viral genome to dsDNA. At that time, both the 5' and the 3' ends of the viral genome are converted to long terminal repeats (LTR), which play important roles during virus replication.[101]) Many approaches have been used for treatment and/or prevention of HIV infection; however, the virus always develops rapid drug resistance. New strategies are underway to develop better therapy to deal with this issue. One of the current directions in the anti HIV therapy is the use of different kinds of NA-based molecules to target different parts in the HIV genome [45]. For example, five phosphothioates (28-mers) AS-ONs were designed to target different regions of the HIV-1 genome. This approach resulted in the inhibition of early HIV infection in cell culture [102]; however it did not achieve similar results in chronically infected cells. One possible explanation is the degradation of these oligonucleotides by the cellular nucleases [102]. Several studies have designed siRNAs and expressed shRNAs targeting most HIV genes including; tat, rev, pol, nef, vif, env, vpr, and the LTR [103-105]. Meanwhile, some host cell genes involved in HIV replication have also been targeted with siRNAs molecules such as; NFkB, CD4 receptors and CXCR4 and CCR5 as co receptors for HIV, and showed similar inhibitory effect on the HIV replication [44, 106, 107]. According to the bioinformatics studies, the HIV genome encodes 5 pre-miRNA candidates, which are further processed into 10 mature miRNAs [108]. The same study showed the presence of several hundred cellular RNAs, which could be targeted by those viral miRNAs. According to their parameters for target selection, they suggested that every miRNA possibly targets 50 to 100 cellular RNAs. These virus-encoded miRNAs are beneficial to the viral replication and their immune evasion strategies [108]. HIV Nef encodes microRNA N367 (miR-N367), which has a unique function at both the transcriptional and translational levels, rather than at the post-transcriptional level [56]. This is mainly due to the suppression of HIV promoter activity [56]. Downregulation of the Nef gene usually results in inhibition of HIV replication. This may lead to production of low-pathogenic strains of HIV or may favor HIV latent infection. Silencing of these viral miRNAs using specific chemicals such as antagomirs (AMO), could potentially have a therapeutic effect on HIV and could be one of the most promising trends in anti-HIV therapy [48, 109]. Furthermore, the AmiRNAs have been used to inhibit the production of HIV-1 variants. This approach offered high mutation tolerance in the HIV 3' UTR in comparison to other shRNAs molecules [110]. Meanwhile, it also showed promising results in controlling the HIV infection even with some mismatches in their target sequence. This strategy will overcome some of the viral escape mutant problems that are frequently encountered in most of the HIV therapy.

3.A.5. Respiratory Syncytial Virus (RSV)

RSV is one of the major causes of respiratory diseases, especially in young children, elderly, and the immunocompomized patients [111]. RSV is an enveloped, negative, single-strand RNA virus. The viral genome encodes 10 proteins, the viral genome is organized in the following order 3'(leader)-NS1-NS2-N-P-M-SH-G-F-22K-L-(trailer) 5' [112, 113]. There are three main viral proteins required to form the functional transcription complex (L, N and P). The phosphoprotein (p) is the smallest component of the RdRp complex and is important in the transcription of the L gene [114]. Most vaccines and antiviral therapeutic strategies have been shown to be ineffective in protecting people against such virus [115, 116]. Earlier study on NA-based drug development is the design of short 2',5'-oligoadenylates (2-5A) antisense molecules targeting the RNase L and used to inhibit RSV replication. This strategy inhibited RSV replication 50-90 times more than the anti-RSV chemical therapy, such as ribavirin, did [117]. This anti-RSV 2-5A- antisense chimera is called NIH351 and only a single dose was enough to induce a marked inhibition of RSV replication in cell lines of both human and monkey origins [117]. Another approach is the use of anti-P dsRNA of RSV, which resulted in 90 % reduction of P protein production in A549 cells [118]. To test this hypothesis *in vivo*, Bitko and his colleagues used Balb/C mice to establish a model for the RSV infection. They designed several specific siRNAs targeting the P gene and administered them intranasally to the Balb/C mice. Four hours later, they challenged the mice with RSV using the same route of administration for infection, too. According to this study, two siRNAs led to 99.89-99 % protection against RSV challenging; at the same time, markedly decreased the RSV titer in the pulmonary tissues [119]. The same group also studied the effect of silencing other genes on viral infectivity and pathogenesis. When they targeted the F gene using specific siRNAs, the resulting viruses lost their cell fusion ability (syncytium formation) *in vivo*. This resulted in inhibition of the virus transfer from cell to cell and minimized the severity of the diseases produced [118]. Furthermore, intranasal instillation of siRNA targeting the P gene in mice for 12 hours, then RSV infection was carried out. The obtained results showed marked reduction in the RSV titer in the lung in comparison to the scrambled siRNA-treated mice. This effect was in a dose dependant manner according to the siRNA concentration [120]. Moving toward clinical trials for the anti-RSV prophylaxes and therapy, some studies used siRNAs targeting the N gene, called ALN-RSV01, which has shown promising results both *in vitro* and *in vivo* [121].

3.A.6. Coxsackieviruses

Coxsackievirus, especially coxsackievirus B3 (CVB3), is the most common cause of viral myocarditis in humans [122]. CVB3 belongs to the genus Enteroviruses in the family *Picornaviridae.* The viral genome is a single stranded positive sense RNA molecule, which serves as mRNA for translation to produce a long single polyprotein [123]. The viral encoded proteases 2A and 3C process this polyprotein to produce capsid proteins (VP1-VP4) and 7 nonstructural proteins, including the RNA-dependant RNA polymerase 3D [124]. The latest trends in anti CVB therapy have focused on a third generation of AS-ON and RNAi as a strategy. Yuan and co-workers employed morpholino oligomers targeting different regions of the 5' and 3'UTRs of the sense and antisense strands of CVB3 genome and found that the IRES is the best site for targeting and achieved a 3-log10 and 2-log10 reduction of CVB3 particle formation in HeLa cells and in mouse heart, respectively [125].The RNAi strategies include application of siRNAs targeting CVB3 nonstructural proteins 2A, 2C, 3C, 3D and structural protein VP1 [125-128]. In our laboratory, we first reported the successful suppression (>92%) of CVB3 replication in HeLa cells with siRNAs targeting viral protease 2A RNA. We also found that the antiviral effect was disrupted by mutations to the central region of the strand, and that mismatch was tolerated near the 3' end but not the 5' end of the siRNA [125]. Further, the siRNA effect is mediated by the antisense strand to the viral genome rather than the sense strand complimentary to the viral negative strand of the replicating intermediate. This effectiveness of CVB3 2A as a gene target were further conformed in a study using a mouse model in which the systemically administered siRNA demonstrated a significant reduction in the viral replication and tissue injury, as well as an increase in the survival rate [126]. Recently, we tested a packaging RNA (pRNA) vector (a component of the bacterial phage nano-motor) for target delivery of siRNA. By conjugation of a folate ligand to the pRNA vector, we specifically delivered the siRNAs targeting CVB3 2A to HeLa cells and HL-1 cardiomyocytes that can express folate receptors [129]. In addition to transfection of mature siRNAs, over expression of shRNAs with plasmids, double expression plasmid or recombinant viral vectors also demonstrated the success in inhibition of expression of CVB3 3D, VP1 and 2C [130, 131, 126] as well as CVB3 cellular receptor gene (CAR)[128, 132] These studies all showed a marked reduction of CVB3 replication and some of them achieved a similar result in animal models [133-135].

3.A.7. Rabies Virus

Rabies virus is one of the most fatal viral diseases affecting animals and humans. The virus belongs to the family *Rhabdoviridae* and genus Lyssavirus. The viral genome is single non- segmented negative sense RNA. It encodes five genes which produce the viral proteins including nucleoprotein (N), phosphoprotein (P), matrix protein (M), glycoprotein (G) and viral RNA polymerase (L) [138]. The current therapy of rabies virus mainly depends on using different drugs such as ribavirin, ketamine and midazole; however these drugs showed minimal therapeutic effects [139]. Brandao and his colleagues studied the effect of siRNA targeting the N protein of rabies virus *in vitro* in BHK-21 cells and achieved a five-time reduction in the virus titer when compared to the non-treated cells (140). In another attempt to inhibit rabies virus replication, several amiRNAs were designed and used for this purpose [59]. In this study they used AmiRNA-expressing vector against different strains of rabies virus and showed that single amiRNA against the nucleocapsid mRNA of the rabies virus strain (CVS) resulted in a decrease of the viral genome expression up to 90% (59). The same study used multiple amiRNA constructs to target either single or multiple sequences in the mRNA of nucleoprotein. Meanwhile, in case of using single amiRNA they founded any mismatches especially in the seeding region will result in reduction in the activity of this amiRNA. This was in contrast to using a construct that carried multiple gene targeting molecules, which can tolerate some mismatches without losing its efficacy in inhibiting the virus replication [59].

3.B. DNA Viruses

In this section we will highlight the progress of using different NA-based antiviral approaches for different DNA viruses such as (HBV, HSV, HCMV, HPV, and SV40).

3.B.1. Hepatitis B Virus (HBV)

HBV infection is one of the most common global health concerns. More than 350 million people are diagnosed to be HBV carriers, with about one million deaths every year [141, 142]. The current therapy for the HBV is the combination between the IFN-α, some nucelosides such as Lamivudine and some nucleotides such as adefovir. Such an approach is highly costive for the patients; requiring several doses due to the short term of its action plus many side effects triggered by such therapy [143-145]. There is an urgent need for the development of other alternative therapeutic approaches. Using different NA-based approaches targeting different gene of HBV showed a great progress [146-153]. HBV belongs to the genus Orthohepadnavirus in the family *Hepadnaviridae*. It is a DNA virus and its envelope, surrounded by the nucleocapsid or the core of the virus. The viral genome encodes four long open reading frames. The pre-S (pre-surface and surface) fragment encodes three viral surface antigens. The preC (precore-core) region encodes the hepatitis B core antigen. The P coding region encodes the viral polymerase. The X region encodes the viral X protein, which is responsible for the modulation of the virus host interaction [141, 158]. The modified phosphorothioate form of the AS-ON was used to inhibit the HBV replication in cells stably transfected with HBV protein. This approach was successful in inhibiting both the HBV replication and in inhibiting the production of the viral proteins [159, 160]. To test the above approach *in vivo*, the HBV transgenic mice with hepatocytes having a similar level of HBV replication to that of the HBV chronically infected patients were examined. Suppression of HBV replication lasted for at least 26 days after treatment in these transgenic mice [153].

HBV-X protein is very important in establishing the hepatocellular carcinoma triggered by the HBV through activating many promoters [161]. Targeting this key gene by different

NA-based approaches may offer a new powerful strategy for HBV therapy. Several studies used different siRNA molecules to target different HBV genes as a mean of controlling the virus replication both *in vitro* and *in vivo* [146-148, 150, 163]. Another study designed seven siRNAs targeting different conserved regions in the HBV genome surface (S), polymerase (P) or pre-core (PreC) region. Those molecules targeting S and PreC gene showed high degree of suppression of HBV gene expression and called siRNA-1 and siRNA-7 respectively. Both siRNAs induced alteration in the expression of several cellular genes, especially those involved in the immune response against viral infection in HepG2.2.15 cell line. They also founded 18 genes were markedly downregulated in both siRNA-1 and siRNA-7. Moreover, of the 18 downregulated genes 7 of the genes normally upregulated due to HBV infection were found to be downregulated due to this treatment, suggesting the possibility of involvement of those 7 genes in the virus host interaction [136]. During the HBV replication, the double strand (ds) relaxed circular DNA is subjected to several modifications to produce mature virus particles. The genome is changed into what is called a crucial intermediate-covalently closed circular DNA (cccDNA). This cccDNA was proved to play important role in the drug resistance and virus persistence [150]. Thus, targeting this cccDNA sequence will interrupt the HBV replication and may act as an interesting therapeutic strategy for HBV. The siRNA designed to target this cccDNA sequence resulted in marked inhibition in the HBV replication [150]. Although most bioinformatics predictions indicate that HBV encodes only one miRNA, several studies failed to identify any cellular genes regulated by this miRNA [166]. On the other hand, cellular miRNAs may play a role in the pathogenesis of HBV. It has been recently shown that seven cellular miRNAs can target HBV polymerase and surface antigen ORFs. One of those miRNAs is the has-miR-125a-5p. This miRNA showed a potent inhibitory effect on the HBV protein translation, including the surface antigen in three cell lines of liver origin [152]. In addition, AmiRNAs have been also used to inhibit the HBV replication. Three vector-based AmiRNAs targeting the HBV S coding region have been tested and successfully inhibited the secretion of HBV Ags as well as a reduction in the copy numbers of the HBV DNA [148].

3.B.2. Herpesviruses

Herpesviruses are group of large ds-DNA viruses and belong to the family *Herpesviridae*. There are ten virus-encoded glycoproteins embedded in the viral envelope. Those proteins play different roles during the virus life cycle including replication, spread and the immune evasion [168]. The family includes three groups called alphaherpesvirus, betaherpesvirus and gammaherpesvirus. Within this family, eight viruses have been identified to cause many diseases in humans: herpes simplex type 1 (HSV-1), herpes simplex type 2 (HSV-2), cytomegalovirus (CMV), Epstein - Barr virus (EBV), human herpesvirus 6, 7 and 8 (HHV-6, 7, and 8) [167]. In this section we will discuss different NA-based antiviral strategies against HSV1, HSV2 and HCMV.

3.B.2.1. Herpes Simplex Viruses 1 and 2 (HSV-1, and HSV-2)

Herpes Simplex viruses are a group of viruses that belong to the family *Herpesviridae*. Both HSV-1 and HSV-2 are responsible for several diseases including cold sores and genital herpes, respectively, in adult population. It has been recently reported that HSV-1 may cause eye infection, which may result in blindness and in rare cases HSV-1 may cause encephalitis, especially in immunocompromized patients [169]. Although the current therapeutic strategy for most HSV-1 mainly depends on the use of some drugs such as acyclovir and ganciclovir, this always results in the development of drug resistance strain of HSV-1 [170]. The NA-based approaches have been used to inhibit HSV-1 and HSV-2 infection both *in vitro and in vivo* [171-181]. The M1GS ribozymes were used to treat the mRNAs of HSV-1, HCMV, and BCR-ABL *in vitro*. This study showed a marked reduction in the expression of these mRNAs [178]. The hammerhead ribozymes were also designed to target the HSV-1 late gene UL20. The antiviral effect of this ribozyme was tested using different strains of HSV-1 including the wild type virus as well as some drug resistant strains. The treatment using this ribozyme resulted in 90 % protection against the lethal HSV-1. This study confirmed the potential therapeutic roles of these ribozyme molecules as an effective therapy against different strains of HSV-1 [174]. Another approach designed siRNAs targeting the glycoprotein E (involved in the cell to cell spread and immune evasion [182]) of HSV-1 *in vitro*. This resulted in great inhibition in the HSV-1 glycoprotein expression level and diminished its effect during viral infection [171]. HSV-2 infection is characterized by high morbidity rate and acts as a predisposing factor for the HIV infection [183]. In an attempt to prevent the sexual transmission of the HSV-2, siRNA targeting HSV-2 UL27 and UL29 genes (encode the envelope glycoprotein and the DNA binding protein respectively). The siRNA molecules were administered by vaginal instillation. This resulted in the silencing of those particular genes in the vagina and ectocervix for at least nine days [177]. Both DNA IV ligase and its co-factor XRCC4 play important roles during HSV replication. They are probably involved in the packaging of the replicative DNA during the active phase of infection. Isabella and Per Elias designed siRNAs targeting these factors and founded that silencing the DNA ligase IV and XRCC4 resulted in a 100-fold reduction of the virus yield and produced tiny plaques. This was in contrast to other siRNA molecules targeting DNA ligase I or III. This confirms the specificity of this siRNA target DNA ligase IV and its effect on the virus replication [176]. One of the major concerns of using this siRNA *in vivo* is the short duration of its action. Another study tried to overcome this problem by using the cholesterol conjugated siRNA. This approach was successful in silencing the HSV-2 receptor gene (nectin-1) for up to two weeks in the vagina without triggering inflammation or inducing interferon [179]. Another study designed two siRNAs (siRNA-1 targeting VP16 gene and siRNA-4 targeting DNA polymerase gene) of the HSV-1. This approach showed marked reduction in the HSV-1 replication by almost 2-log10 and - log10, respectively. Meanwhile it resulted also in the reduction in the virus plaque formation by 85% and 70 %, respectively. The expression levels of the mRNAs of VP16 and DNA polymerase showed great reduction [180]. Another siRNA molecule targeting the UL39 gene of HSV-1, which is responsible for the expression of the ICP6 (ribonucleotide reductase), achieved inhibition of HSV-1 replication *in vitro* [181]. The hairpin loop-structured 54-mer oligonucelotides were designed and used to target the UL5 gene (encodes the helicase/primase complex) of HSV-1, this approach was more efficient in the inhibition of the HSV-1 replication than siRNA targeting the same region [137].

3.B.2.2. Human Cytomegalovirus (HCMV)

HCMV belongs to the subfamily Betaherpesvirinae of the family *Herpesviridae*. The viral genome is linear double stranded DNA and 235 kb in length. It is enveloped and the viral genome is surrounded by an icosahedral capsid. This is in addition to several outer layers composed of viral protein, called tegument [138]. HCMV poses significant health problem especially for immunocompromised patients [139]. The virus genome has a unique organization in which two domains are inversely in relative to each other. This usually results in the production of four genomic isomers within the virus particle. Those two domains are long (L) and short (S). Each domain has central unique fragment designated as (U_L and U_S) respectively. These unique region are usually flanked by repeated sequence which may reside at the end of the genome and called (TR_L and TR_S) or in the interior of each fragment and then called (IR_L and IR_S) so the virus genome organization is as follow TR_L-U_L-IR_L-IR_S-TR_S [140]. Ribozymes, especially the RNase P class, including M1GS, have been used to target and inhibit the HCMV replication. This ribozyme designed to target the overlapping fragment of mRNA that code for the major transcription factors IE1 and IE2 (essential region for the viral replication and gene expression). According to this study, cells expressing M1GS ribozyme infected with HCMV resulted in potent inhibition of the virus replication by 150 to 3000 fold (141). Different siRNA molecules have been designed to target important genes in the HCMV and reduced the virus replication [142, 143]. Duan and his colleagues designed siRNA molecules targeting the UL122 gene which is responsible for the activation of many HCMV genes the early and late genes. These siRNA molecules showed great inhibition in the mRNA of UL122 genes by 82 % in vitro [142]. The DNA based external guide sequence called (mininEGSs) has been used to silence some HCMV genes. In this study, a mini-form of AS-ON, only 12 nucleotides (12 AS-ONs), was also designed to target the HCMV UL49 gene in HeLa cells. Using this approach marked inhibition of the UL49 gene up 67 % in comparison to the mock and control miniEGSs was also reported. This may represent a new therapeutic strategy for the HCMV especially this miniEGSs is shorter than any other oligonucelotides based approaches [144]. It has been recently reported that HCMV encodes 15 miRNAs [48]. The most commonly expressed three miRNAs during the active phase of HCMV infection are miR-UL23-5p, miR-UL23-3p, and miR-US24. The miR-UL112 also plays important role in establishing latent phase of HCMV infection by targeting the histocompatibility complex (MHC) class I associated proteins, especially the MHC class I–related chain B (MICB). Furthermore, it regulates early viral protein expression, such as immediate early protein (IE)-72. This IE72 is a key mediator in the shift from the latent to the active phase of viral infection, because it suppresses IE1. Downregulation of UL114 protein, using miR-UL112-1, results in inhibition of viral DNA replication and subsequently triggers the latent phase of infection, making the virus able to evade the host immune system [48, 57, 145-147].

3.B.3. Human Papillomavirus (HPV)

HPV is one of the major causes of a wide variety of cancers, especially in organs that have squamous epithelial cells [148, 149]. The developed cancer ranges in size from small warts or papillomas, to invasive carcinomas (148). HPV is classified according to the severity of the disease and the type of the cancer they produce into high risk (HR) and low risk (LR). The HR virus types are usually associated with massive invasive cancer, while the LR type viruses usually cause mild lesions in the form of genital or skin warts [150]. Among those virus types, HPV 16 and HPV 18 are the most common HR viruses and responsible for at least 80% of the HPV induced invasive cancer lesions [150].

The HPV genome is circular DNA, about 8 kb in length. It encodes 6 early genes (E1, E2, E3, E4, E5, E6, and E7) plus two late genes (L1 and L2). The expression of both E6 and

E7 genes induces cancer formation *in vitro* in different squamous epithelial cells. This was the idea behind the discovery of the HPV induced cervical carcinoma (151). HPV therapy initially focused on the anti-cancer, not on anti HPV. This was mainly based on the surgical removal of the skin warts or lesions. HPV vaccines started to be used for the prophylactic purposes using virus like particles (VLP). Although this vaccine offered a good protection umbrella against the HPV, it was lacking in therapeutic potential. Several classes of vaccines have been developed against the HPV 16 E6 and E7, such as the protein /peptide based or the DNA based vaccines.

This approach was tested in both healthy and patients with invasive cancer. Those vaccines were able to induce high level of both humoral and cytotoxic T cell responses, however; it had limited effect on the regression of the already developed tumor [152]. This was one of the reasons why those vaccines did not continue to the phase II and III clinical trials. This was in addition to the high cost of the DNA vaccines [152]. With the identification of HPV oncogenes especially E6 and E7 new therapeutic strategies have been developed using different NA-based approaches targeting those genes such as ribozymes, antisense molecules, siRNA, shRNA and miRNAs [153-157]. Targeting the E6 and E7 genes by complementary antisense resulted in a reduction in cell growth and loss of the typical morphology in the cancer cells, in both cervical and oral cell lines [156]. Another study showed that targeting E6 and E7 using different oligonucleotides had anti-proliferative effect on the primary tumors [158].

The modified form of the oligonucleotides (phosphorothioate) had been used also to target the E6 and E7 genes of HPV in CaSki and SiHa cells. This treatment resulted in the inhibition of the cell proliferation *in vitro* as well as reduction in the tumor size of the SiHa cells implanted into nude mice [156, 157]. Using adenovirus vector to deliver the antisense of E6/E7 genes showed a great inhibition of the cell proliferation *in vitro* as well as complete inhibition of the tumor production *in vivo* [159, 160].

Another approach in the control of HPV is the use of ribozymes. It has been used to target and cleave the HPV E6/E7 genes which resulted in the inhibition of the HPV induced tumor formation [121]. Another hammerhead ribozyme (Rz170) has been designed to target the E6E7 of the HPV 16. This was useful approach to inhibit the cell proliferation as well as induction of apoptosis. This was in addition to the inhibition in the tumor formation *in vivo* in nude mice [161]. Several studies used siRNA to silence the HPV E6 and E7 genes and most of them showed great inhibitory effects on the cell proliferation and they also induced apoptosis [155, 162-164]. Even the direct injection of the E6/E7 siRNA to the HPV induced subcutaneous tumor resulted in the regression of this tumor [165].

Several studies claimed that it is unlikely that most strains of HPV could produce miRNAs during their replication [49] however, HPV31 may encodes some viral miRNAs at very early stage of the infection but these miRNAs are degraded in case of the latent infection [49]. It has been shown that miRNA-34a is usually downregulated during HPV infection. This miRNA targets some p53 downstream genes and lead to the inhibition of cell cycle progression at the G2 phase and further induce apoptosis. Restoring the expression level of this miRNA during HPV infection may represent a new therapeutic strategy for such virus [166].

4. Advantages of Using NA Based Antiviral Agents

NA-based antiviral strategy including (Ribozymes, aptamers, oligonucleotides, siRNA, shRNA, and miRNA) is one of the most promising gene therapy approaches for infectious diseases including viruses (Table 2) [167]. They can be designed and used for the prevention and or treatment of many viral diseases (Table 1). This approach may represent an ideal antiviral strategy because most viral genes are unique and do not share homology to the cellular genes [168]. The major advantage of most of these molecules is they can be easily designed *in vitro* according to the Watson-Crick base pairing rules or can be easily separated and isolated from libraries according to the SELEX protocol [169]. They may also be designed for intracellular and extracellular targets [170]. Another advantage for the different NA-based molecules is their small size which renders them less immunogenic molecules when compared to other peptide or protein based drugs [169]. There is also a possibility of targeting almost any gene with this technology, regardless of the function of this gene or their encoded protein structure [171]. This approach will enable us to silence any viral gene of interest, especially those involved in the viral virulence and pathogenesis. Furthermore, their production is very much easier than that of conventional drugs, as they are mainly produced by chemical synthesis, making their large scale production inexpensive [170]. Aptamers are unique the NA-based antiviral approach because they work on the protein level leading to alteration in the function of the target protein. Those targeted proteins lost their function upon aptamer treatment [171]. The most interesting feature of aptamers is their ability to inhibit the function of one domain of certain protein without disrupting its three dimensional structures [171]. The early clinical trials of using aptamers as antiviral therapy revealed they are safe, well tolerated and showed no significant side effects after their use [16].

5. Problems Associated with Using NA Based Antiviral Therapy and Potential Solutions

Although the NA-based antiviral therapy has many advantages over the conventional therapy [3, 169, 172, 173], several concerns still exist and many questions remain to be answered before using this approach on a large scale as antiviral therapy, especially *in vivo*. One of the major concerns is the stability of these molecules *in vivo*, the serum half life of some of these molecules is relatively very short, ranging from seconds to several minutes [169]. To overcome this big concern, several modifications in the base, ribose or phosphate group of this polymer have been made [3]. Another concern is the fast rate of renal clearance of these molecules; this may be easily resolved by increasing the molecular weight of these polymers by different approaches such as conjugation of these molecules with other chemicals and /or carriers such as liposomes, and polyethylene glycol (PEG) [174]. Some of these molecules may result in the induction of strong innate immune response in addition to saturation of certain endogenous pathways, as in the case of using shRNAs [175]. Using ribozymes as antiviral therapy is also associated with many challenges, especially rapid degradation by the cellular nucleases. Introducing some modifications on those ribozymes such as 2`ribose with allyl group showed substantial increases in nuclease activity of such ribozyme molecules [176]. Many problems exist while using siRNA for antiviral therapy, such as non specific gene silencing or the off- target effect, as well as immunoactivation [177-180]. Meanwhile, several approaches had been made to improve the action of siRNA and minimize its associated pitfalls [181-183]. In order to enhance the cellular uptake and reduce nuclease degradation of siRNA molecules, several chemical modifications in the siRNA duplex have been applied, including modifications to the sugar backbone and bases of the oligonucleotides. Another approach is the conjugation of the siRNA molecules with other lipid or peptide moieties [93, 184-191]. Delivery of siRNA to the target tissues and organs also represents one of the greatest challenges of their therapeutic application. The non viral vectors have been widely used for the purpose of siRNA delivery both in vitro and *in vivo* models with great success [192-196]. The chemically modified encapsulated siRNA, such as stable nucleic acid particles (SNALPs), have been used to treat many viruses, such as Ebola and HBV. This approach was superior to the non-modified siRNA molecules in response to the virus challenge in mouse and non-human primate models. The chemically modified siRNA treated group was resistant to the viral challenge; longer half-life time of these siRNA also observed in the same group. Furthermore, a reduction in the frequency of siRNA treatment was also achieved [197-200]. Another concern associated with siRNA as anti-viral therapy is the generation of viral escape mutants [201]. Viruses may evade the effect of the siRNA targeting by mutations in the siRNA target sequences. To overcome this problem, several siRNA libraries were screened and the most promising siRNA candidates targeting the most conserved regions in the viral genome were selected, minimizing the possibility of the viral escape mutations. Another solution is to design siRNA targeting host cell genes involved in the replication of those viruses. One of the best examples was the silencing CD4 gene using specific siRNA molecule which resulted in marked inhibition of the HIV replication [44].

Conclusion

Although our knowledge about the host-virus interaction is expanding dramatically, we still face many obstacles for the development of safe, stable and specific therapy for different viral diseases. We are still challenged by the emergence of new viruses such as SARSCoV and the re-emergence of other virus variants from time to time, such as different types of influenza viruses. More than 1450 NA-based therapies are currently in clinical trials. About 60 % out of them are still in the early phases, however 3% have moved to the phase III trials. We believe that there will be robust preclinical and clinical trails on their way to develop effective, stable and safe NA-based antiviral therapy for several viral diseases in near future. Some drug companies' believe that by 2018, most of the NA-based drugs in the late stages of clinical trials will come to the market. This will be achieved after addressing all the concerns about their safety and efficacy. This is in addition to optimization of the nucleic acid delivery system which may result in the production of novel polymers or lipopolymer complexes which may help in carrying larger DNA molecules to their target tissues. We believe that this expectation is very possible. Given the immense interest in NA-based gene target research and the rapid progress made in this field and other areas, such as bioinformatics analysis of the gene target for drug design, high throughput screening of the drug candidates and nano-biotechnology for drug delivery, the coming year will likely see a huge increase in the number of clinical trials. The realization of this goal in combating emerging and reemerging viral diseases faces a bright future.

Acknowledgments

This work was supported by grants from the Canadian Institutes of Health Research and the Heart and Stroke Foundation of BC and Yukon. Dr. Maged Gomaa Hemida is a recipient of the CIHR-IMPACT postdoctoral training fellowship. Xin Ye is supported by a UGF Award from the University of British Columbia.

The authors have no conflicts of interest that are directly relevant to the content of this work.

References

[1] Cherry J. D. The chronology of the 2002-2003 S. A. R. S. mini pandemic. *Paediatr. Respir. Rev.* 2004 Dec.;5(4):262-9.

[2] Saxena S. K., Mishra, N. and Saxena, R. Advances in antiviral drug discovery and development: Part II: Advancements in antiviral drug development. *Future Virology.* 2009;4(3):209-15.

[3] Kurreck J. Antisense technologies. Improvement through novel chemical modifications. *Eur. J. Biochem.* 2003 Apr.;270(8):1628-44.

[4] Stephenson M. L., Zamecnik P. C. Inhibition of Rous sarcoma viral R. N. A. translation by a specific oligodeoxyribonucleotide. *Proc. Natl. Acad. Sci. US.* 1978 Jan.;75(1): 285-8.

[5] Zamecnik P. C., Stephenson M. L. Inhibition of Rous sarcoma virus replication and cell transformation by a specific oligodeoxynucleotide. *Proc. Natl. Acad. Sci. US.* 1978 Jan.;75(1):280-4.

[6] Cherry S. What have RNAi screens taught us about viral-host interactions? *Curr. Opin. Microbiol.* 2009 Aug.;12(4):446-52.

[7] Jarald E., Edwin, S., Dubey, P., Tiwari, A., and Thakre, V. Nucleic acid drugs: a novel approach. *African Journal of Biotechnology.* 2004 Dec. 3(12):662-6.

[8] Schubert S., and Kurreck, J. Ribozyme- and deoxyribozyme-strategies for medical applications. *Curr. Drug Targets.* 2004 Nov.;5(8):667-81.

[9] Bramlage B., Luzi E., Eckstein F. HIV-1 L. T. R. as a target for synthetic ribozyme-mediated inhibition of gene expression: site selection and inhibition in cell culture. *Nucleic Acids Res.* 2000 Nov. 1;28(21):4059-67.

[10] Rossi J. J., Sarver N., R. N. A. enzymes (ribozymes) as antiviral therapeutic agents. *Trends Biotechnol.* 1990 Jul.;8(7):179-83.

[11] Lo K. M., Biasolo M. A., Dehni G., Palu G., Haseltine W. A. Inhibition of replication of HIV-1 by retroviral vectors expressing tat-antisense and anti-tat ribozyme R. N. A. *Virology.* 1992 Sep.;190(1):176-83.

[12] Yamada O., Kraus G., Leavitt M. C., Yu M., Wong-Staal F. Activity and cleavage site specificity of an anti-HIV-1 hairpin ribozyme in human T cells. *Virology*. 1994 Nov. 15;205(1):121-6.

[13] Yamada O., Yu M., Yee J. K., Kraus G., Looney D., Wong-Staal F. Intracellular immunization of human T cells with a hairpin ribozyme against human immunodeficiency virus type 1. *Gene Ther.* 1994 Jan.; 1(1):38-45.

[14] Gatto B., Palumbo M., Sissi C. Nucleic acid aptamers based on the G-quadruplex structure: therapeutic and diagnostic potential. *Curr.Med. Chem.* 2009;16(10):1248-65.

[15] Rimmele M. Nucleic acid aptamers as tools and drugs: recent developments. *Chembiochem*. 2003 Oct. 6;4(10):963-71.

[16] Gopinath S. C. Antiviral aptamers. *Arch. Virol*. 2007;152(12):2137-57.

[17] Tombelli S., Minunni M., Mascini M. Analytical applications of aptamers. *Biosens Bioelectron*. 2005 Jun. 15;20(12):2424-34.

[18] Ng E. W., Shima D. T., Calias P., Cunningham E. T., Jr., Guyer D. R., Adamis A. P. Pegaptanib, a targeted anti-VEGF aptamer for ocular vascular disease. *Nat. Rev. Drug Discov*. 2006 Feb.;5(2):123-32.

[19] Chen H., Gold L. Selection of high-affinity R. N. A. ligands to reverse transcriptase: inhibition of cDNA synthesis and RNase H activity. *Biochemistry.* 1994 Jul. 26;33(29):8746-56.

[20] Jeon S. H., Kayhan B., Ben-Yedidia T., Arnon R. A. D. N. A. aptamer prevents influenza infection by blocking the receptor binding region of the viral hemagglutinin. *J. Biol. Chem*. 2004 Nov. 12;279(46):48410-9.

[21] Lochrie M. A., Waugh S., Pratt D. G., Jr., Clever J., Parslow T. G., Polisky B. In vitro selection of RNAs that bind to the human immunodeficiency virus type-1 gag polyprotein. *Nucleic Acids Res*. 1997 Jul. 15;25(14):2902-10.

[22] Rieger A., Nassal M. Distinct requirements for primary sequence in the 5'- and 3'-part of a bulge in the hepatitis B virus R. N. A. encapsidation signal revealed by a combined in vivo selection/in vitro amplification system. *Nucleic Acids Res*. 1995 Oct. 11;23(19): 3909-15.

[23] Umehara T., Fukuda K., Nishikawa F., Kohara M., Hasegawa T., Nishikawa S. Rational design of dual-functional aptamers that inhibit the protease and helicase activities of H. C. V. NS3. *J. Biochem.* 2005 Mar.;137(3):339-47.

[24] Wang J., Jiang H., Liu F. In vitro selection of novel R. N. A. ligands that bind human cytomegalovirus and block viral infection. *R. N. A*. 2000 Apr.;6(4):571-83.

[25] Haasnoot J., Berkhout B. Nucleic acids-based therapeutics in the battle against pathogenic viruses. *Handb Exp. Pharmacol*. 2009(189):243-63.

[26] Herdewijn P. Heterocyclic modifications of oligonucleotides and antisense technology. *Antisense Nucleic Acid Drug Dev*. 2000 Aug.; 10(4):297-310.

[27] Matsukura M., Shinozuka K., Zon G., Mitsuya H., Reitz M., Cohen J. S., et al. Phosphorothioate analogs of oligodeoxynucleotides: inhibitors of replication and cytopathic effects of human immunodeficiency virus. *Proc. Natl. Acad. Sci. US*. 1987 Nov.; 84(21): 7706-10.

[28] Crooke S. T. Progress in antisense technology: the end of the beginning. *Methods Enzymol.* 2000;313:3-45.

[29] Elayadi A. N., Corey D. R. Application of P. N. A. and L. N. A. oligomers to chemotherapy. *Curr. Opin. Investig Drugs*. 2001 Apr.; 2(4):558-61.

[30] Arzumanov A., Walsh A. P., Rajwanshi V. K., Kumar R., Wengel J., Gait M. J. Inhibition of HIV-1 Tat-dependent trans activation by steric block chimeric 2'-O-methyl/LNA oligoribonucleotides. *Biochemistry*. 2001 Dec. 4;40(48):14645-54.

[31] Li X., Mueller S., Wimmer E. Inhibition of hepatitis C virus IRES-mediated translation by oligonucleotides. *Virus Res*. 2009 Dec.; 146(1-2):29-35.

[32] Wu Y., Zhang G., Li Y., Jin Y., Dale R., Sun L. Q., et al. Inhibition of highly pathogenic avian H5N1 influenza virus replication by R. N. A. oligonucleotides targeting NS1 gene. *Biochem. Biophys. Res. Commun*. 2008 Jan. 11;365(2):369-74.

[33] Sample R., Bryan L., Long S., Majji S., Hoskins G., Sinning A., et al. Inhibition of iridovirus protein synthesis and virus replication by antisense morpholino oligonucleotides targeted to the major capsid protein, the 18 kDa immediate-early protein, and a viral homolog of R. N. A. polymerase II. *Virology*. 2007 Feb. 20;358(2): 311-20.

[34] Torrence P. F., Gupta N., Whitney C., Morrey J. D. Evaluation of synthetic oligonucleotides as inhibitors of West Nile virus replication. *Antiviral Res*. 2006 Jun.;70(2):60-5.

[35] Tallet-Lopez B., Aldaz-Carroll L., Chabas S., Dausse E., Staedel C., Toulme J. J. Antisense oligonucleotides targeted to the domain IIId of the hepatitis C virus I. R. E. S. compete with 40S ribosomal subunit binding and prevent in vitro translation. *Nucleic Acids Res*. 2003 Jan. 15; 31(2): 734-42.

[36] Pinskaia M. D., Brodin P., Romanova E. A., Volkov E. M., Mouscadet J. F., Gottikh M. V. [Inhibition of integration of human immunodeficiency virus D. N. A., modified by oligonucleotides]. *Mol. Biol.* (Mosk.). 2000 Nov.-Dec.;34(6):1039-45.

[37] Fire A., Xu S., Montgomery M. K., Kostas S. A., Driver S. E., Mello C. C. Potent and specific genetic interference by double-stranded R. N. A. in Caenorhabditis elegans. *Nature*. 1998 Feb. 19;391(6669): 806-11.

[38] Elbashir S. M., Harborth J., Lendeckel W., Yalcin A., Weber K., Tuschl T. Duplexes of 21-nucleotide RNAs mediate R. N. A. interference in cultured mammalian cells. *Nature*. 2001 May 24; 411(6836):494-8.

[39] Elbashir S. M., Lendeckel W., Tuschl T., R. N. A. interference is mediated by 21- and 22-nucleotide RNAs. *Genes Dev*. 2001 Jan. 15; 15(2):188-200.

[40] Haasnoot J., Berkhout B., R. N. A. interference: its use as antiviral therapy. *Handb Exp. Pharmacol*. 2006(173):117-50.

[41] Tan F. L., Yin J. Q. RNAi, a new therapeutic strategy against viral infection. *Cell Res*. 2004 Dec.;14(6):460-6.

[42] Semizarov D., Frost L., Sarthy A., Kroeger P., Halbert D. N., Fesik S. W. Specificity of short interfering RNA determined through gene expression signatures. *Proc. Natl. Acad. Sci. US*. 2003 May 27; 100(11):6347-52.

[43] Rao D. D., Vorhies J. S., Senzer N., Nemunaitis J. siRNA vs. shRNA: similarities and differences. *Adv. Drug Deliv. Rev*. 2009 Jul. 25;61(9): 746-59.

[44] Novina C. D., Murray M. F., Dykxhoorn D. M., Beresford P. J., Riess J., Lee S. K., et al. siRNA-directed inhibition of HIV-1 infection. *Nat. Med*. 2002 Jul.;8(7):681-6.

[45] Aagaard L., Rossi J. J. RNAi therapeutics: principles, prospects and challenges. *Adv. Drug Deliv. Rev*. 2007 Mar. 30;59(2-3):75-86.

[46] Cullen B. R. Viral and cellular messenger R. N. A. targets of viral microRNAs. *Nature*. 2009 Jan. 22;457(7228):421-5.

[47] Scaria V., Hariharan M., Pillai B., Maiti S., Brahmachari S. K. Host-virus genome interactions: macro roles for microRNAs. *Cell Microbiol.* 2007 Dec.;9(12):2784-94.

[48] Moens U. Silencing viral microR. N. A. as a novel antiviral therapy? *J. Biomed. Biotechnol.* 2009;2009:419539.

[49] Cai X., Li G., Laimins L. A., Cullen B. R. Human papillomavirus genotype 31 does not express detectable microR. N. A. levels during latent or productive virus replication. *J. Virol.* 2006 Nov.;80(21):10890-3.

[50] Denli A. M., Tops B. B., Plasterk R. H., Ketting R. F., Hannon G. J. Processing of primary microRNAs by the Microprocessor complex. *Nature.* 2004 Nov. 11;432(7014): 231-5.

[51] Gregory R. I., Yan K. P., Amuthan G., Chendrimada T., Doratotaj B., Cooch N., et al. The Microprocessor complex mediates the genesis of microRNAs. *Nature.* 2004 Nov. 11;432(7014):235-40.

[52] Han J., Lee Y., Yeom K. H., Kim Y. K., Jin H., Kim V. N. The Drosha-DGCR8 complex in primary microRNA processing. *Genes Dev.* 2004 Dec. 15;18(24):3016-27.

[53] Cai X., Hagedorn C. H., Cullen B. R. Human microRNAs are processed from capped, polyadenylated transcripts that can also function as mRNAs. *R. N. A.* 2004 Dec.;10(12): 1957-66.

[54] Cullen B. R. Viruses and microRNAs. *Nat. Genet.* 2006 Jun.;38 Suppl.: S25-30.

[55] Kim V. N. Small RNAs: classification, biogenesis, and function. *Mol. Cells.* 2005 Feb. 28;19(1):1-15.

[56] Omoto S., Fujii Y. R. Regulation of human immunodeficiency virus 1 transcription by nef microRNA. *J. Gen. Virol.* 2005 Mar.;86(Pt 3):751-5.

[57] Pfeffer S., Sewer A., Lagos-Quintana M., Sheridan R., Sander C., Grasser F. A., et al. Identification of microRNAs of the herpesvirus family. *Nat. Methods.* 2005 Apr.;2(4):269-76.

[58] Sullivan C. S., Grundhoff A. T., Tevethia S., Pipas J. M., Ganem D. SV40-encoded microRNAs regulate viral gene expression and reduce susceptibility to cytotoxic T cells. *Nature.* 2005 Jun. 2;435(7042):682-6.

[59] Jopling C. L., Yi M., Lancaster A. M., Lemon S. M., Sarnow P. Modulation of hepatitis C virus RNA abundance by a liver-specific MicroRNA. *Science.* 2005 Sep. 2;309(5740):1577-81.

[60] Li L., Liu J., Diao Z., Shu D., Guo P., Shen G. Evaluation of specific delivery of chimeric phi29 pRNA/siRNA nanoparticles to multiple tumor cells. *Mol. Biosyst.* 2009 Nov.;5(11):1361-8.

[61] Israsena N., Supavonwong P., Ratanasetyuth N., Khawplod P., Hemachudha T. Inhibition of rabies virus replication by multiple artificial microRNAs. *Antiviral Res.* 2009 Oct.;84(1):76-83.

[62] Bouvier N. M., Palese P. The biology of influenza viruses. *Vaccine.* 2008 Sep. 12;26 Suppl. 4:D49-53.

[63] Englund J. A. Antiviral therapy of influenza. *Semin Pediatr Infect Dis.* 2002 Apr.;13(2):120-8.

[64] Saravolac E. G., Wong J. P. Recent Patents on development of nucleic acid-based antiviral drugs against seasonal and pandemic influenza virus infections. *Recent Pat Antiinfect Drug Discov.* 2007 Jun.;2(2):140-7.

[65] Wong J. P., Christopher M. E., Salazar A. M., Dale R. M., Sun L. Q., Wang M. Nucleic acid-based antiviral drugs against seasonal and avian influenza viruses. *Vaccine.* 2007 Apr. 20;25(16):3175-8.

[66] Ge Q., Eisen H. N., Chen J. Use of siRNAs to prevent and treat influenza virus infection. *Virus Res.* 2004 Jun. 1;102(1):37-42.

[67] Lazarev V. N., Shmarov M. M., Zakhartchouk A. N., Yurov G. K., Misurina O. U., Akopian T. A., et al. Inhibition of influenza A virus reproduction by a ribozyme targeted against PB1 mRNA. *Antiviral Res.* 1999 May;42(1):47-57.

[68] Leiter J. M., Agrawal S., Palese P., Zamecnik P. C. Inhibition of influenza virus replication by phosphorothioate oligodeoxynucleotides. *Proc. Natl. Acad. Sci. US.* 1990 May;87(9):3430-4.

[69] Spurgers K. B., Sharkey C. M., Warfield K. L., Bavari S. Oligonucleotide antiviral therapeutics: antisense and RNA interference for highly pathogenic R. N. A. viruses. *Antiviral Res.* 2008 Apr.;78(1): 26-36.

[70] Hatta T., Takai K., Nakada S., Yokota T., Takaku H. Specific inhibition of influenza virus R. N. A. polymerase and nucleoprotein genes expression by liposomally endocapsulated antisense phosphorothioate oligonucleotides: penetration and localization of oligonucleotides in clone 76 cells. *Biochem. Biophys. Res. Commun.* 1997 Mar. 17;232(2): 545-9.

[71] Khaliq S., Khaliq S. A., Zahur M., Ijaz B., Jahan S., Ansar M., et al. RNAi as a new therapeutic strategy against H. C. V. *Biotechnol. Adv.* 2010 Jan.-Feb.;28(1):27-34.

[72] Feld J. J., Hoofnagle J. H. Mechanism of action of interferon and ribavirin in treatment of hepatitis C. *Nature.* 2005 Aug. 18;436(7053): 967-72.

[73] Tsukiyama-Kohara K., Iizuka N., Kohara M., Nomoto A. Internal ribosome entry site within hepatitis C virus R. N. A. *J. Virol.* 1992 Mar.; 66(3):1476-83.

[74] Lin C., Lindenbach B. D., Pragai B. M., McCourt D. W., Rice C. M. Processing in the hepatitis C virus E2-NS2 region: identification of p7 and two distinct E2-specific products with different C termini. *J. Virol.* 1994 Aug.;68(8):5063-73.

[75] Lin C., Pragai B. M., Grakoui A., Xu J., Rice C. M. Hepatitis C virus NS3 serine proteinase: trans-cleavage requirements and processing kinetics. *J. Virol.* 1994 Dec.;68(12):8147-57.

[76] Brown-Driver V., Eto T., Lesnik E., Anderson K. P., Hanecak R. C. Inhibition of translation of hepatitis C virus R. N. A. by 2-modified antisense oligonucleotides. *Antisense Nucleic Acid Drug Dev.* 1999 Apr.;9(2):145-54.

[77] Jubin R., Vantuno N. E., Kieft J. S., Murray M. G., Doudna J. A., Lau J. Y., et al. Hepatitis C virus internal ribosome entry site (I. R. E. S.) stem loop IIId contains a phylogenetically conserved G. G. G. triplet essential for translation and I. R. E. S. folding. *J. Virol.* 2000 Nov.; 74(22):10430-7.

[78] Michel T., Martinand-Mari C., Debart F., Lebleu B., Robbins I., Vasseur J. J. Cationic phosphoramidate alpha-oligonucleotides efficiently target single-stranded D. N. A. and R. N. A. and inhibit hepatitis C virus IRES-mediated translation. *Nucleic Acids Res.* 2003 Sep. 15;31(18):5282-90.

[79] Wakita T., Moradpour D., Tokushihge K., Wands J. R. Antiviral effects of antisense R. N. A. on hepatitis C virus R. N. A. translation and expression. *J. Med. Virol.* 1999 Mar.;57(3):217-22.

[80] Macejak D. G., Jensen K. L., Jamison S. F., Domenico K., Roberts E. C., Chaudhary N., et al. Inhibition of hepatitis C virus (H. C. V.)-R. N. A.-dependent translation and replication of a chimeric H. C. V. poliovirus using synthetic stabilized ribozymes. *Hepatology*. 2000 Mar.;31(3):769-76.

[81] Kapadia S. B., Brideau-Andersen A., Chisari F. V. Interference of hepatitis C virus R. N. A. replication by short interfering RNAs. *Proc. Natl. Acad. Sci. US*. 2003 Feb. 18;100(4):2014-8.

[82] McCaffrey A. P., Meuse L., Pham T. T., Conklin D. S., Hannon G. J., Kay M. A., R. N. A. interference in adult mice. *Nature*. 2002 Jul. 4;418(6893):38-9.

[83] Randall G., Grakoui A., Rice C. M. Clearance of replicating hepatitis C virus replicon RNAs in cell culture by small interfering RNAs. *Proc. Natl. Acad. Sci. US*. 2003 Jan. 7;100(1):235-40.

[84] Wilson J. A., Jayasena S., Khvorova A., Sabatinos S., Rodrigue-Gervais I. G., Arya S., et al. R. N. A. interference blocks gene expression and R. N. A. synthesis from hepatitis C replicons propagated in human liver cells. *Proc. Natl. Acad. Sci. US*. 2003 Mar. 4;100(5): 2783-8.

[85] Wilson J. A., Richardson C. D. Induction of R. N. A. interference using short interfering R. N. A. expression vectors in cell culture and animal systems. *Curr. Opin. Mol Ther*. 2003 Aug.;5(4):389-96.

[86] Yokota T., Sakamoto N., Enomoto N., Tanabe Y., Miyagishi M., Maekawa S., et al. Inhibition of intracellular hepatitis C virus replication by synthetic and vector-derived small interfering RNAs. *E. M. B. O. Rep*. 2003 Jun.;4(6):602-8.

[87] Ray R. B., Kanda T. Inhibition of H. C. V. replication by small interfering R. N. A. *Methods Mol. Biol*. 2009;510:251-62.

[88] Lanford R. E., Hildebrandt-Eriksen E. S., Petri A., Persson R., Lindow M., Munk M. E., et al. Therapeutic silencing of microRNA-122 in primates with chronic hepatitis C virus infection. *Science*. 2010 Jan. 8;327(5962):198-201.

[89] Pfeffer S., Baumert T. F. Antagonizing microRNA-122 and treatment of hepatitis C virus infection. *Hepatology*. 2010 Apr.;51(4):1461-3.

[90] Young D. D., Connelly C. M., Grohmann C., Deiters A. Small molecule modifiers of microRNA miR-122 function for the treatment of hepatitis C virus infection and hepatocellular carcinoma. *J. Am. Chem. Soc*. 2010 Jun. 16;132(23):7976-81.

[91] Lu A., Zhang H., Zhang X., Wang H., Hu Q., Shen L., et al. Attenuation of S. A. R. S. coronavirus by a short hairpin R. N. A. expression plasmid targeting R. N. A.-dependent R. N. A. polymerase. *Virology*. 2004 Jun. 20;324(1):84-9.

[92] Marra M. A., Jones S. J., Astell C. R., Holt R. A., Brooks-Wilson A., Butterfield Y. S., et al. The Genome sequence of the SARS-associated coronavirus. *Science*. 2003 May 30;300(5624):1399-404.

[93] Elmen J., Thonberg H., Ljungberg K., Frieden M., Westergaard M., Xu Y., et al. Locked nucleic acid (L. N. A.) mediated improvements in siRNA stability and functionality. *Nucleic Acids Res*. 2005;33(1):439-47.

[94] Li T., Zhang Y., Fu L., Yu C., Li X., Li Y., et al. siRNA targeting the leader sequence of SARS-CoV inhibits virus replication. *Gene Ther*. 2005 May;12(9):751-61.

[95] Shi Y., Yang D. H., Xiong J., Jia J., Huang B., Jin Y. X. Inhibition of genes expression of S. A. R. S. coronavirus by synthetic small interfering RNAs. *Cell Res*. 2005 Mar.;15(3):193-200.

[96] Zhao G., Ni B., Jiang H., Luo D., Pacal M., Zhou L., et al. Inhibition of severe acute respiratory syndrome-associated coronavirus infection by equine neutralizing antibody in golden Syrian hamsters. *Viral Immunol.* 2007 Spring;20(1):197-205.

[97] Zhou L., Ni B., Luo D., Zhao G., Jia Z., Zhang L., et al. Inhibition of infection caused by severe acute respiratory syndrome-associated coronavirus by equine neutralizing antibody in aged mice. *Int. Immunopharmacol.* 2007 Mar.;7(3):392-400.

[98] Zhang Y., Li T., Fu L., Yu C., Li Y., Xu X., et al. Silencing SARS-CoV Spike protein expression in cultured cells by R. N. A. interference. *F. E. B. S. Lett.* 2004 Feb. 27;560(1-3):141-6.

[99] Li B. J., Tang Q., Cheng D., Qin C., Xie F. Y., Wei Q., et al. Using siRNA in prophylactic and therapeutic regimens against S. A. R. S. coronavirus in Rhesus macaque. *Nat. Med.* 2005 Sep.;11(9):944-51.

[100] Frankel A. D., Young J. A. HIV-1: fifteen proteins and an R. N. A. *Annu. Rev. Biochem.* 1998;67:1-25.

[101] Weinberg M. S., Morris K. V. Are viral-encoded microRNAs mediating latent HIV-1 infection? *D. N. A. Cell Biol.* 2006 Apr.;25(4):223-31.

[102] Lisziewicz J., Sun D., Klotman M., Agrawal S., Zamecnik P., Gallo R. Specific inhibition of human immunodeficiency virus type 1 replication by antisense oligonucleotides: an in vitro model for treatment. *Proc. Natl. Acad. Sci. US.* 1992 Dec. 1;89(23):11209-13.

[103] Coburn G. A., Cullen B. R. Potent and specific inhibition of human immunodeficiency virus type 1 replication by R. N. A. interference. *J. Virol.* 2002 Sep.;76(18):9225-31.

[104] Jacque J. M., Triques K., Stevenson M. Modulation of HIV-1 replication by R. N. A. interference. *Nature.* 2002 Jul. 25;418(6896):435-8.

[105] Lee N. S., Dohjima T., Bauer G., Li H., Li M. J., Ehsani A., et al. Expression of small interfering RNAs targeted against HIV-1 rev transcripts in human cells. *Nat. Biotechnol.* 2002 May;20(5):500-5.

[106] Capodici J., Kariko K., Weissman D. Inhibition of HIV-1 infection by small interfering RNA-mediated R. N. A. interference. *J. Immunol.* 2002 Nov. 1;169(9):5196-201.

[107] Park W. S., Miyano-Kurosaki N., Hayafune M., Nakajima E., Matsuzaki T., Shimada F., et al. Prevention of HIV-1 infection in human peripheral blood mononuclear cells by specific R. N. A. interference. *Nucleic Acids Res.* 2002 Nov. 15;30(22):4830-5.

[108] Bennasser Y., Le S. Y., Yeung M. L., Jeang K. T. HIV-1 encoded candidate micro-RNAs and their cellular targets. *Retrovirology.* 2004;1:43.

[109] Hemida M. G., Ye X., Thair S., Yang D. Exploiting the therapeutic potential of microRNAs in viral diseases: expectations and limitations. *Mol. Diagn Ther.* 2010 Oct. 1;14(5):271-82.

[110] Liu Y. P., Gruber J., Haasnoot J., Konstantinova P., Berkhout B. RNAi-mediated inhibition of HIV-1 by targeting partially complementary viral sequences. *Nucleic Acids Res.* 2009 Oct.;37(18): 6194-204.

[111] Ebbert J. O., Limper A. H. Respiratory syncytial virus pneumonitis in immunocompromised adults: clinical features and outcome. *Respiration.* 2005 May-Jun.;72(3):263-9.

[112] Welliver R. C. Review of epidemiology and clinical risk factors for severe respiratory syncytial virus (R. S. V.) infection. *J. Pediatr.* 2003 Nov.;143(5 Suppl.):S112-7.

[113] Welliver R. C. Respiratory syncytial virus and other respiratory viruses. *Pediatr. Infect Dis. J.* 2003 Feb.;22(2 Suppl.):S6-10; discussion S-2.

[114] Yu Q., Hardy R. W., Wertz G. W. Functional cDNA clones of the human respiratory syncytial (R. S.) virus N., P., and L. proteins support replication of RS virus genomic RNA analogs and define minimal trans-acting requirements for R. N. A. replication. *J. Virol.* 1995 Apr.;69(4): 2412-9.

[115] Falsey A. R. Respiratory syncytial virus infection in adults. *Semin Respir Crit. Care Med.* 2007 Apr.;28(2):171-81.

[116] Murata Y., Falsey A. R. Respiratory syncytial virus infection in adults. *Antivir. Ther.* 2007;12(4 Pt B):659-70.

[117] Player M. R., Barnard D. L., Torrence P. F. Potent inhibition of respiratory syncytial virus replication using a 2-5A-antisense chimera targeted to signals within the virus genomic R. N. A. *Proc. Natl. Acad. Sci. US.* 1998 Jul. 21;95(15):8874-9.

[118] Bitko V., Barik S. Phenotypic silencing of cytoplasmic genes using sequence-specific double-stranded short interfering R. N. A. and its application in the reverse genetics of wild type negative-strand R. N. A. viruses. *B. M. C. Microbiol.* 2001;1:34.

[119] Bitko V., Musiyenko A., Shulyayeva O., Barik S. Inhibition of respiratory viruses by nasally administered siRNA. *Nat. Med.* 2005 Jan.;11(1):50-5.

[120] Zhang W., Tripp R. A. R. N. A. interference inhibits respiratory syncytial virus replication and disease pathogenesis without inhibiting priming of the memory immune response. *J. Virol.* 2008 Dec.;82(24): 12221-31.

[121] Alvarez R., Elbashir S., Borland T., Toudjarska I., Hadwiger P., John M., et al. R. N. A. interference-mediated silencing of the respiratory syncytial virus nucleocapsid defines a potent antiviral strategy. *Antimicrob Agents Chemother.* 2009 Sep.;53(9):3952-62.

[122] Muir P., Kammerer U., Korn K., Mulders M. N., Poyry T., Weissbrich B., et al. Molecular typing of enteroviruses: current status and future requirements. The European Union Concerted Action on Virus Meningitis and Encephalitis. *Clin. Microbiol Rev.* 1998 Jan.; 11(1):202-27.

[123] Stanway G. Structure, function and evolution of picornaviruses. *J. Gen. Virol.* 1990 Nov;.71 (Pt 11):2483-501.

[124] Marchant D., Si X., Luo H., McManus B., Yang D. The impact of CVB3 infection on host cell biology. *Curr. Top Microbiol Immunol.* 2008;323: 177-98.

[125] Yuan J., Cheung P. K., Zhang H. M., Chau D., Yang D. Inhibition of coxsackievirus B3 replication by small interfering RNAs requires perfect sequence match in the central region of the viral positive strand. *J. Virol.* 2005 Feb.;79(4):2151-9.

[126] Merl S., Michaelis C., Jaschke B., Vorpahl M., Seidl S., Wessely R. Targeting 2A protease by R. N. A. interference attenuates coxsackieviral cytopathogenicity and promotes survival in highly susceptible mice. *Circulation.* 2005 Apr. 5;111(13): 1583-92.

[127] Racchi G., Klingel K., Kandolf R., Grassi G. Targeting of protease 2A genome by single and multiple siRNAs as a strategy to impair CVB3 life cycle in permissive HeLa cells. *Methods Find Exp Clin. Pharmacol.* 2009 Mar.;31(2):63-70.

[128] Werk D., Schubert S., Lindig V., Grunert H. P., Zeichhardt H., Erdmann V. A., et al. Developing an effective R. N. A. interference strategy against a plus-strand R. N. A. virus: silencing of coxsackievirus B3 and its cognate coxsackievirus-adenovirus receptor. *Biol Chem.* 2005 Sep.;386(9):857-63.

[129] Zhang H. M., Su Y., Guo S., Yuan J., Lim T., Liu J., et al. Targeted delivery of anti-coxsackievirus siRNAs using ligand-conjugated packaging RNAs. *Antiviral Res.* 2009 Sep.;83(3):307-16.

[130] Kim J. Y., Chung S. K., Hwang H. Y., Kim H., Kim J. H., Nam J. H., et al. Expression of short hairpin RNAs against the coxsackievirus B3 exerts potential antiviral effects in Cos-7 cells and in mice. *Virus Res.* 2007 Apr.;125(1):9-13.

[131] Nygardas M., Vuorinen T., Aalto A. P., Bamford D. H., Hukkanen V. Inhibition of coxsackievirus B3 and related enteroviruses by antiviral short interfering R. N. A. pools produced using phi6 R. N. A.-dependent R. N. A. polymerase. *J. Gen. Virol.* 2009 Oct.;90(Pt 10):2468-73.

[132] Fechner H., Pinkert S., Wang X., Sipo I., Suckau L., Kurreck J., et al. Coxsackievirus B3 and adenovirus infections of cardiac cells are efficiently inhibited by vector-mediated R. N. A. interference targeting their common receptor. *Gene Ther.* 2007 Jun.;14(12):960-71.

[133] Crocker S. J., Frausto R. F., Whitmire J. K., Benning N., Milner R., Whitton J. L. Amelioration of coxsackievirus B3-mediated myocarditis by inhibition of tissue inhibitors of matrix metalloproteinase-1. *Am. J. Pathol.* 2007 Dec.;171(6):1762-73.

[134] Tan E. L., Wong A. P., Poh C. L. Development of potential antiviral strategy against coxsackievirus B4. *Virus Res.* 2010 Jun.;150(1-2):85-92.

[135] Yuan J., Cheung P. K., Zhang H., Chau D., Yanagawa B., Cheung C., et al. A phosphorothioate antisense oligodeoxynucleotide specifically inhibits coxsackievirus B3 replication in cardiomyocytes and mouse hearts. *Lab Invest.* 2004 Jun.;84(6): 703-14.

[136] Guo Y., Guo H., Zhang L., Xie H., Zhao X., Wang F., et al. Genomic analysis of anti-hepatitis B virus (H. B. V.) activity by small interfering R. N. A. and lamivudine in stable H. B. V.-producing cells. *J. Virol.* 2005 Nov.;79(22):14392-403.

[137] Falkenhagen A., Heinrich J., Moelling K. Short hairpin-loop-structured oligodeoxynucleotides reduce HSV-1 replication. *Virol J.* 2009;6:43.

[138] Dolan A., Cunningham C., Hector R. D., Hassan-Walker A. F., Lee L., Addison C., et al. Genetic content of wild-type human cytomegalovirus. *J. Gen. Virol.* 2004 May;85(Pt 5):1301-12.

[139] McGregor A. Current and new cytomegalovirus antivirals and novel animal model strategies. *Inflamm Allergy Drug Targets.* 2010 Sep.;9(4): 286-99.

[140] Borst E. M., Messerle M. Analysis of human cytomegalovirus oriLyt sequence requirements in the context of the viral genome. *J. Virol.* 2005 Mar.;79(6):3615-26.

[141] Trang P., Kim K., Liu F. Developing RNase P ribozymes for gene-targeting and antiviral therapy. *Cell Microbiol.* 2004 Jun.;6(6):499-508.

[142] Duan Q. J., Tao R., Hu M. F., Shang S. Q. Efficient inhibition of human cytomegalovirus UL122 gene expression in cell by small interfering RNAs. *J. Basic Microbiol.* 2009 Dec.;49(6):531-7.

[143] Wiebusch L., Truss M., Hagemeier C. Inhibition of human cytomegalovirus replication by small interfering RNAs. *J. Gen. Virol.* 2004 Jan.;85(Pt 1):179-84.

[144] Zeng Z., Li H., Li Y., Cui Y., Zhou Q., Zou Y., et al. Effective inhibition of human cytomegalovirus gene expression by D. N. A.-based external guide sequences. *Acta Biochim. Biophys. Sin* (Shanghai). 2009 May; 41(5):389-98.

[145] Grey F., Meyers H., White E. A., Spector D. H., Nelson J. A human cytomegalovirus-encoded microR. N. A. regulates expression of multiple viral genes involved in replication. *PLoS Pathog.* 2007 Nov.; 3(11):e163.
[146] Grey F., Nelson J. Identification and function of human cytomegalovirus microRNAs. *J. Clin. Virol.* 2008 Mar.;41(3):186-91.
[147] Murphy E., Vanicek J., Robins H., Shenk T., Levine A. J. Suppression of immediate-early viral gene expression by herpesvirus-coded microRNAs: implications for latency. *Proc. Natl. Acad. Sci. US.* 2008 Apr. 8;105(14):5453-8.
[148] zur Hausen H. Papillomavirus infections--a major cause of human cancers. *Biochim. Biophys Acta.* 1996 Oct. 9;1288(2):F55-78.
[149] zur Hausen H. Roots and perspectives of contemporary papillomavirus research. *J. Cancer Res. Clin. Oncol.* 1996;122(1):3-13.
[150] Bharti A. C., Shukla S., Mahata S., Hedau S., Das B. C. Anti-human papillomavirus therapeutics: facts and future. *Indian J. Med. Res.* 2009 Sep.;130(3):296-310.
[151] Munger K., Phelps W. C., Bubb V., Howley P. M., Schlegel R. The E6 and E7 genes of the human papillomavirus type 16 together are necessary and sufficient for transformation of primary human keratinocytes. *J. Virol.* 1989 Oct.;63(10):4417-21.
[152] Greenstone H. L., Nieland J. D., de Visser K. E., De Bruijn M. L., Kirnbauer R., Roden R. B., et al. Chimeric papillomavirus virus-like particles elicit antitumor immunity against the E7 oncoprotein in an HPV16 tumor model. *Proc. Natl. Acad. Sci. US.* 1998 Feb. 17;95(4): 1800-5.
[153] Alvarez-Salas L. M., Cullinan A. E., Siwkowski A., Hampel A., DiPaolo J. A. Inhibition of HPV-16 E6/E7 immortalization of normal keratinocytes by hairpin ribozymes. *Proc. Natl. Acad. Sci. US.* 1998 Feb. 3;95(3):1189-94.
[154] Bai L., Wei L., Wang J., Li X., He P. Extended effects of human papillomavirus 16 E6-specific short hairpin RNA on cervical carcinoma cells. *Int. J. Gynecol. Cancer.* 2006 Mar.-Apr.;16(2):718-29.
[155] Jiang M., Milner J. Selective silencing of viral gene expression in H. P. V.-positive human cervical carcinoma cells treated with siRNA, a primer of R. N. A. interference. *Oncogene.* 2002 Sep. 5;21(39):6041-8.
[156] Steele C., Cowsert L. M., Shillitoe E. J. Effects of human papillomavirus type 18-specific antisense oligonucleotides on the transformed phenotype of human carcinoma cell lines. *Cancer Res.* 1993 May 15;53 (10 Suppl.):2330-7.
[157] Tan T. M., Ting R. C. In vitro and in vivo inhibition of human papillomavirus type 16 E6 and E7 genes. *Cancer Res.* 1995 Oct. 15;55(20):4599-605.
[158] Madrigal M., Janicek M. F., Sevin B. U., Perras J., Estape R., Penalver M., et al. In vitro antigene therapy targeting HPV-16 E6 and E7 in cervical carcinoma. *Gynecol Oncol.* 1997 Jan.;64(1):18-25.
[159] Hamada K., Alemany R., Zhang W. W., Hittelman W. N., Lotan R., Roth J. A., et al. Adenovirus-mediated transfer of a wild-type p53 gene and induction of apoptosis in cervical cancer. *Cancer Res.* 1996 Jul. 1;56(13) :047-54.
[160] Hamada K., Sakaue M., Alemany R., Zhang W. W., Horio Y., Roth J. A., et al. Adenovirus-mediated transfer of HPV 16 E6/E7 antisense R. N. A. to human cervical cancer cells. *Gynecol. Oncol.* 1996 Nov.;63(2):219-27.

[161] Zheng Y., Zhang J., Rao Z. Ribozyme targeting HPV16 E6E7 transcripts in cervical cancer cells suppresses cell growth and sensitizes cells to chemotherapy and radiotherapy. *Cancer Biol. Ther.* 2004 Nov.; 3(11):1129-34; discussion 35-6.
[162] Butz K., Ristriani T., Hengstermann A., Denk C., Scheffner M., Hoppe-Seyler F. siRNA targeting of the viral E6 oncogene efficiently kills human papillomavirus-positive cancer cells. *Oncogene.* 2003 Sep. 4;22(38):5938-45.
[163] Gu W., Putral L., Hengst K., Minto K., Saunders N. A., Leggatt G., et al. Inhibition of cervical cancer cell growth in vitro and in vivo with lentiviral-vector delivered short hairpin R. N. A. targeting human papillomavirus E6 and E7 oncogenes. *Cancer Gene Ther.* 2006 Nov.; 13(11):1023-32.
[164] Yamato K., Yamada T., Kizaki M., Ui-Tei K., Natori Y., Fujino M., et al. New highly potent and specific E6 and E7 siRNAs for treatment of HPV16 positive cervical cancer. *Cancer Gene Ther.* 2008 Mar.;15(3):140-53.
[165] Niu X. Y., Peng Z. L., Duan W. Q., Wang H., Wang P. Inhibition of H. P. V. 16 E6 oncogene expression by R. N. A. interference in vitro and in vivo. *Int. J. Gynecol Cancer.* 2006 Mar.-Apr.;16(2):743-51.
[166] Wang X., Wang H. K., McCoy J. P., Banerjee N. S., Rader J. S., Broker T. R., et al. Oncogenic H. P. V. infection interrupts the expression of tumor-suppressive miR-34a through viral oncoprotein E6. *R. N. A.* 2009 Apr.;15(4):637-47.
[167] Bunnell B. A., Morgan R. A. Gene therapy for infectious diseases. *Clin. Microbiol. Rev.* 1998 Jan.;11(1):42-56.
[168] Alama A., Barbieri F., Cagnoli M., Schettini G. Antisense oligonucleotides as therapeutic agents. Pharmacol Res. 1997 Sep.; 36(3):171-8.
[169] Mescalin A., and Restle, T. Oligomeric Nucleic acid antivirals. *Molcules.* 2011;16:1271-96.
[170] Lopez-Fraga M., Wright N., Jimenez A., R. N. A. interference-based therapeutics: new strategies to fight infectious disease. *Infect Disord Drug Targets.* 2008 Dec.;8(4): 262-73.
[171] Prasad S. C., and Roy, I. Nucleic acid based therapeutic molcules. *C. R. I. P. S.* 2008;9(3):49-55.
[172] Castanotto D., Rossi J. J. The promises and pitfalls of RNA-interference-based therapeutics. *Nature.* 2009 Jan. 22;457(7228):426-33.
[173] Schubert S., Grunert H. P., Zeichhardt H., Werk D., Erdmann V. A., Kurreck J. Maintaining inhibition: siRNA double expression vectors against coxsackieviral RNAs. *J. Mol. Biol.* 2005 Feb. 18;346(2):457-65.
[174] Ryan S. M., Mantovani G., Wang X., Haddleton D. M., Brayden D. J. Advances in PEGylation of important biotech molecules: delivery aspects. *Expert Opin Drug Deliv.* 2008 Apr.;5(4):371-83.
[175] Jackson A. L., Linsley P. S. Recognizing and avoiding siRNA off-target effects for target identification and therapeutic application. *Nat. Rev. Drug Discov.* 2010 Jan.;9(1):57-67.
[176] James H. A., Gibson I. The therapeutic potential of ribozymes. *Blood.* 1998 Jan. 15;91(2):371-82.
[177] Jackson A. L., Bartz S. R., Schelter J., Kobayashi S. V., Burchard J., Mao M., et al. Expression profiling reveals off-target gene regulation by RNAi. *Nat. Biotechnol.* 2003 Jun.;21(6):635-7.

[178] Marques J. T., Williams B. R. Activation of the mammalian immune system by siRNAs. *Nat Biotechnol.* 2005 Nov.;23(11):1399-405.

[179] Scacheri P. C., Rozenblatt-Rosen O., Caplen N. J., Wolfsberg T. G., Umayam L., Lee J. C., et al. Short interfering RNAs can induce unexpected and divergent changes in the levels of untargeted proteins in mammalian cells. *Proc. Natl. Acad. Sci. US.* 2004 Feb. 17;101(7): 1892-7.

[180] Sioud M. Induction of inflammatory cytokines and interferon responses by double-stranded and single-stranded siRNAs is sequence-dependent and requires endosomal localization. *J. Mol. Biol.* 2005 May 20;348(5): 1079-90.

[181] Chiu Y. L., Rana T. M. RNAi in human cells: basic structural and functional features of small interfering R. N. A. *Mol Cell.* 2002 Sep.; 10(3):549-61.

[182] Kim D. H., Behlke M. A., Rose S. D., Chang M. S., Choi S., Rossi J. J. Synthetic dsRNA Dicer substrates enhance RNAi potency and efficacy. *Nat. Biotechnol.* 2005 Feb.;23(2):222-6.

[183] Reynolds A., Leake D., Boese Q., Scaringe S., Marshall W. S., Khvorova A. Rational siRNA design for R. N. A. interference. *Nat. Biotechnol.* 2004 Mar.;22(3):326-30.

[184] Braasch D. A., Jensen S., Liu Y., Kaur K., Arar K., White M. A., et al. R. N. A. interference in mammalian cells by chemically-modified R. N. A. *Biochemistry.* 2003 Jul. 8;42(26):7967-75.

[185] Cheng K., Ye Z., Guntaka R. V., Mahato R. I. Enhanced hepatic uptake and bioactivity of type alpha1(I) collagen gene promoter-specific triplex-forming oligonucleotides after conjugation with cholesterol. *J. Pharmacol. Exp. Ther.* 2006 May;317(2):797-805.

[186] Czauderna F., Fechtner M., Dames S., Aygun H., Klippel A., Pronk G. J., et al. Structural variations and stabilising modifications of synthetic siRNAs in mammalian cells. *Nucleic Acids Res.* 2003 Jun. 1;31(11):2705-16.

[187] Hall A. H., Wan J., Shaughnessy E. E., Ramsay Shaw B., Alexander K. A., R. N. A. interference using boranophosphate siRNAs: structure-activity relationships. *Nucleic. Acids Res.* 2004;32(20):5991-6000.

[188] Jacobson I. M. Therapeutic options for chronic hepatitis B: considerations and controversies. *Am. J. Gastroenterol.* 2006;101 Suppl. 1:S13-8.

[189] Lorenz C., Hadwiger P., John M., Vornlocher H. P., Unverzagt C. Steroid and lipid conjugates of siRNAs to enhance cellular uptake and gene silencing in liver cells. *Bioorg. Med. Chem. Lett.* 2004 Oct. 4;14(19):4975-7.

[190] Muratovska A., Eccles M. R. Conjugate for efficient delivery of short interfering R. N. A. (siRNA) into mammalian cells. *F. E. B. S. Lett.* 2004 Jan. 30;558(1-3):63-8.

[191] Simeoni F., Morris M. C., Heitz F., Divita G. Insight into the mechanism of the peptide-based gene delivery system M. P. G.: implications for delivery of siRNA into mammalian cells. *Nucleic Acids Res.* 2003 Jun. 1;31(11):2717-24.

[192] Choi Y., Thomas T., Kotlyar A., Islam M. T., Baker J. R., Jr. Synthesis and functional evaluation of DNA-assembled polyamidoamine dendrimer clusters for cancer cell-specific targeting. *Chem. Biol.* 2005 Jan.;12(1):35-43.

[193] Han S., Mahato R. I., Sung Y. K., Kim S. W. Development of biomaterials for gene therapy. *Mol. Ther.* 2000 Oct.;2(4):302-17.

[194] Mahato R. I., Rolland A., Tomlinson E. Cationic lipid-based gene delivery systems: pharmaceutical perspectives. *Pharm. Res.* 1997 Jul.;14(7):853-9.

[195] Santel A., Aleku M., Keil O., Endruschat J., Esche V., Fisch G., et al. A novel siRNA-lipoplex technology for R. N. A. interference in the mouse vascular endothelium. *Gene Ther.* 2006 Aug.;13(16):1222-34.

[196] Zhang C., Tang N., Liu X., Liang W., Xu W., Torchilin V. P. siRNA-containing liposomes modified with polyarginine effectively silence the targeted gene. *J. Control Release.* 2006 May 15;112(2):229-39.

[197] Daddario-DiCaprio K. M., Geisbert T. W., Stroher U., Geisbert J. B., Grolla A., Fritz E. A., et al. Postexposure protection against Marburg haemorrhagic fever with recombinant vesicular stomatitis virus vectors in non-human primates: an efficacy assessment. *Lancet.* 2006 Apr. 29;367(9520):1399-404.

[198] Geisbert T. W., Hensley L. E., Kagan E., Yu E. Z., Geisbert J. B., Daddario-DiCaprio K., et al. Postexposure protection of guinea pigs against a lethal ebola virus challenge is conferred by R. N. A. interference. *J. Infect. Dis.* 2006 Jun. 15;193(12):1650-7.

[199] Morrissey D. V., Lockridge J. A., Shaw L., Blanchard K., Jensen K., Breen W., et al. Potent and persistent in vivo anti-HBV activity of chemically modified siRNAs. *Nat Biotechnol.* 2005 Aug.;23(8):1002-7.

[200] Zimmermann T. S., Lee A. C., Akinc A., Bramlage B., Bumcrot D., Fedoruk M. N., et al. RNAi-mediated gene silencing in non-human primates. *Nature.* 2006 May 4;441(7089):111-4.

[201] Gitlin L., Andino R. Nucleic acid-based immune system: the antiviral potential of mammalian R. N. A. silencing. *J. Virol.* 2003 Jul.;77(13): 7159-65.

[202] Gopinath S. C., Balasundaresan D., Akitomi J., Mizuno H. An R. N. A. aptamer that discriminates bovine factor IX from human factor IX. *J. Biochem.* 2006 Nov.;140(5): 667-76.

[203] Gopinath S. C., Misono T. S., Kawasaki K., Mizuno T., Imai M., Odagiri T., et al. An R. N. A. aptamer that distinguishes between closely related human influenza viruses and inhibits haemagglutinin-mediated membrane fusion. *J. Gen. Virol.* 2006 Mar.; 87(Pt 3):479-87.

[204] Abe T. M. T., Hatta T., Miyano-Kurosaki N., Fujiwara M., Takai K., Shigeta S., Yokota T., Takaku H. Antisense therapy of influenza. *Eur. J. Pharm. Sci.* 2001;13(1):61-9.

[205] Tompkins S. M., Lo C. Y., Tumpey T. M., Epstein S. L. Protection against lethal influenza virus challenge by RNA interference in vivo. *Proc. Natl. Acad. Sci. US.* 2004 Jun. 8;101(23):8682-6.

[206] McCown M., Diamond M. S., Pekosz A. The utility of siRNA transcripts produced by R. N. A. polymerase i in down regulating viral gene expression and replication of negative- and positive-strand R. N. A. viruses. *Virology.* 2003 Sep. 1;313(2):514-24.

[207] Song L., Liu H., Gao S., Jiang W., Huang W. Cellular microRNAs inhibit replication of the H1N1 influenza A virus in infected cells. *J. Virol.* 2010 Sep.;84(17):8849-60.

[208] Aldaz-Carroll L., Tallet B., Dausse E., Yurchenko L., Toulme J. J. Apical loop-internal loop interactions: a new R. N. A. – R. N. A. recognition motif identified through in vitro selection against R. N. A. hairpins of the hepatitis C virus mRNA. *Biochemistry.* 2002 May 7;41(18):5883-93.

[209] Bellecave P., Andreola M. L., Ventura M., Tarrago-Litvak L., Litvak S., Astier-Gin T. Selection of D. N. A. aptamers that bind the R. N. A.-dependent R. N. A. polymerase of

hepatitis C virus and inhibit viral R. N. A. synthesis in vitro. *Oligonucleotides*. 2003;13(6):455-63.

[210] Biroccio A., Hamm J., Incitti I., De Francesco R., Tomei L. Selection of R. N. A. aptamers that are specific and high-affinity ligands of the hepatitis C virus R. N. A.-dependent R. N. A. polymerase. *J. Virol*. 2002 Apr.;76(8):3688-96.

[211] Hwang B., Cho J. S., Yeo H. J., Kim J. H., Chung K. M., Han K., et al. Isolation of specific and high-affinity R. N. A. aptamers against NS3 helicase domain of hepatitis C virus. *R. N. A.* 2004 Aug.;10(8):1277-90.

[212] Hugle T., Cerny A. Current therapy and new molecular approaches to antiviral treatment and prevention of hepatitis C. *Rev. Med. Virol.* 2003 Nov.-Dec.;13(6):361-71.

[213] Wakita T., Wands J. R. Specific inhibition of hepatitis C virus expression by antisense oligodeoxynucleotides. In vitro model for selection of target sequence. *J. Biol. Chem.* 1994 May 13;269(19): 14205-10.

[214] Wilson J. A., Richardson C. D. Hepatitis C virus replicons escape R. N. A. interference induced by a short interfering R. N. A. directed against the NS5b coding region. *J. Virol*. 2005 Jun.;79(11):7050-8.

[215] Zhang J., Yamada O., Sakamoto T., Yoshida H., Iwai T., Matsushita Y., et al. Down-regulation of viral replication by adenoviral-mediated expression of siRNA against cellular cofactors for hepatitis C virus. *Virology*. 2004 Mar. 1;320(1):135-43.

[216] Ahn D. G., Jeon I. J., Kim J. D., Song M. S., Han S. R., Lee S. W., et al. R. N. A. aptamer-based sensitive detection of S. A. R. S. coronavirus nucleocapsid protein. *Analyst*. 2009 Sep.;134(9):1896-901.

[217] Shum K. T., Tanner J. A. Differential inhibitory activities and stabilisation of D. N. A. aptamers against the S. A. R. S. coronavirus helicase. *Chembiochem*. 2008 Dec. 15;9(18):3037-45.

[218] Fukushima A., Fukuda N., Lai Y., Ueno T., Moriyama M., Taguchi F., et al. Development of a chimeric D. N. A. – R. N. A. hammerhead ribozyme targeting S. A. R. S. virus. *Intervirology*. 2009;52(2):92-9.

[219] Shi Y., Luo H., Jia J., Xiong J., Yang D., Huang B., et al. Antisense downregulation of SARS-CoV gene expression in Vero E6 cells. *J. Gene Med*. 2005 Jan.;7(1):97-107.

[220] He M. L., Zheng B., Peng Y., Peiris J. S., Poon L. L., Yuen K. Y., et al. Inhibition of SARS-associated coronavirus infection and replication by R. N. A. interference. *J. A. M. A.* 2003 Nov. 26;290(20):2665-6.

[221] Zhao P., Qin Z. L., Ke J. S., Lu Y., Liu M., Pan W., et al. Small interfering R. N. A. inhibits SARS-CoV nucleocapsid gene expression in cultured cells and mouse muscles. *F. E. B. S. Lett.* 2005 Apr. 25; 579(11):2404-10.

[222] Lai S. H., Stein D. A., Guerrero-Plata A., Liao S. L., Ivanciuc T., Hong C., et al. Inhibition of respiratory syncytial virus infections with morpholino oligomers in cell cultures and in mice. *Mol. Ther.* 2008 Jun.;16(6):1120-8.

[223] Barik S. Control of nonsegmented negative-strand R. N. A. virus replication by siRNA. *Virus Res*. 2004 Jun. 1;102(1):27-35.

[224] Fischer A. J., Wohlford-Lenane, C. L., Sinn, P. L., Jia, H. P., Varga, S. M., Davidson, B. L., McCray, B. P. RNAi Applications for Respiratory Epithelia: Delivery and Efficacy. *Molecular Therapy*. 2005;11:S317.

[225] Boiziau C., Dausse E., Yurchenko L., Toulme J. J., D. N. A. aptamers selected against the HIV-1 trans-activation-responsive R. N. A. element form R. N. A. – D. N. A. kissing complexes. *J. Biol. Chem.* 1999 Apr. 30;274(18):12730-7.
[226] Khati M., Schuman M., Ibrahim J., Sattentau Q., Gordon S., James W. Neutralization of infectivity of diverse R5 clinical isolates of human immunodeficiency virus type 1 by gp120-binding 2'F-RNA aptamers. *J. Virol.* 2003 Dec.;77(23):12692-8.
[227] Pileur F., Andreola M. L., Dausse E., Michel J., Moreau S., Yamada H., et al. Selective inhibitory D. N. A. aptamers of the human RNase H1. *Nucleic Acids Res.* 2003 Oct. 1;31(19):5776-88.
[228] Yamamoto R., Katahira M., Nishikawa S., Baba T., Taira K., Kumar P. K. A novel R. N. A. motif that binds efficiently and specifically to the Ttat protein of H. I. V. and inhibits the trans-activation by Tat of transcription in vitro and in vivo. *Genes Cells.* 2000 May;5(5):371-88.
[229] Taylor N. R., Rossi J. J. Ribozyme-mediated cleavage of an HIV-1 gag R. N. A.: the effects of nontargeted sequences and secondary structure on ribozyme cleavage activity. *Antisense Res. Dev.* 1991 Summer; 1(2):173-86.
[230] Arzumanov A., Walsh A. P., Liu X., Rajwanshi V. K., Wengel J., Gait M. J. Oligonucleotide analogue interference with the HIV-1 Tat protein-TAR R. N. A. interaction. Nucleosides *Nucleotides Nucleic Acids.* 2001 Apr.-Jul.;20(4-7):471-80.
[231] Galderisi U., Cipollaro M., Cascino A. Clinical trials of a new class of therapeutic agents: antisense oligonucleotides. *Expert Opin. Emerg. Drugs.* 2001 Apr.;6(1):69-79.
[232] Vickers T., Baker B. F., Cook P. D., Zounes M., Buckheit R. W., Jr., Germany J., et al. Inhibition of H. I. V. – L. T. R. gene expression by oligonucleotides targeted to the TAR element. *Nucleic Acids Res.* 1991 Jun. 25;19(12):3359-68.
[233] Boden D., Pusch O., Lee F., Tucker L., Ramratnam B. Human immunodeficiency virus type 1 escape from R. N. A. interference. *J. Virol.* 2003 Nov.;77(21):11531-5.
[234] Unwalla H. J., Li M. J., Kim J. D., Li H. T., Ehsani A., Alluin J., et al. Negative feedback inhibition of HIV-1 by TAT-inducible expression of siRNA. *Nat. Biotechnol.* 2004 Dec.;22(12):1573-8.
[235] Wang J., Bakkers J. M., Galama J. M., Bruins Slot H. J., Pilipenko E. V., Agol V. I., et al. Structural requirements of the higher order R. N. A. kissing element in the enteroviral 3'UTR. *Nucleic Acids Res.* 1999 Jan. 15;27(2):485-90.
[236] Brandao P. E., Castilho, J. G., Fahl, W., Carnieli, P., Oliveira, R. Short-interfering RNAs as antiviral against Rabies. *The Brazilian Journal of Infectious Disease.* 2007;11(2):224-5.
[237] Tan T. M., Zhou L., Houssais S., Seet B. L., Jaenicke S., Peter F., et al. Intracellular inhibition of hepatitis B virus S gene expression by chimeric D. N. A. – R. N. A. phosphorothioate minimized ribozyme. *Antisense Nucleic Acid Drug Dev.* 2002 Aug.;12(4):257-64.
[238] Wands J. R., Geissler M., Putlitz J. Z., Blum H., von Weizsacker F., Mohr L., et al. Nucleic acid-based antiviral and gene therapy of chronic hepatitis B infection. *J. Gastroenterol Hepatol.* 1997 Oct.;12(9-10):S354-69.
[239] Giladi H., Ketzinel-Gilad M., Rivkin L., Felig Y., Nussbaum O., Galun E. Small interfering R. N. A. inhibits hepatitis B virus replication in mice. *Mol. Ther.* 2003 Nov.;8(5):769-76.

[240] Hamasaki K., Nakao K., Matsumoto K., Ichikawa T., Ishikawa H., Eguchi K. Short interfering RNA-directed inhibition of hepatitis B virus replication. *F. E. B. S. Lett.* 2003 May 22;543(1-3):51-4.

[241] Chen Y., Du D., Wu J., Chan C. P., Tan Y., Kung H. F., et al. Inhibition of hepatitis B virus replication by stably expressed shRNA. *Biochem. Biophys Res. Commun.* 2003 Nov. 14;311(2):398-404.

[242] Ren X. R., Zhou L. J., Luo G. B., Lin B., Xu A. Inhibition of hepatitis B virus replication in 2.2.15 cells by expressed shRNA. *J. Viral Hepat.* 2005 May;12(3): 236-42.

[243] Liu J., Lewin A. S., Tuli S. S., Ghivizzani S. C., Schultz G. S., Bloom D. C. Reduction in severity of a herpes simplex virus type 1 murine infection by treatment with a ribozyme targeting the UL20 gene R. N. A. *J. Virol.* 2008 Aug.;82(15):7467-74.

[244] Bryant K. F., Cox J. C., Wang H., Hogle J. M., Ellington A. D., Coen D. M. Binding of herpes simplex virus-1 US11 to specific R. N. A. sequences. *Nucleic Acids Res.* 2005;33(19):6090-100.

[245] Kean J. M., Kipp S. A., Miller P. S., Kulka M., Aurelian L. Inhibition of herpes simplex virus replication by antisense oligo-2'-O-methylribonucleoside methylphosphonates. *Biochemistry.* 1995 Nov. 14;34(45):14617-20.

[246] Bhuyan P. K., Kariko K., Capodici J., Lubinski J., Hook L. M., Friedman H. M., et al. Short interfering RNA-mediated inhibition of herpes simplex virus type 1 gene expression and function during infection of human keratinocytes. *J. Virol.* 2004 Oct.;78(19):10276-81.

[247] Palliser D., Chowdhury D., Wang Q. Y., Lee S. J., Bronson R. T., Knipe D. M., et al. An siRNA-based microbicide protects mice from lethal herpes simplex virus 2 infection. *Nature.* 2006 Jan. 5;439(7072): 89-94.

[248] Kaiser N., Lischka P., Wagenknecht N., Stamminger T. Inhibition of human cytomegalovirus replication via peptide aptamers directed against the nonconventional nuclear localization signal of the essential viral replication factor pUL84. *J. Virol.* 2009 Nov.;83(22):11902-13.

[249] Bai Z., Li L., Wang B., Liu Z., Liu H., Jiang G., et al. Inhibition of human cytomegalovirus infection by IE86-specific short hairpin R. N. A.-mediated R. N. A. interference. *Biosci. Biotechnol. Biochem.* 2010;74(7):1368-72.

[250] Tao R., Hu M., Duan Q., Shang S. Efficient inhibition of human cytomegalovirus D. N. A. polymerase expression by small hairpin R. N. A. in vitro. *Curr. Microbiol.* 2008 Nov.;57(5):395-400.

[251] Huang Y., Kong Y., Wang Y., Qi G., Lu C. Stable expression of anti-HPV 16 E7-ribozyme in CV-1 cell lines. *Chin J. Biotechnol.* 1996; 12(4):215-20.

[252] Nauenburg S., Zwerschke W., Jansen-Durr P. Induction of apoptosis in cervical carcinoma cells by peptide aptamers that bind to the HPV-16 E7 oncoprotein. *FASEB J.* 2001 Mar.;15(3):592-4.

[253] Lea J. S., Sunaga N., Sato M., Kalahasti G., Miller D. S., Minna J. D., et al. Silencing of H. P. V. 18 oncoproteins With R. N. A. interference causes growth inhibition of cervical cancer cells. *Reprod. Sci.* 2007 Jan.;14(1):20-8.

[254] Qi Z., Xu X., Zhang B., Li Y., Liu J., Chen S., et al. Effect of simultaneous silencing of HPV-18 E6 and E7 on inducing apoptosis in HeLa cells. *Biochem. Cell Biol.* 2010 Aug.;88(4):697-704.

In: Medical and Biological Frontiers Research Compendium ISBN: 978-1-62417-022-5
Editor: Tsisana Shartava

Chapter 2

The Role of Platelet-Rich Plasma Injections in Achilles Tendonoses

Wasim Khan*[*1] and Umile Giuseppe Longo[2#]
[1]University College London Institute of Orthopaedics and Musculoskeletal Science, London, UK
[2]Campus Bio-Medico University, Rome, Italy

Abstract

Tendon disorders include Achilles tendonoses and are common. Achilles tendonosis has poor results with conservative surgery and many patients eventually require surgical management. There has been an increasing interest in the use of platelet rich plasma for Achilles tendonosis supported by the fact that it is a less invasive treatment option with a good safety profile, and the availability of new devices for outpatient preparation and delivery. It is thought that platelet rich plasma injection for Achilles tendonosis is effective because of the high concentration of platelets it delivers. Although recent reviews report promising results of the use of platelet rich plasma in tendonosis, a recent systematic review of randomised controlled trials showed that platelet rich plasma was not more efficacious than placebo for Achilles tendonosis. There is only limited evidence in the literature supporting the use of platelet rich plasma in Achilles tendonosis, and it is based on animal studies and clinical studies with limitations. There is only one high quality randomised control study that compared platelet rich plasma with control saline injection in Achilles tendonosis, and showed no significant difference between both groups. Control subjects may have responded to saline injections as active therapy as these produce some local trauma and bleeding, and this has shown to have a stimulatory effect on the tendon. Injection of any fluid invariably changes the pressure-volume relationship within a given anatomical space and can potentially destroy pathological vascular and neural growth. We conclude that platelet rich plasma injection in Achilles

* Corresponding Author: Mr Wasim S Khan, Clinical Lecturer, University College London Institute of Orthopaedics and Musculoskeletal Science, Royal National Orthopaedic Hospital, Stanmore, London, HA7 4LP, U. K. Telephone number: +44 (0) 7971 190720. Fax number: +44 (0) 20 8570 3864. E-mail address: *wasimkhan@doctors.org.uk*.

Orthopaedic Specilaist, Campus Bio-Medico University, Via Alvaro del Portillo, 200, 00128 Trigoria Rome, Italy.

tendonosis is effective not because of the high concentration of platelets it delivers, but due to the local injection effects of percutaneous tenotomy, local bleeding and changes in pressure-volume relationship.

Introduction

Tendon disorders account for around 40% of all sports-related injuries [1]. Tendonosis is a tendon disorder characterised by the clinical triad of pain, swelling and decreased activity [2]. The Achilles tendon has inherent poor healing properties [3] and patients with Achilles tendonosis generally do not improve with a wait-and-see approach [4]. As the results with conservative treatment with Achilles tendonosis have been disappointing, 25%-45% of patients eventually require surgical management [2].

Platelet Rich Plasma (PRP) is a volume of the plasma fraction from autologous blood with a platelet concentration almost four times the baseline [5,6]. Autologous activated platelets are proposed to be a source of growth factors that in turn control cell fate including cell growth, differentiation and the synthesis of functional proteins facilitating tendon repair [7]. Procedures are described where platelets are derived from whole blood using simple cell-separating systems [8,9]. There is general acceptance of PRP as it offers a less invasive treatment option and when initially proposed, was supported by basic sciences research and animal studies. It use continues to grow encouraged by its safety as well as the availability of new devices for outpatient preparation and delivery of PRP. There is increasing interest and use of PRP for Achilles tendonosis in orthopaedics, rheumatology and sports medicine clinical setting [8-12]. It is thought that PRP injection for Achilles tendonosis is effective because of the high concentration of platelets it delivers.

Although recent reviews report promising results of the use of PRP in tendonosis [8,10,11], a recent systematic review of randomised controlled trials published in Lancet showed that PRP was not more efficacious than placebo for Achilles tendonosis [13]. There is only limited evidence in the literature suggesting that PRP affects outcome in Achilles tendonosis, and it consists of animal studies or clinical studies with limitations.

A study on rabbits suggested that PRP enhances neovascularisation which may accelerate the healing process and promotes scar tissue of better histological quality [14]. In the study, the Achilles tendon was transacted transversely and either PRP or saline was injected in the tendon mass. Although immunohistochemical staining at one and two weeks showed greater angiogenesis and better organised collagen fibres in the PRP group, at four weeks the number of the newly formed vessels were significantly reduced compared to the control. In a follow-up study, the same group suggested that PRP may affect tendon healing by altering TGF-beta1 expression [15]. PRP treatment resulted in a TGF-beta1 expression upregulation during the first two weeks but a downregulation in the following two weeks. In this study, no other genes were examined. These studies had a number of limitations. They were based on an animal model that has not been validated for tendonosis and the rabbit tendons in this study were transacted with a transverse incision. There was also limited follow-up of only four weeks and the results were variable.

In a sheep acute Achilles tendon rupture model study, an acellular porcine dermal patch with a PRP fibrin matrix was shown to augment tendon repair compared with a control group [16]. After 24 weeks, biomechanical and histological testing was performed and showed no significant elongation, no fibrosis and healing occurred with new tendon fibres across the separation and peripheral integration of the patch to the tendon fibres. In an earlier animal study looking at the effects of platelets on Achilles tendon regenerates in rats following transaction, tensile testing at 14 days showed improved repair [17]. In an *in vitro* and sheep model study, cultured tendon cells seeded on platelet-rich matrix showed enhanced proliferation, and synthesised more angiogenic factor, VEGF compared to platelet-poor matrix [18]. There was no difference in type I collagen or the angiogenic factor HGF. Infiltration in sheep tendon was performed to assess the in vivo cellular and vascular effects of each treatment. The results showed that the injection of pre-clotted plasma within tendons increased cellular density and promoted neovascularization.

There have been a number of clinical studies looking at the effect of PRP in Achilles tendonosis but they have been limited as they were either uncontrolled or had limitations in their design. In a recent study autologous PRP was injected into 15 Achilles tendons of 14 patients with Acilles tendonosis [19]. The patients were followed-up with physical and imaging evaluations at 6 weeks, and at 3, 6, and 18 months. Although the study showed a statistically significant improvement in the American Orthopedic Foot and Ankle Society (AOFAS) scale and the validated Victorian Institute of Sport Assessment- Achilles (VISA-A) scale, there was no control group. In another case report, a 34-year old competitive athlete underwent autologous PRP injections into an Achilles tendon lesion on three occasions, seven days apart, followed by a progressive rehabilitation programme [20]. The patient managed to return to competitive sport after 64 days, and tissue repair was confirmed by magnetic resonance and ultrasound imaging. In a case-control study, six athletes underwent open suture repair for Achilles tendon rupture in conjunction with a preparation rich in platelet growth factors and were compared with six athletes from a retrospective historical group who underwent open repair only [21]. The study group recovered their range of motion earlier and took less time to take up gentle running and resume training activities. The cross-section area in the study group was less than the control. The study was limited in that the control group was a retrospective historical group and the authors acknowledged the need for a randomised clinical trial.

There is only one high quality randomised control double-blinded study that performed a sample size calculation to ensure appropriate power, lost no patients to follow-up and used a validated disease-specific outcome measure [22]. The study compared eccentric exercises with either a PRP or control saline injection in Achilles tendonosis. The mean VISA-A questionnaire score improved significantly after 24 weeks in the PRP group by 21.7 points and in the saline group by 20.5 points. The increase was not significantly different between both groups. The authors conclude that among patients with chronic Achilles tendonosis who were treated with eccentric exercises, a PRP injection compared with a saline injection did not result in greater improvement in pain and activity. The authors provide two possible explanations for no obvious benefit in the PRP group compared with the saline group:

1. Eccentric exercises, with proven efficacy, were undertaken by both groups.
2. Substantial placebo effect following saline injection due to heightened expectations following invasive treatment.

A likely explanation is that the control subjects responded to saline injections as active therapy. Tendons heal at a slow rate partially due to poor vascularisation [23]. The saline injections do produce some local trauma and bleeding, and this has shown to have a stimulatory effect on the tendon. In an uncontrolled study, 75 athletes with chronic Achilles tendonosis underwent ultrasound-guided percutaneous longitundinal tenotomy after failed conservative management [24]. Of the 63 patients reviewed, 47 rated their outcome excellent or good. Multiple percutaneous longitudinal tenotomies in the management of Achilles tendonosis have shown excellent or good results in 37 of 52 patients [25]. In another study, dry needling in nine healthy subjects resulted in an increase in the blood volume and oxygen saturation for 30 minutes when measured using red laser lights [26]. Autologous blood through injection or by bleeding is likely to result in the release of cellular and humoral mediators that stimulate a repair cascade. In an uncontrolled study, 28 patients with lateral epicondylitis who had failed previous nonsurgical treatments were injected with autologous blood [27]. At follow-up after 9.5 months, 22 patients had complete resolution of their symptoms. The pain score reduced from 7.8 to 2.3 and the Nirschl stage decreased from 6.5 to 2.0. The remaining six patients needed two or three injections and ended up with scores less than 0.9.

Injection of any fluid invariably changes the pressure-volume relationship within a given anatomical space. A study on 30 patients with chronic Achilles tendonosis who failed an eccentric exercise programme were injected with 10 mL of 0.5% bupivacaine hydrochloride, 25 mg of hydrocortisone acetate, and 40 mL of 0.9% NaCl saline solution [28]. The 21 patients who responded showed a significant improvement of pain and function scores at four weeks with VISA-A score improving from 45 points to 76 points at a mean follow-up of 30 weeks. These local mechanical effects were hypothesised to destroy pathological vascular and neural growth. In a later study by the same group, 11 athletes with chronic Achilles tendonosis who had previously failed nonoperative treatment were injected with the same solution under real time ultrasound guidance [29]. After a 2.9 week follow-up, the grade of neovascularisation reduced from 3 to 1.1, the maximal tendon diameter decreased from 8.7 to 7.6 mm, and the VISA-A scores improved from 46.3 to 84.1. All changes were statistically significant. Similar beneficial effects with high volume injections have also been described with chronic patellar tendonosis [30]

We conclude that PRP injection in Achilles tendonosis is likely to be effective not because of the high concentration of platelets it delivers, but due to the local injection effects of percutaneous tenotomy, local bleeding and changes in pressure-volume relationship.

References

[1] Järvinen T. A., Kannus P., Maffulli N., Khan K. M. Achilles tendon disorders: etiology and epidemiology. *Foot Ankle Clin.* 2005;10:255-66.

[2] Alfredson H. Chronic midportion Achilles tendinopathy: an update on research and treatment. *Clin. Sports Med.* 2003;22:727-41.

[3] Kader D., Sakena A., Movin T., Magulli N. Achilles tendinopathy: some aspects of basic science and clinical management. *Br. J. Sports Med.* 2002;36:239-49.

[4] Rompe J. D., Nafe B., Furia J. P., Maffulli N. Eccentric loading, shock-wave treatment, or a wait-and-see policy for tendinopathy of the main body of tendo Achillis: a randomised controlled trial. *Am. J. Sports Med.* 2007;35:374-83.

[5] Pietrzak W., Eppley B. Scientific foundations platelet rich plasma: biology and new technology. *J. Craniofac. Surg.* 2005;16:1043-54.

[6] Rees J. D., Maffulli N., Cook J. Management of tendinopathy. *Am. J. Sports Med.* 2009;37:1855-67.

[7] Anitua E., Sanchez M., Nurden A. T., et al. New insights into and novel applications for platelet-rich fibrin therapies. *Trends Biotechnol.* 2006;24:227-34.

[8] Sampson S., Gerhardt M., Mandelbaum B. Platelet rich plasma injection grafts for musculoskeletal injuries: a review. *Curr. Rev. Musculoskelet Med.* 2008;1:165-74.

[9] Dohan Ehrenfest D. M., Rasmusson L., Albrektsson T. Classification of platelet concentrates: from pure platelet-rich plasma (P-PRP) to leucocyte- and plateletrich fibrin (L-PRF). *Trends Biotechnol* 2009;27:158-67.

[10] Mishra A., Woodall J. Jr, Vieira A. Treatment of tendon and muscle using platelet-rich plasma. *Clin. Sports Med.* 2009;28:113-25.

[11] Sánchez M., Anitua E., Orive G., Mujika I., Andia I. Platelet-rich therapies in the treatment of orthopaedic sport injuries. *Sports Med* 2009;39:345-54.

[12] Alsousou J., Thompson M., Hulley P., Noble A., Willett K. The biology of platelet-rich plasma and its application in trauma and orthopaedic surgery: a review of the literature. *J. Bone Joint Surg.* 2009;91B:987-96.

[13] Coombes B. K., Bisset L., Vicenzino B. Efficacy and safety of corticosteroid injections and other injections for management of tendinopathy: a systematic review of randomised controlled trials. *Lancet.* 2010 Oct. 21. [Epub ahead of print].

[14] Lyras D. N., Kazakos K., Verettas D. et al. The influence of platelet-rich plasma on angiogenesis during the early phase of tendon healing. *Foot Ankle Int.* 2009;30:1101-6.

[15] Lyras D. N., Kazakos K., Tryfonidis M. et al. Temporal and spatial expression of TGF-beta1 in an Achilles tendon section model after application of platelet-rich plasma. *Foot Ankle Surg.* 2010;16:137-41.

[16] Sarrafian T. L., Wang H., Hackett E. S. et al. Comparison of Achilles tendon repair techniques in a sheep model using a cross-linked acellular porcine dermal patch and platelet-rich plasma fibrin matrix for augmentation. *J. Foot Ankle Surg.* 2010;49:128-34.

[17] Virchenko O., Aspenberg P. How can one platelet injection after tendon injury lead to a stronger tendon after 4 weeks? Interplay between early regeneration and mechanical stimulation. *Acta Orthop.* 2006;77:806-12.

[18] Anitua E., Sanchez M., Nurden A. T. et al. Autologous fibrin matrices: a potential source of biological mediators that modulate tendon cell activities. *J. Biomed. Mater Res. A* 2006;77:285-93.

[19] Gaweda K., Tarczynska M., Krzyzanowski W. Treatment of achilles tendinopathy with platelet-rich plasma. *Int. J. Sports Med.* 2010;31:577-83.

[20] Filardo G., Presti M. L., Kon E., Marcacci M. Nonoperative biological treatment approach for partial Achilles tendon lesion. *Orthopedics* 2010;33:120-3.

[21] Sánchez M., Anitua E., Azofra J., Andía I., Padilla S., Mujika I. Comparison of surgically repaired Achilles tendon tears using platelet-rich fibrin matrices. *Am. J. Sports Med.* 2007;35:245-51.

[22] de Vos R. J., Weir A., van Schie H. T. et al. Platelet-rich plasma injection for chronic Achilles tendinopathy: a randomized controlled trial. *J. A. M. A.* 2010;303:144-9.

[23] Fenwick S. A., Hazlelman B. L., Riley G. P. The vasculature and its role in the damaged and healing tendon. *Arthritis Res* 2002;4:252-60.

[24] Testa V., Capasso G., Benazzo F., Maffulli N. Management of Achilles tendinopathy by ultrasound-guided percutaneous tenotomy. *Med. Sci. Sports Exerc.* 2002;34:573-80.

[25] Maffulli N., Testa V., Capasso G., Bifulco G., Binfield P. M. Results of percutaneous longitudinal tenotomy for Achilles tendinopathy in middle- and long-distance runners. *Am. J. Sports Med.* 1997;25:835-40.

[26] Kubo K., Yajima H., Takayama M., Ikebukuro T., Mizoguchi H., Takakura N. Effects of acupuncture and heating on blood volume and oxygen saturation of human Achilles tendon in vivo. *Eur. J. Appl. Physiol.* 2010;109:545-50.

[27] Edwards S. G., Calandruccio J. H. Autologous blood injections for refractory lateral epicondylitis. *J. Hand Surg*. 2003;28A:272-8.

[28] Chan O., O'Dowd D., Padhiar N. et al. High volume image guided injections in chronic Achilles tendinopathy. *Disabil. Rehabil.* 2008;30:1697-1708.

[29] Humphrey J., Chan O., Crisp T. et al. The short-term effects of high volume image guided injections in resistant non-insertional Achilles tendinopathy. *J. Sci. Med. Sport* 2010;13:295-8.

[30] Crisp T., Khan F., Padhiar N. et al. High volume ultrasound guided injections at the interface between the patellar tendon and Hoffa's body are effective in chronic patellar tendinopathy: A pilot study. *Disabil. Rehabil.* 2008;30:1625-34.

In: Medical and Biological Frontiers Research Compendium ISBN: 978-1-62417-022-5
Editor: Tsisana Shartava

Chapter 3

Advances in Tissue Engineering Applications for Ligament Repair

Mamun Al-Rashid[#1] ***and Wasim S. Khan***[*2]
[1]Barking Havering and Redbridge N. H. S. Trust, London, UK
[2]University College London Institute of Orthopaedics and Musculoskeletal Sciences, Stanmore, UK

Abstract

Ligament injuries form a significant proportion of musculoskeletal injuries with resulting disability and mobidity to patients worldwide. Current treatment regimens may not result in the ligament achieving its pre-injury characteristics or function. The use of mesenchymal stem cells to repair injured ligament tissue is an emerging novel technique, that holds great promise due to its unique characteristics. This review highlights these characteristics, and what makes mesenchymal stem cells so amenable to use in tissue engineering in the arena of ligament regeneration. It discusses the current research evidence and clinical trials in the application of mesenchymal stem cells in ligament injury and the future challenges and potential of this exciting and expanding area of functional tissue engineering.

Introduction

Ligament injuries form a significant proportion of muskuloskeletal injuries. Treatment of these injuries currently follows two routes: conservative involving rehabilitation and pain relief or surgical repair vs. reconstruction. Even when ligament healing does occur following the use of either of these treatment modalities, it may not result in the ligament achieving its

---

Department of Trauma and Orthopaedics, Barking Havering and Redbridge N. H. S. Trust, London, U. K.
* Corresponding Author: Clinical Lecturer, University College London Institute of Orthopaedics and Musculoskeletal Science, Royal National Orthopaedic Hospital, Stanmore, U. K. Tel: +44 (0) 7971 190720. Fax number: +44 (0) 20 8570 3864. E-mail address: *wasimkhan@doctors.org.uk*.

pre-injury characteristics or function. [1] The inability of the ligament to self repair in certain circumstances and the relative inefficiency of current treatment regimens has propelled increasing interest in the search for novel alternatives. One such promising alternative is the use of stem cells to repair injured ligament tissue either through direct application or in conjunction with scaffolding. [2]

This review provides a current snap shot of what is known about mesenchymal stem cells, their unique characteristics and how this fits into augmenting ligament healing and regeneration; the highlights of the clinical translation trials and the challenges that lay ahead along with its future potential.

Unique Properties of Mesenchymal Stem Cells

Stem cells are cells that have the ability to self-renew and differentiate into many different tissue types, including cartilage, bone, adipose tissue, tendon and ligament. There are several sources of stem cells embryonic stem cells, umbilical cord stem cells and adult stem cells. Most current interest is focused on adult stem cells, due to its easier accessability and practicality of use in the clinical environment. Adult stem cells are undifferentiated cells, found in differentiated tissues, it can renew itself and become specialised to the cell types of the tissue from which it originated. Sources of adult stem cells have been found in the bone marrow, blood stream, cornea and retina of the eyes, the dentine, liver, skin, pancreas and gastro intestinal tract. In contrast to the embryonic stem cells, these are not capable of forming all the cells of the body that is they are not pleuripotent. Bone marrow contains two main cell types: haematopoietic cells and stromal cells. The stem cells from non haematopoietic tissues are referred as mesenchymal cells because of their ability to differentiate as mesenchymal or stromal cells. Mesenchymal stem cells (MSC) are easily obtainable form bone marrow by means of minimally invasive approach and can be expanded in culture and encouraged to differentiate into the desired lineage. This differentiation can be achieved by the application of bioactive signaling molecules, specific growth factors. The transforming growth factor beta (TGF-beta) superfamily member proteins such as the bone morphogenetic proteins (BMPs) are the most important factors of chondrogenic and osteogenic differentiation of mesenchymal stem cells. BMP 2, 4 and 7 in particular is thought to play an important role in chondrogenic and osteogenic differentiation proteins. MSCs may be identified by virtue of its expression of different molecules as CD105, CD73, and are negative for the haematopoietic markers CD34, CD45, and CD14. [4]

Studies have demonstrated that MSCs when transplanted systemically are able to migrate to sites of injury in animals, surggesting that MSCs possess migratory capacity [5]. However the mechanisms underlying the migration remain unknown. Chemokine receptors and their ligands and adhesion molecules play an important role in tissue-specific homing of leukocytes. It is postulated that these may contribute to the migratory process. Another unique characteristic is that the immune phenotype of MSCs (widely described as MHC I^{+}, MHC II^{-}, $CD40^{-}$, $CD80^{-}$, $CD86^{-}$) is regarded as nonimmunogenic and, therefore,transplantation into an allogeneic host may not require immunosuppression. MSCs are also thought to regulate immune responses such as the regulation of antibody production by B Cells, alterations in

T cell subtypes,and immune tolerance of allogenic transplants[4]. These characteristics make MSCs promising vehicles for gene therapy, cell therapy and tissue engineering.

MSCs in Tissue Engineering of Ligament Repair

Ligaments function to support bone, and thus facilitate skeletal motion. It therefore possesses significant stiffness, strength, and also an element of elasticity [6] Repair process of ligamentous tissues is a complex process and remodeling of the healing tissue can require long periods of convalescence to achieve biomechanical levels necessary for optimal function of the tissue. Current ligament tissue engineering trials have incorporated cells into the structural materials to enhance extracellular matrix production, promote growth factors via genetic engineering of the cells, and recruit endogenous cells to the site of repair [7]. Terminally differentiated fibroblasts or chondrocytes from different sources have been used in most of these designs.

Initial experiments using MSCs to regenerate musculoskeletal tissues began with autologous MSCs suspended in a type 1 collagen matrix.[8] Several studies looking at the effects of MSC concentration on the kinetics, have shown increasing cell concentration related to increased rate of contraction of tissue. [9] Other studies have shown that MSC gene expression may be altered and the composition of collagen types in the matrix changed when a cyclical load is applied.[10] In experiments where human MSC/collagen gel constructs were subject to cycles of tension to model the effects of tensile forces in vivo, structural changes were evident in the cycled tissue as compared to static tension as early as 24 hours. Histologically, cycled tissue demonstrated collagen fibre organisation, parallel to the long axis of the tensile loading with an alignment of crimp patterns that was not evident in the static constructs. [11] Additionally these MSCs produced increased amounts of collagen type vi, which is associated with repairing connective tissues and with the early maturation of normal tendon and ligamentous tissues.[10] This discovery that MSCs were able to organise the structure of collagen in vitro, led to testing whether MSCs could organise a biocompatible implant, that when implanted in vivo would result in early structural organisation and gains in biomechanical function. A series of studies subsequently have shown that biomechanically, tendinous tissues implanted with MSCs consistently led to significant improvements in the structural and material properties compared to controls. A study labeled MSCs with a fluorescent cell surface molecular marker on a collagen construct which were tensioned, and implanted the constructs in patellar tendon defects of rabbits [12]. The cells were found in the repaired central part of the patella, and these MSC loaded tissues were 58% stronger and 51% stiffer than the natural repair process of scar tissue formed in the control group at 12 weeks and 174% stronger and 183% stiffer at 26 weeks post op. However there still remains paucity of data as to how to stimulate specifically the ligamentogenic differentiation amongst MSCs. One recent study suggests that transducting MSC and anterior cruciate ligament fibroblasts with adcnoviral vectors encoding the human cDNA for bone morphogenetic protein (BMP) 12 and BMP 13 can lead to ligamentogenic differentiation of these cells. [13]. Another animal study found that coating autologous hamstring tendon grafts with mesenchymal stem cells, in Anterior cruciate ligament reconstruction, resulted in healing by an intervening zone of cartilage resembling the chondral enthesis of normal anterior cruciate ligament insertions rather than collagen fibres and scar tissue. Mesenchymal stem cell enhanced anterior cruciate ligament reconstructions performed significantly better than controls on biomechanical testing [14].

Future Developments and Challenges

While progress has been made in generating engineered tissues for ligament replacements such as the anterior cruciate ligament, in model systems, several challenges still remain. These include the choice of suitable scaffold, the density and differentiation state of mesenchymal stem cells, the biomechanical environment required for optimal in vitro generation. Also to consider are the parameters required for successful engrafting, and factors that optimise ligamentogenic differentiation of mesenchymal stem cells. The clinical use of mesenchymal stem cells is an emerging field with exciting potential. Critical to its progress lies in the development of functional tissue engineering. Where the in vivo mechanical environment acting on the tissue is determined and then the tissue-engineered constructs from bone-marrow derived mesenchymal stem cells and collagen scaffolds, is preconditioned. These tissue engineered constructs are therefore subjected to the optimum mechanical signals to improve repair outcome significantly. This coupled with identifying specific molecular factors to stimulate MSCs to attain ligamentogenic differentiation hold great promise.

References

[1] Hoffman A., Gross G., Tendon and ligament engineering in the adult organisms: mesenchymal stem cells and gene-therapeutic approaches. *International Orthopaedics* 2007 31:791-797.

[2] Pittenger M., Vanguri P., Simonetti D., Young R. Adult mesenchymal stem cells: Potential for muscle and tendon regeneration and use in gene therapy. *J. Musculoskel Neuron. Interact.* 2002; 2(4):309-320.

[3] Howard D., Buttery L., Shakesheff K., Roberts S. Tissue engineering: strategies, stem cells and scaffolds. *Journal of Anatomy* 2008 July; 213(1):66-72.

[4] Chamberlain G., Fox J., Ashton B., Middleton J. Concise Review: Mesenchymal Stem Cells: Their Phenotype, Differentiation Capacity, Immunological Features, and Potential for Homing. *Stem Cells*. Volume 25, Issue 11, pages 2739-2749, November 2007.

[5] Gao J., Dennis J. E., Muzic R. F. et al. The dynamic in vivo distribution of bone marrow-derived mesenchymal stem cells after infusion. *Cells Tissues Organs* 2001; 169:12–20.

[6] Sharma P., Maffulli N. Biology of tendon injury: healing, modeling and remodeling. *J. Musculoskelet Neuronal. Interact.* 6:181-190.

[7] Best T. M., Garrett W. E. Basic science of soft tissue muscle and tendon. In: DeLee J. C. (ed) *Orthopaedic sports medicine*. W. B. Saunders, Philadelphia, US; 1994:25-45.

[8] Woo S. L., Hildebrand K., Watanabe N., Fenwick J. A., Papageorgiou C. D., Wang J. H. Tissue engineering of ligament and tendon healing. *Clin. Orthop.* 1999; 367(Suppl.):S312-323.

[9] Young R. G., Butler D. L., Weber W., Caplan A. I., Gordon S. L., Fink D. J. The use of mesenchymal stem cells in Achilles tendon repair. *J. Orthop. Res.* 1998; 16:406-413.

[10] Archambault M. P., Peter S. J., Young R. Y. Effects of cyclic tension on matrix synthesis and tissue formation in a three-dimensional culture system. *Transactions of the 46th Annual Meeting,Orthopaedic Research Society,* 2000; Poster No. 0636.

[11] Awad HA, Butler DL, Harris MT, Ibrahim RE, Wu Y, Young RG, Kadiyala S, Boivin GP. In vitro characterization of mesenchymal stem cell-seeded collagen scaffolds for tendon repair: Effects of initial seeding density on contraction kinetics. *J. Biomed. Mater. Res.* 2000; 51:233-240.

[12] Awad HA, Butler DL, Boivin GP, Dressler MR , Smith FNL, Young RG. Effects of implant seeding density on MSC-mediated repair of patellar tendon injuries. *Transactions of the 46th Annual Meeting*, Orthopaedic Research Society, 2000; No. 048.

[13] Haddad-Weber M.,Prager P., Kunz M. BMP12 and BMP13gene transfer induce ligamentogenic differentiation in mesenchymal progenitor and anterior cruciate ligament cells. *Cytotherapy,* July 2010, vol./is. 12/4(505-513), 1465-3249;1477-2566(July 2010).

[14] Jit- Kheng Lim, Hui J., Li L. .I., Thambvah A., Goh J., Eng-Hin Lee Enhancement of tendon graft osteointegration using mesenchymal stem cells in a rabbit model of anterior cruciate ligament reconstruction. *Arthroscopy: The Journal of Arthroscopic and Related SurgeryVolume* 20, Issue 9 Pages 899-910, November 2004.

In: Medical and Biological Frontiers Research Compendium ISBN: 978-1-62417-022-5
Editor: Tsisana Shartava

Chapter 4

Advances in Ceramic Bearings for Total Hip Replacements

Paul Whittingham-Jones and Wasim S. Khan*
University College London Institute of Orthopaedics and Musculoskeletal Science,
Royal National Orthopaedic Hospital, Stanmore, London, UK

The search for the perfect bearing in hip arthroplasty remains elusive with all combinations proving over time to have their own idiosyncrasies, benefits and problems. It has become increasingly clear that it is the bearing couple which presents the major obstacle to increasing the longevity of hip arthroplasties. Over the years the femoral stem has evolved and most available prostheses in wide usage can boast survival data far in excess of what may have been expected a few deacades ago. Similarly although the debate over fixation methods of the acetabular component persists, expected survival of the shell is unlikely to be limited by wear. The use of ceramics as either ceramic on ceramic (COC) or ceramic on polyethylene (COP) has been a popular choice of surgeons worldwide during a period which has seen significant improvements in materials manufacture and machining tolerances. At the time of writing Ceramic on Metal is also undergoing trial.

Using COC or COP can be an attractive option; particularly in younger and more active patients with the likelihood of much improved longevity [1]. Over recent years there has been increased focus on Metal-on-metal (MOM) articulations and metal ion levels due to wear and corrosion. Any factor resulting in high metal ion levels appears to be associated with an increased failure rate. Young females are one risk factor for failure, possibly due to their small size, and are therefore more likely to receive COC or COP bearings as a primary hip arthroplasty [2] COC or COP have the potential advantage of excellent wear characteristics from high wettablilty, scratch resistance and hardness – only diamond being harder. [3] Zirconia rates 8.5 on Mohs scale of mineral hardness with diamond rating 10. Ceramics are

* Corresponding Author: Mr Wasim S Khan, Clinical Lecturer, University College London Institute of Orthopaedics and Musculoskeletal Science, Royal National Orthopaedic Hospital, Stanmore, London, HA7 4LP, UK. Telephone number: +44 (0) 7971 190720. Fax number: +44 (0) 20 8570 3864. E-mail address: wasimkhan@doctors.org.uk.

inorganic, crystalline materials whose popularity in hip arthroplasty is growing - ceramic femoral heads are likely to overtake metallic heads in the National Joint Registry of England and Wales in numbers used.

In vitro testing of volumetric wear have been demonstrated as low as $0.01mm^3$/million cycles with MOM articulations achieving $1.23mm^3$/million cycles and in vivo testing showed markedly reduced chromium ion production [4,5]. Such couples appear to be highly biocompatible, not having been implicated in osteolysis, the development of pseudo-tumours, ALVAL or other distant effects which remain a concern with bearings involving metal. The manufacture of ceramics for hip prostheses has evolved over the last three decades, seeing advances in materials such as the addition of zirconium to alumina ceramic and the change of the design of the femoral taper from 14/16 to 12/14mm, allowing for a thicker ceramic head. [6, 7, 8, 9, 10].

Alumina or aluminium oxide was employed for hip bearings in the 1970s by Boutin. In earlier usage an industrial standard of alumina was employed but resulted in a fracture rate as high as 13%. [11]. Currently, a third generation of alumina ceramic is employed which utilizes a reduced grain size and hot isostatic pressing for increased density and hence strength. Zirconia or Zirconium oxide represents an alternative to alumina which was developed to reduce the risk of component fracture. Zirconia has demonstrable increases in toughness and strength when compared to Alumina. Zirconia appears to display these improved properties due to phase transformations. Zirconia can exist as monoclinic, tetragonal or cubic structures, depending on temperature. At temperatures less than 1170^0 C the monoclinic structure persists which is not inherently strong. With the addition however of other metals it is stabilized and becomes useful. The addition of Magnesium, Calcium or Yttrium is seen in different industries such as in the production of ceramic knives. Yttrium oxide is added in joint replacements to stabiles the structure. Surface roughness is comparable to alumina but volumetric wear rates have shown improvements [12].

As time has passed the literature has highlighted certain issues around the use of ceramics, namely squeaking and more significantly prosthesis fracture. Much work has been done by manufacturers and recent examples have tested burst strength of 98kN – much greater than the minimum recommendation of 48kN by the United States Food and Drug Administration. Previous manufacturing processes did not monitor accuracy of taper tolerances or roughness of the trunion [13]. The reported incidence of ceramic fracture is as little as 0% to 0.004%. The potentially devastating consequences mandate reviewing strategies available to surgeons in the avoidance of ceramic fracture and also how to manage fractures when they do occur [14].

Factors at the time of insertion of the prostheses which should mitigate fracture risk include correct placement of both the femoral and acetabular components. Malpositioning may result in edge loading and the generation of high contact stresses. A ceramic head must be gently screwed or tapped onto the femoral trunion as point loading through any defect may cause fracture [15]. Following implantation many surgeons also advocate the avoidance of high impact activities despite the increased tolerances [16].

When fractures of ceramic do occur they appear to be a sudden and unpredictable result of fatigue failure; although excessive trauma may still produce fractures. On presentation the clinician must have a high index of suspicion as such fractures can remain occult on standard X-Ray imaging- the role of the stress radiograph has been suggested [14]. Furthermore, fractures of ceramic components can remain asymptomatic: one report being of a fracture discovered at revision for sepsis [17]. A number of cases in the literature emphasise the serious effects of persistent ceramic debris on the survival of a revision hip arthroplasty and the potential for catastrophic wear which can result in harmful circulating levels of implant-derived metal ions. The results described are massive metallosis and polyethylene debris with associated acceleration in wear [15].

In 2009, The Lancet reported the disturbing case of a patient who had undergone MOP revision for a fractured ceramic femoral head. The result was elevated serum metal ions.(Table 1, case 1) [18]. The effects of the ions proved catastrophic, resulting in blindness, deafness, cranial nerve dysfunction, hypothyroidism and the loss of ambulation due to lower limb hyposthenia.

Another case report of a similar sequence of events resulted in even higher levels of serum cobalt (Table 1, case 2), possibly the highest ever recorded in humans [19]. A further case with fracture of the ceramic liner, reported polyneuropathy and serum cobalt levels higher than those reported with MOM bearings. (Table 1, case 3) [20]. Analyses agree that median levels of 1.7 μg/litre (Co) and 2.3 μg/litre (Cr) are typical for patients with well functioning unilateral MOM hip arthroplasty, which is ten-fold higher than the median levels in individuals without metallic implants [21].

It seems in these cases that high levels of Cobalt and Chromium have been produced from orthopaedic implants that have had devastating consequences. The mechanism for ion generation in these cases is likely to involve accelerated third body wear between the polyethylene acetabular liner and metal femoral head due to persisting ceramic micro-debris. Once the polyethylene liner has completely worn through, the cobalt-chromium femoral head articulated with the titanium acetabular cup and caused catastrophic wear of both components [1, 15, 22].

Undoubtedly one of the main advantages of ceramic as a bearing is its' inherent hardness; it is also this property which mandates fastidious technique when revising components following ceramic fracture.

A new ceramic head placed on an undamaged trunion has been shown to be effective but this is likely to be against manufacturers' advice and warranty, moreover any microscopic damage will by definition remain unseen at the time of revision [22]. Thus, surgeons should use metal trunion sleeves, revision ceramic heads with factory fitted metal taper linings, or consider revising the femoral stem.

Since even a radical synovectomy is unlikely to eradicate all microdebris, high density polyethylene would be an unsafe option likely to produce early failure. It is therefore sensible to insert another COC couple. Furthermore, revision should not be delayed as any debris from fracture will persist within the joint until it is removed and can affect either the stem or cup leading to metallosis or bony destruction. The advice therefore is to immobilize the patient and revise all parts urgently, including a radical synovectomy and capsular excision [23]. If the stem is well fixed, it may be preserved if a modular design allows only change of the trunion.

Regardless of how careful the procedure, there is always a risk of ceramic microparticles persisting, hence the need for full appreciation of the problems, fastidious preoperative planning of revision surgery and meticulous technique at operation.

Table 1. Clinical details of reported cases

Clinical detail	Case 1	Case 2	Case 3
Presentation history	11 months post MOP revision for ceramic head fracture	4 months post MOP revision for ceramic head fracture	2 years post MOP revision for ceramic liner fracture
Plasma ion concentration / µg/litre	Cobalt 549* Chromium 54*	Cobalt 625* Chromium 81*	Cobalt ℘400 Chromium 221
Hypothyroidism	Y	Y	Y
Cranial nerve dysfunction	Y	Y	Y
Peripheral neuropathy (confirmed slowing on conduction studies)	Y	Y	Y
Convulsion	N	Y	N
Blindness and deafness	Y	N	N
Altered echocardiography	N	Y	N
Weight loss (unexplained >10 Kg) Eczema Nail discolouration Dysguesia	not reported	Y	Not reported

* 1 parts per billion = 1 µg/litre = 1 ng/ml.

As ceramic materials and manufacture improve, so their popularity will rise which will herald an increased burden of ceramic component fractures. It is imperative that surgeons are aware of this in order to identify patients with this problem and manage them appropriately. As a bearing in hip arthroplasty, ceramics likely represent the future but as ever it remains incumbent upon the surgeon to maintain a full understanding of material properties.

References

[1] BE Bierbaum, J Nairus, D Kuesis, JC Morrison, and D Ward. Ceramic-on-ceramic bearings in total hip arthroplasty. *Clin. Orthop. Relat Res.*, Dec 2002; (405) 158-63.

[2] S. Glyn-Jones, H. Pandit,, Y.-M. Kwon, H. Doll, H. S. Gill, BEng,D. W. Murray. Risk factors for inflammatory pseudotumour formation following hip resurfacing. *Journal of Bone and Joint Surgery* - British Volume, Vol 91-B, Issue 12, 1566-1574.

[3] G Willmann. Ceramics for total hip replacement--what a surgeon should know. *Orthopedics,* Feb 1998; 21(2): 173-7.

[4] Firkins PJ, Tipper JL, InghamE, Stone MH, Farrar R, Fisher J. A novel low wearing differential hardness, cermic-on-metal hip joint prosthesis. *J. Biomechanics*. 34:1291-8.

[5] Isaac GH, Brockett C, Breckon A et al (2009) Ceramic-on-metal bearings in total hip replacement. *Jounal of Bone and Joint Surgery Br.* 91-B: 1134-41.

[6] Früh HJ, Willmann G, Pfaff HG. Wear characteristics of ceramic-on-ceramic for hip endoprostheses. *Biomaterials.* 1997 Jun;18(12):873-6.

[7] Willmann G, Früh HJ, Pfaff HG. Wear characteristics of sliding pairs of zirconia (Y-TZP) for hip endoprostheses. *Biomaterials*. 1996 Nov;17(22):2157-62.

[8] Wirganowicz PZ, Thomas BJ. Massive osteolysis after ceramic on ceramic total hip arthroplasty. A case report. *Clin. Orthop. Relat Res*. 1997 May;(338):100-4.

[9] Yoon TR, Rowe SM, Jung ST, Seon KJ, Maloney WJ. Osteolysis in association with a total hip arthroplasty with ceramic bearing surfaces. *J. Bone Joint Surg. Am*. 1998 Oct;80(10):1459-68.

[10] Hannouche D, Nich C, Bizot P, Meunier A, Nizard R, Sedel L. Fractures of ceramic bearings: history and present status. *Clin. Orthop. Relat. Res*. 2003 Dec;(417):19-26.

[11] Knahr K, Bohler M, Frank P, Plenk H, Salzer M. Survival analysis of an uncemented ceramic acetabular componentin total hip replacement. *Arch. Orthop Trauma Surg*. 106: 297-300.

[12] Kumar P, Oka M, Ikeuchi K, Shimzu K, Yamamuro T, Okumura H, Kotoura Y. Low wear rate of UHMWPE against zirconia ceramic (Y-PSZ) in comparison to alumina ceramic andSUS 316L alloy. *J. Biomed. Mater Res*. 25:813-28.

[13] Sedel L. Evolution of alumina-on-alumina implants: a review. *Clin. Orthop*. 2000;379:48-54.

[14] Willmann G. Ceramic femoral head retrieval data. *Clin. Orthop. Relat Res*. 2000 Oct;(379):22-8.

[15] J. Allain, D. Goutallier, M. C. Voisin, and S. Lemouel Failure of a Stainless-Steel Femoral Head of a Revision Total Hip Arthroplasty Performed after a Fracture of a Ceramic Femoral Head. A Case Report. J. *Bone Joint Surg. Am.,* Sep 1998; 80: 1355 - 1360.

[16] Simon JA, Dayan AJ, Ergas E, Stuchin SA, Di Cesare PE. Catastrophic failure of the acetabular component in a ceramic-polyethylene bearing total hip arthroplasty. *J. Arthroplasty* 1998;13:108-13.

[17] Sariali E, Stewart T, Mamoudy P, Jin Z, Fisher J. Undetected Fracture of an Alumina Ceramic on Ceramic Hip Prosthesis. *J. Arthroplasty*. 2009 Jul 3.

[18] MC Rizzetti, P Liberini, G Zarattini, S Catalani, U Pazzaglia, P Apostoli, and A Padovani. Loss of sight and sound. Could it be the hip? *Lancet,* Mar 2009; 373(9668): 1052.

[19] M Oldenburg, R Wegner, and X Baur. Severe cobalt intoxication due to prosthesis wear in repeated total hip arthroplasty. *J. Arthroplasty*, Aug 2009; 24(5): 825.e15-20.

[20] Ikeda T, Takahashi K, Kabata T, Sakagoshi D, Tomita K, YamadaM. Polyneuropathy caused by cobalt-chromium metallosis after total hip replacement. *Muscle Nerve*. 2010;42(1):140-3.

[21] Winship PD, Faria N, Skinner JA, Hart AJ, Powell JJ. The determination of cobalt and chromium in whole blood sampled from metal-metal and metal-polyethylene hip articulation patients by DRC-ICP-MS. In: Collery P, ed. *Metal ions in biology and medicine*. Vol. 10. Corsica: John Libbey Eurotext, 2008:27-33.

[22] Sedel L, Willmann G. *Reliability and long-term results of ceramics in orthopaedics*. pp 117. Stuttgart: Georg Thieme, 1999. ISBN: 3-13-118481-7.

[23] H.R. Dürr. Problemfall Keramikbruch. Was ist zu tun? *Orthopäde* 2009 38:698–703.

In: Medical and Biological Frontiers Research Compendium
Editor: Tsisana Shartava
ISBN: 978-1-62417-022-5

Chapter 5

Liver Metastases of Colorectal Carcinoma: Magnetic Resonance Imaging Techniques and New Developments

Kenneth Coenegrachts*
Department of Radiology, AZ St.-Jan Brugge-Oostende AV, Belgium

Abstract

The early detection of (especially malignant) focal liver lesions is of utmost importance. For example, the resection of liver metastases of some malignancies (including colorectal cancer) has been shown to improve the survival of the patients. Exact knowledge of the number, size, and regional distribution of colorectal liver metastases is essential to determine their resectability. Almost all colorectal liver metastases larger than 10mm are demonstrated with current imaging techniques but the detection of smaller colorectal liver metastases is still relatively poor.

One of the advantages of Magnetic Resonance Imaging (MRI) of the liver is the better soft tissue contrast (compared to other radiologic modalities), which reveals better detection and characterization of the colorectal liver metastases in question. Developments in MRI hardware and software and the availability of novel MRI contrast agents have further improved the diagnostic yield of MRI in lesion detection and characterization. Although the primary modalities for liver imaging are ultrasound and Computed Tomography, recent studies have suggested that MRI is the most sensitive method for detecting small colorectal liver metastases and MRI is now considered the pre-operative standard.

Two recent developments in MRI sequences for the upper abdomen comprise (unenhanced) diffusion-weighted imaging (DWI) and T1-weighted keyhole-based dynamic contrast-enhanced MRI (T1w DCE MRI).

DWI using low b-values, allows improved detection ($b=10s/mm^2$) of (especially) small (<10mm) colorectal liver metastases because of the black-blood effect and thus is

* Phone: ++32 50 45 21 03 - Fax: ++32 50 45 21 46, E-mail: kenneth.coenegrachts@azbrugge.be.

useful as a road map sequence. The black-blood effect facilitates detection of colorectal liver metastases by better differentiation between vascular branches, colorectal liver metastases and surrounding liver parenchyma. Using higher b-values, the calculation of Apparent Diffusion Coefficient (ADC) value, true diffusion coefficient (D) and the perfusion fraction f has been used for the characterization of focal liver lesions. The true diffusion coefficient D is a parameter for the (patho)physiologic molecular diffusion of focal liver lesions. It therefore permits characterization of tissues and pathologic conditions. The perfusion fraction f is a parameter for the (patho)physiologic microperfusion of focal liver lesions.

T1w keyhole-based DCE MRI enables perfusion imaging of the liver with high temporal and spatial resolution with full liver coverage. T1w keyhole-based DCE MRI (4D THRIVE sequence) improves the evaluation of focal liver lesions by providing multiple arterial and venous phases and allows the calculation of parametric maps displaying different perfusion parameters using pharmacokinetic models. The use of 4D THRIVE with parametric mapping enables spatially matching tumour vascular characteristics such as blood volume, blood flow, permeability and leakage space. Parametric maps therefore have the advantage that they can be used in clinical practice and might also be useful for follow-up purposes (e.g. during therapy in an oncological setting).

Introduction

The incidence of liver metastases is approximately 40% in patients with colorectal cancer [1]. In the United States, approximately 50,000 cases of colorectal liver metastases are seen annually [2]. Metastatic disease to the liver is a very common clinical situation in oncology. The liver is one of the most common sites of metastatic spread of epithelial cancers, second only to regional lymph nodes. The true prevalence of metastatic disease is unknown, but approximately 20%-25% of patients with colorectal cancer have liver metastases at the time of diagnosis. Studies based on autopsy results showed that up to 70% of colon cancer patients have liver metastases at autopsy [3]. Further, Morana et al. [4] have shown in cadaver studies of primary colorectal carcinoma that on average at least one liver metastasis less than 10mm in diameter is missed for each detected liver metastasis larger than 10mm.

The early detection of liver metastases is of utmost importance in patients with cancer. In general, the presence of (relatively extended) liver metastases indicates non-resectability of the primary tumour for oncologic reasons [5], except for tumour palliation (i.e. to relieve obstruction of the gastrointestinal tract). In these patients, chemotherapy is the method of choice. Chemotherapy can also be used to decrease tumour load to allow subsequent surgical treatment. In many cases, chemotherapy is also used after surgery or ablation therapy as neo-adjuvant therapy. Resection of liver metastases of some malignancies (including colorectal cancer) has been shown to improve the survival of the patients [6]. The presence of limited synchronous colorectal liver metastases (i.e. occurring at the time of diagnosis of the primary tumour) or metachronous colorectal metastases (occurring after diagnosis of the primary tumour) warrants surgical resection [5].

Exact knowledge of the number, size, and regional distribution of liver metastases is essential to determine their resectability. In patients with liver metastases from colorectal cancer, hepatic resection has proven survival benefits and is curative in a small proportion of cases. Patients whose metastases are small, few in number and metachronous have the best prognosis, but there is now good evidence that patients with more extensive disease can benefit from resection [7-10]. The number, size and distribution of lesions are no longer limiting factors, provided all lesions are removed with adequate tumour-free margins and there is sufficient normal liver to maintain liver function postoperatively. Based on the number and localization of the liver metastases and considering all other clinical parameters of the patient, only about 30% of colorectal patients with liver metastases may undergo resection. However, the 5-year survival of these patients is between 30% and 48% in comparison to a survival of less than 5% of patients with liver metastases not amenable to liver surgery [6, 11-13].

In recent years, together with the progress that has been made in systemic chemotherapy, there has been an increasing tendency for use of hepatic arterial infusion chemotherapy (HAIC) to be limited to patients at high risk of liver function aggravation due to a large volume of liver metastases and to patients who had not responded well to the standard therapies of FOLFIRI and FOLFOX and whose liver metastases could not be suppressed. For this reason, it is desirable to be able to evaluate the response to HAIC as soon as possible. In addition, 5-FU is the key drug in HAIC delivered through the catheter port [14], but patients who have undergone FOLFIRI and/or FOLFOX have often become resistant to 5-FU, and early evaluation of the response to HAIC would also aid in regimen selection.

Imaging

It is the task of imaging to evaluate the liver to assess the presence or absence of liver metastases in surgical candidates and to evaluate the success of chemotherapy or ablation therapy in others. Incomplete resection of colorectal liver metastases does not prolong survival [3], so knowledge of the exact extent of intra-hepatic disease is crucially important in determining patient management and outcome. Almost all liver metastases larger than 10mm are demonstrated with current imaging techniques but the detection of smaller liver metastases is still relatively poor [15-19].

US, CT, PET(/CT)

Transabdominal UltraSonography (US) is widely used to assess the liver, but has some limitations: it needs considerable operator expertise and often reveals equivocal results in patients with (chemotherapy-induced) fatty infiltration of the liver [20]. Contrast-Enhanced (CE)-US has increased potential in characterizing malignant and benign focal liver lesions compared with baseline US. CE-US increased diagnostic confidence in the detection and characterization of liver metastases compared with standard US [21]. Real-time CE-US is particularly advantageous in detecting small liver metastases, even when compared to CE-Multi-Slice Computed Tomography (MSCT) and Magnetic Resonance Imaging (MRI) [21-24]. CE-US with sulphur hexafluoride (Sonovue®) is comparable with CE-MSCT in the characterization of focal liver lesions [25, 26]. Limitations of CE-US are essentially the same as those of US and are related to the presence of bowel gas and to the patient's body habitus [27]. Among radiologic imaging techniques, US and CE-US is a relatively cheap technique and therefore is used in many general radiology departments [28, 29]. However, for accurate oncological staging, US examinations often are complemented by other imaging techniques.

Diagnostic problem cases using US are then often referred for a CT or MRI examination. With the introduction of MSCT imaging, the use of MSCT in oncologic patients to search for lung, liver, and lymph node metastases in the body has substantially increased [30, 31].

The development of MSCT has substantially increased patient throughput allowing volume coverage of the whole thorax and abdomen in one breath-hold. However, even using MSCT, the sensitivity and discrimination between small liver metastases and liver cysts is inferior compared to MRI [30]. For the evaluation of lung metastases, imaging can be limited to chest radiography. In doubtful cases or potential candidates for surgery, CT of the chest can be performed [32].

A few studies have assessed the effect of chemotherapy on the sensitivity of MSCT – all showed a significant decrease in sensitivity of MSCT [33-35]. Several articles described difficulties with lesion delineation on CT after chemotherapy, due to diminished lesion-to-liver contrast [36, 37].

Furthermore, there is a limited understanding of the role of MRI in the preoperative assessment of patients with colorectal liver metastases and neo-adjuvant chemotherapy. There are several articles that assessed the influence of chemotherapy on the sensitivity of MSCT. All articles showed a significant decline of 15–22% post-chemotherapy, resulting in poor sensitivities of 54–65% [33-35].

Most colorectal liver metastases showing complete response at MSCT still contain viable tumour cells at pathological examination (30–83%), mainly in the periphery of the initial tumour area [37,38]. Therefore, there is an ongoing discussion whether it is necessary to include the initial tumour area in the resection specimen or to operate on the images provided after neo-adjuvant chemotherapy.

Fluoro-18-DeoxyGlucose Positron Emission Tomography (FDG-PET) has been reported to be superior to CT for the detection of liver metastases from colorectal cancer [39-42] and was found to be the most sensitive non-invasive imaging modality for the detection of liver metastases [42, 43]. FDG-PET has also been described as the most accurate imaging technique to detect extrahepatic disease [32, 42, 44]. Direct comparison between MRI and FDG-PET has been limited, but would be critical for optimization of imaging at diagnosis and during follow-up.

Combined Positron Emission Tomography/Computed Tomography (PET/CT) images have significant advantages over either technique alone because it provides both functional and anatomical data. The most significant additional information provided by PET/CT relates to the accurate detection of distant metastases. PET/CT should be performed on selected patients with possible but inconclusive metastatic lesions with CT [45]. The incremental value of integrated FDG-PET/CT imaging compared with either technique alone in a study by Roman et al. resulted in incremental diagnostic value of integrated PET/CT imaging in 27% and incremental impact on management in 12.5% of patients [46]. In a study by Wiering et al. FDG-PET was clearly superior to CT in predicting extrahepatic disease in patients with colorectal liver metastases [44].

Magnetic Resonance Imaging

MRI is still limited in anatomic coverage, although the recent introduction of multichannel MRI coils with wider coverage and the moving-table MRI technique has re-established the competitiveness of MRI with MSCT with regard to patient throughput. One of the advantages of MRI in liver imaging is the better soft tissue contrast, which reveals better characterization of focal liver lesions in question. The development of liver-specific MRI contrast agents has further improved the diagnostic yield of MRI in lesion detection and characterization [47]. Although the primary modalities for liver imaging are US and CT, recent studies have suggested that CE-MRI is the most sensitive method for detecting small liver metastases and MRI is now considered the preoperative standard [48-53]. Developments in MRI hardware and software and the availability of novel MRI contrast agents have improved small focal liver lesion detection [3]. During previous years, MRI enhanced with SuperParamagnetic IronOxide (SPIO) probably has been considered the most sensitive method for detecting liver metastases [3]. In the few studies which have compared the different liver specific agents, SPIO-enhanced MRI has demonstrated varying degrees of superiority, particularly for small focal liver lesions [54, 55].

Furthermore, the importance using ferucarbotran (SPIO contrast agent) by bolus injection and providing the opportunity to obtain dynamic T1w images has been described [3]. Ward et al. [3] has found early T1 enhancement on 3D fat-suppressed T1w Gradient Echo images to be particularly valuable for depicting small focal liver lesions. The T1 effect is considerably less than occurs with extracellular fluid gadolinium-based contrast agents but this is often beneficial in the context of metastatic disease.

Liver and vessels often have a similar signal intensity which produces a virtual blank canvas against which small liver metastases are extremely conspicuous and reliably distinguished from vessels. The combination of thin-slice 3D T1w and T2w imaging after SPIO increases diagnostic confidence and is more accurate for small focal liver lesion detection than delayed T2w imaging alone [3].

Gadolinium-ethoxybenzyl-diethylenetriamine pentaacetic acid (Gd-EOB-DTPA, Bayer Schering Pharma AG, Berlin, Germany) is a paramagnetic, hydrophilic, ionic, highly water-soluble and therefore bolus-injectable magnetic resonance imaging (MRI) contrast agent. It allows combined dynamic imaging and hepatocyte-specific imaging in one examination [56, 57].

In the hepatocyte phase, hepatic lesions lacking normally functioning hepatocytes, including cysts, haemangioma and metastasis, are imaged as a defect of hepatocyte-selective enhancement compared with normal parenchyma, and evaluation of vascularity and hepatocyte-specific uptake enables accurate detection and characterisation of focal liver lesions [58].

Therefore, Gd-EOB-DTPA-enhanced MRI may be superior to standard imaging using gadolinium chelates or MSCT, especially for the detection of small hepatic metastases and differential diagnosis of hypervascular lesions [59].

New Developments in MRI Sequences for the Liver

1. Diffusion-Weighted Imaging (DWI)(Single Shot Spin Echo Echo Planar Imaging (SS SE-EPI Sequence))

Diffusion-weighted MRI is sensitive to molecular diffusion due to random and microscopic translational motion of molecules, known as Brownian motion. Random motion in the field gradient produces incoherent phase shifts that results in signal attenuation. Flowing spins induce the same attenuation effect; the pseudorandom organization of the moving spins at the voxel level, such as perfusion, can also be considered to be an incoherent motion, and this effect can induce much larger signal attenuation than the diffusion effect on an image with very low Motion-Probing Gradients (MPGs) [60, 61]. The strength of the applied MPG increases with increasing b-value (expressed in s/mm^2). On the basis of this theory, the Apparent Diffusion Coefficient (ADC) value calculated from the images with no and low MPGs (ADC_{low}) is considered to be more strongly influenced by the flowing spins (microcirculation) than molecular diffusion. The true diffusion coefficient (D) can be obtained from the calculation from images with the higher b-values [60, 61]. D as measured at IntraVoxel Incoherent Motion (IVIM) MRI is a true parameter of molecular diffusion [60, 61]. It therefore permits characterization of tissues and pathologic conditions. Furthermore, the perfusion fraction f as measured at IVIM MRI is the (microperfusion) deviation factor representing the fractional volume (of spins) occupied in the voxel by flowing spins (= sum of the spins in the microcirculation and spins in turbulent flow) [62].

During recent years, diffusion-weighted imaging (using Echo Planar Imaging (EPI) sequence with low b-values) of the liver has been proven useful for the detection of focal liver lesions because of the black-blood effect when using low b-values. The black-blood effect renders blood vessels black while focal liver lesions remain bright. The use of the black-blood effect for facilitating detection of focal liver lesions - by better differentiation between small vascular branches and small focal liver lesions - has been described previously [63]. This black-blood effect has proven to be useful in detecting (especially smaller (<10 mm)) focal liver lesions [64-67]. We also recommend starting each MRI examination of the upper abdomen with the SS SE-EPI sequence (using respiratory-triggering to optimize the SNR). The SS SE-EPI sequence can then be used as a road map sequence to guide the rest of the MRI examination.

Respiratory-triggered SS SE-EPI is preferred for liver MRI as respiratory-triggering increases the Signal-to-Noise Ratio (SNR) and helps to avoid false-negative but also false-positive (due to noise) results. In our experience [64], for focal liver lesion detection a b-value of b=10s/mm^2 is to be preferred over b=20 or 50 s/mm^2.

Diffusion-weighted imaging (using SS SE-EPI with low and high b-values) of the liver seems promising for the characterization of focal liver lesions by calculating D, f and ADC_{low} [60-62, 68, 69].

Therapy-induced changes assessed by DWI (using also high b-values) comprise effective anticancer treatment results in tumour lysis, loss of cell membrane integrity, increased extracellular space, and, therefore, an increase in water diffusion [70, 71].

Current models of tumour response postulate cell swelling to occur soon after initiation of anticancer therapy, which can lead to a transient decrease in tumour ADC [72-74]. Later, this is followed by cell necrosis and lysis, resulting in an increase in ADC. Animal studies assessing very early cellular changes have also noted a decrease in intratumoural ADC in the first 36 hours after commencement of anticancer therapy [75, 76].

However, this scheme does not consider the contribution of intravascular perfusion to the diffusion measurement, which may be substantial in tumours as DWI provides simultaneous information on diffusion as well as microperfusion [77, 78]. Hence, therapies that are targeted against tumour vasculature (such as selective internal radiotherapy - SIRT) may result in a reduction in ADC values, especially when DWI were acquired using low b values, which are influenced by tissue perfusion effects [74].

Several authors have reported that tumours with low pretreatment ADC values show a better response to various therapies than those with high ADC [73, 79-81].

The most important issue regarding DWI is non-standardization among MRI manufactures and researchers. Substantial differences in the ADC values of the same normal and diseased organs have been presented [82] by researchers using a different imaging technique. Therefore, standardization of the imaging protocol is fundamental.

Currently, spatial resolution of DWI is possibly not high enough. In order to compensate for the rather limited spatial resolution, qualitative assessment might need superimposition of DWI on corresponding T1- or T2-weighted images, and quantitative assessment may require meticulous ADC measurements for small lesions. Utilization of high-field MRI may be able to solve the issue of limited spatial resolution.

2. T1w Dynamic Contrast-Enhanced (DCE) MRI (4D THRIVE)

Three-phased dynamic contrast-enhanced MR imaging is currently accepted as an important imaging tool for detecting and characterizing tumours in abdominal organs like the liver [83]. The hepatic purely arterial phase is especially important to distinguish fast enhancing lesions from slow contrast uptake in liver parenchyma [84-86]. Also, imaging of the portal venous phase is crucial for characterizing focal liver lesions. However, often the arterial hepatic phase will overlap with enhancement of blood coming from the portal vein in the duration of a 20-second acquisition time typically achieved in three-phased MRI [86]. To address this problem, Beck et al. recently proposed a fast imaging technique called CENTRA Plus [87] or Four-Dimensional T1-weighted High Resolution Imaging with Volume Excitation (4D THRIVE), combining the principles of keyhole imaging with half-Fourier acquisition to achieve a higher temporal resolution with full liver coverage and minor decrease of the spatial resolution. This method is based on a 3D fat-saturated spoiled turbo gradient echo sequence where a fat saturation pre-pulse followed by the acquisition of several profiles is combined with 3D dynamic elliptical centric Keyhole, Half Scan (partial Fourier acquisition) and Sensitivity Encoding (SENSE) to accelerate the acquisition. The elliptical centric keyhole method consists of dynamically acquiring a limited number of central ky-kz-space profiles (disk), and sharing the high spatial resolution information from a single full data set called reference (Figure 1). To further accelerate the technique, an alternating viewsharing technique as described in ref. [88, 89] was applied.

The central ky-kz disk defined by the keyhole percentage hereby is subdivided in three regions, P^+, C and P^-, where P^+ and P^- cover positive and negative peripheral regions in this central disk and C the central region as shown in figure 1.

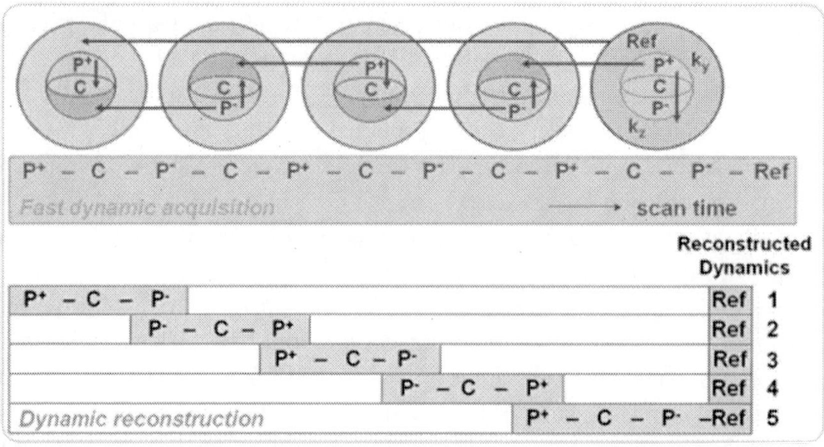

Figure 1. Displays a schematic depiction of the alternating viewsharing technique. The central ky-kz disk defined by the keyhole percentage is subdivided in three regions, P+, C and P-, where P+ and P- cover positive and negative peripheral regions in this central disk and C the central region as shown in figure 1. The central region C is acquired every dynamic scan while regions P+ and P- are shared with subsequent dynamic scans according to an alternating viewsharing scheme: P+-C-P--C-P+-C-P--C-P+-Ref. The P- and P+ parts from subsequent keyhole scans are shared in the reconstruction process.

The central region C is acquired every dynamic scan while regions P^+ and P^- are shared with subsequent dynamic scans according to an alternating viewsharing scheme: P^+-C-P^--C-P^+-C-P^--C-P^+-Ref. The P- and P+ parts from subsequent keyhole scans are shared in the reconstruction process. With this strategy it was shown that the precision of contrast-enhancement sampling could be improved [87].

The 4D THRIVE sequence parameters using 3T MRI for liver imaging that are illustrated (Figure 2) in this chapter are TR/TE= 2.9ms/1.4ms, turbo factor = 46, FOV 375mm x 280 mm, in-plane resolution 2mm, acquisition slice thickness 3mm, reconstruction of 133 slices of 1.5 mm thickness. Acquisition in transverse plane, Sense factor was 2 in the anterior-posterior direction. The keyhole factor was 45% (spatial resolution in phase and slice encoding direction was 3.7 mm) and the viewsharing percentage (P^+ + C)/(P^++C+P^-) was 55% leading to a total acquisition time of 24.8 % with respect to the reference acquisition. A first 3D scan of the whole liver was obtained during breath-hold before injection of contrast agent. During the first four breath-holds after injection, 3 dynamic scans were performed per breath-hold - with 2 keyhole acquisitions acquiring only the central alternating ky-kz parts, P^--C and P^+-C, as shown in figure 1, concluded by a reference acquisition, P^--C-P^+-Ref, that acquires both central and peripheral ky-kz parts. During the last two breath-holds 1 dynamic scan, P^--C-P^+-Ref, was performed. This resulted in 15 dynamic scans in total. The acquisition time of the central part of k-space was 2.7 seconds and the acquisition time of the reference acquisition was 10.8 seconds (10.8s x 45/100 (Keyhole percentage) = 4.9s; 4.9s x 0.55 (viewsharing) = 2.7s). This results in an acquisition time of 16.2 seconds per breath-hold for the first four post-contrast breath-holds, and an acquisition time of 10.8 seconds for the remaining two post-contrast breath-holds. One ml/10 kg (0.05 mmol/kg) body weight of gadolinium-BOPTA (MultiHance®, Bracco, Milan, Italy) was injected as a bolus via the cubital vein immediately followed by 20ml of physiologic saline (NaCl 0,9%) both at 3ml/s using Spectris MR injector (Medrad, Maastricht, The Netherlands). Fluoroscopic imaging was used for bolus tracking. Scanning was started when the contrast agent was filling the right atrium.

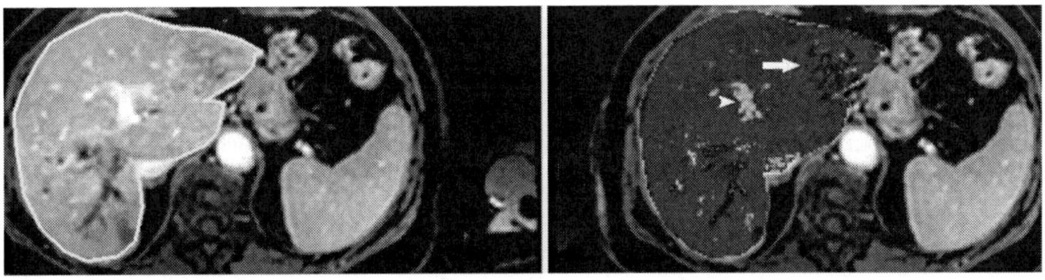

Figure 2. Displays a colorectal liver metastasis in a 68-year-old woman using transverse contrast-enhanced 4D THRIVE. The reference image using 4D THRIVE in delayed phase (on the left) is shown with corresponding automatically calculated perfusion map (on the right). The parametric map shows the colorectal liver metastasis (white arrow) as a heterogenous lesion with ring enhancement. Portal vein is indicated with white arrowhead.

Importantly, this DCE MRI technique offers the potential for assessment of the whole liver volume as part of a routine MR examination including high-resolution anatomical imaging. DCE MRI sequences with high temporal resolution can also be used to generate parametric maps and to compute perfusion and permeability parameters using pharmacokinetic models, with potential benefits in terms of detection, characterization, staging and therapy monitoring [90, 91]. The above mentioned 4D THRIVE sequence is a new development with specialized DCE-MRI protocol. T1-weighted DCE-MRI has already been performed by several study groups. An issue comparable with DWI techniques, is that also for DCE-MRI techniques there is a non-standardization among MRI manufactures and researchers. So, also for DCE-MRI standardization of the imaging protocol is a fundamental issue.

Analysis of Tumour Heterogeneity: Region-of-Interest (ROI) Placements versus Parametric (Pixel) Mapping

Analysis of DCE-MRI data (and other functional data eg. DWI data, glucose metabolism) need to take into account the heterogeneity of tumoural characteristics. Whole tumour ROIs have good signal-to-noise ratio but lack spatial resolution and are unable to evaluate tumour heterogeneity (partial volume effects and calculation of mean perfusion parameters within the ROI). Therefore, whole tumour ROIs may not reflect small areas of rapid change and so may be insensitive to specific perfusion characteristics that might allow characterization of focal liver lesions (and drug action when evaluation of treatment effect of chemotherapy is performed). That explains why many authors have commented that whole tumour ROI assessment may be inappropriate particularly for the evaluation of malignant lesions where heterogeneous areas of enhancement are diagnostically important [92-94]. Parametric mapping (in combination with histogram analysis) has a number of advantages including the appreciation of heterogeneity of enhancement and removal for the need to selectively place user-defined ROIs. The use of parametric mapping is needed for accurate evaluation of the whole liver parenchyma in oncologic staging. Parametric mapping is able to spatially match tumoural vascular characteristics such as blood volume, blood flow, permeability and leakage space. Parametric mapping has the advantage that it can be used in clinical practice because a rather easy visual evaluation of the liver parenchyma is possible and parametric mapping also allows sufficient workflow to use this technique in clinical practice. The placement of ROIs within the liver parenchyma is time-consuming and does not allow accurate and repetitive evaluation of the whole liver parenchyma in a clinically feasible manner. Also for the evaluation of focal liver lesions parametric mapping has the advantage to evaluate each pixel within a focal liver lesion separately rather than calculating mean changes of perfusion parameters of the whole lesion or a part of a lesion which is included within the ROI. A further advantage of parametric mapping is the calculation of parametric maps after registration procedures (the realigning and fusion of different sets of perfusion images). Parametric mapping techniques have the disadvantages of having poor signal-to-noise ratios and require specialist (non-commercially available) software for their generation.

Magnetic Resonance Imaging Characteristics of "Hypovascular" Colorectal Liver Metastases

Lesion detection is size related. When reviewing the literature, a lower threshold for detection is about 1cm [95]. Unfortunately, postmortem assessment of the size of liver metastases has shown that the ratio between metastases larger than 1cm and those smaller than 1cm is approximately 1:1.6 for metastases of colorectal adenocarcinoma and 1:4 for other liver metastases [96]. This clearly indicates that a capacity to accurately detect and characterize metastases smaller than 1cm is necessary.

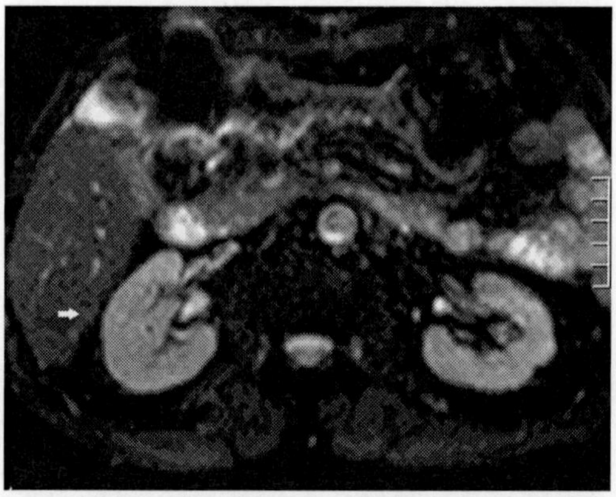

Figure 3a. Displays a transverse SS SE-EPI using b=0s/mm^2 image in a 62-year-old man hardly detecting any visible lesion in the area indicated by the white arrow.

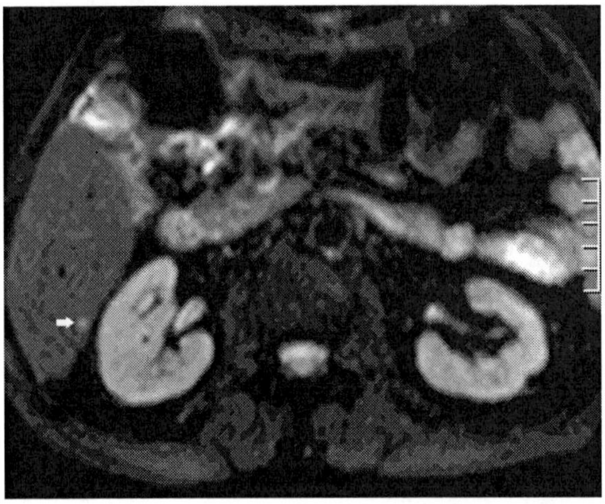

Figure 3b. Displays a transverse SS SE-EPI using b=10s/mm^2 image in a 62-year-old man clearly detecting a colorectal liver metastasis (white arrow).

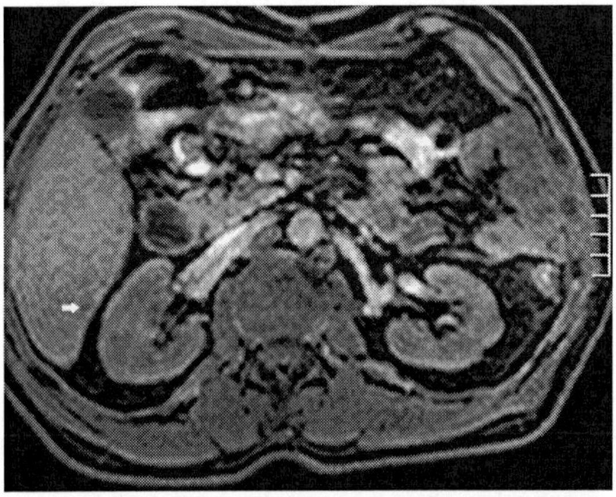

Figure 3c. Displays a transverse fat-suppressed T1w 3D GE image in the portal-venous phase after intravenous injection of SPIO in a 62-year-old man hardly detecting this liver metastasis (white arrow).

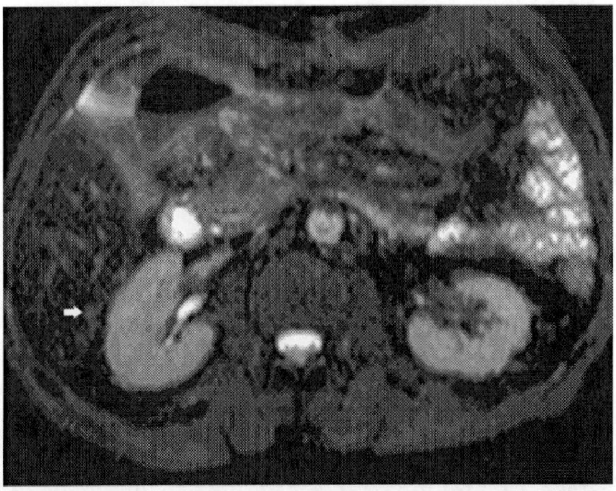

Figure 3d. Displays a transverse SPIO-enhanced T2w TSE (short TE with fat suppression) image in a 62-year-old man hardly detecting this liver metastasis (white arrow).

Detection and characterization of small (<1cm) focal liver lesions using MDCT is inferior to MRI [30]. Furthermore, with the venue of the respiratory-triggered SS SE-EPI sequence, detection of focal liver lesions down to 3mm is even possible using MRI [64]. In a study by Coenegrachts K et al., unenhanced respiratory-triggered SS SE-EPI performed better than SPIO-enhanced MRI (literature gold standard [3]) for detecting so-called hypovascular liver metastases (Figure 3a-d) [64].

Therefore, the SS SE-EPI sequence is ideally suited to be used as the first sequence (road map sequence) during an MRI examination of the liver. In most cases, the respiratory-triggered SS SE-EPI depicts the whole liver with good image quality and excellent Contrast-to-Noise Ratio (CNR). In that case, if no focal liver lesions can be detected using the unenhanced respiratory-triggered SS SE-EPI sequence, then the presence of malignant focal liver lesions is extremely unlikely (high negative predictive value of SS SE-EPI).

The signal intensity of the metastases is moderately increased compared with the surrounding hepatic tissue on T2w images and decreased on unenhanced T1w images [97]. Malignant tumours tend to have margins that are not sharply defined.

Liquefactive necrosis within the metastasis increases signal intensity on T2w images, whereas coagulative necrosis [98], desmoplastic reaction, or calcifications [99] decrease signal intensity on T2w images.

The presence of mucin within metastases can increase the signal intensity on T1w images [100].

On T1w DCE imaging, in the arterial phase “hypovascular” colorectal liver metastases can show a fleeting ring enhancement that blurs the margins of the lesions and corresponds to a desmoplastic reaction, inflammatory infiltration, and vascular proliferation in the tumour-liver parenchyma margin [4]. Enhancement progresses centrally with concomitant peripheral wash-out [4]. In the venous phase, liver metastases are hypo-intense compared with the surrounding liver parenchyma.

During the perfusion phase using SPIO-enhanced T1w GE imaging, ring enhancement is highly suggestive of malignant liver lesions [101]. Metastases do not contain Reticulo-Endothelial System (RES) cells; thus, after SPIO injection the liver metastasis CNR is improved with increased lesion conspicuity and detection compared with unenhanced T2w images [44, 50, 102].

Recent works have described that both Gd-EOB-DTPA-enhanced MRI and DWI are useful for the detection of hepatic metastases [59, 67, 103, 104]. In a study by Shimada K et al. [105], Gd-EOB-DTPA-enhanced MRI yielded better accuracy in the detection of small hepatic metastases than DWI. There was image deterioration owing to artefacts, especially at the upper edge and the lateral segment of the liver on DWI. However, there were three nodules that were better visualised on DWI than on Gd-EOB-DTPA-enhanced MRI. Thus, the addition of DWI may allow improved detection of small hepatic metastases that are difficult to differentiate from thin vessels or small hepatic cysts on Gd-EOB-DTPA-enhanced MRI sequences.

In a study by Löwenthal D et al. [106] late-phase Gd-EOB-DTPA-enhanced images were superior for the detection of FLLs, while DWIs were most valuable for the identification of particularly small metastases. Combined interpretation of unenhanced images resulted in a high diagnostic accuracy for the characterisation of FLLs. The authors of this study suggest that the need for the systematic use of contrast agents for MR imaging of the liver may therefore be reduced.

For the differentiation of small (<10mm) focal liver lesions, the calculation of D, f and ADC_{low} also seems promising. Still, for the characterization of small focal liver lesions more research is needed [62].

Nonetheless, if an operation is planned, the surgeon has an accurate guidance during the operation using Intra-Operative UltraSound (IOUS) to further characterize these small focal liver lesions in those areas where a focal liver lesion is detected with DWI or late-phase Gd-EOB-DTPA-enhanced MRI. This allows the surgeon to locally treat small malignant focal liver lesions with minimally-invasive techniques. This should likely benefit the patients' prognosis by optimizing the removal of all malignant deposits within the liver during one treatment session.

Usefulness of High B-Value DWI in Clinical Practice

There have not been many reports on the use of DWI for early detection of the response to chemotherapy. However, Cui et al. reported that a weak but significant correlation was found between final tumour size reduction and early ADC changes for various systemic chemotherapies against gastric or colorectal hepatic metastases [73]. A study by Marugami N et al. [107] also found a significant positive correlation between %ADC and reduction ratio, and a significant difference in %ADC between the responder and the nonresponder groups in HAIC with 5-FU, a unified regimen against colorectal liver metastases. The fact that HAIC delivers a higher concentration of anticancer drugs to tumours compared with systemic chemotherapy might be the reason that the results in this study showed sharper early ADC changes than the results reported by Cui et al. [107].

Higano et al. reported that the minimum ADC of malignant astrocytomas, preferably when cystic or necrotic components are avoided, can provide additional information regarding clinical malignancy related to posttreatment prognosis [108].

For several reasons the minimum ADC was considered useful for the evaluation of therapeutic monitoring in the present study [107]. First, from the viewpoint of the histological findings of colorectal hepatic metastases, it is well recognized that colorectal hepatic metastases contain necrosis, which is reported in 49% of pathologically proven lesions [98]. Second, from the viewpoint of drug distribution, on CT during arterial injection of contrast material, the peripheral site of colorectal hepatic metastases is enhanced strongly, which means that high concentrations of 5-FU are present in the tumour periphery. The most common pattern seen on ADC maps is the presence of highly cellular components in the tumour periphery and necrotic components in the tumour center; therefore, highly cellular areas correspond to areas of high drug distribution.

As already mentioned, reproducibility is considered to be a significant problem in ADC measurement. To avoid the influence of different MR units and DWI parameters in determining therapeutic monitoring, the relative change ratio of the ADC value before and after treatment can be selected, rather than the ADC value. Also, in future studies, parametric mapping (in combination with histogram analysis) should be performed as a sophisticated method for analysis of tumour heterogeneity.

In clinical studies, researchers have also reported that an early increase in the ADC value after starting therapy suggests a better treatment outcome [70, 73, 109, 110]. Koh et al. [79] also have reported that patients with colorectal liver metastases show an increase in ADC, at least in those who show a partial response to treatment, but not in non-responders. A decrease in ADC during follow-up suggests tumour recurrence [74].

In a study by Dudeck O et al., DWI was able to differentiate tumour response at an early stage following SIRT. As colorectal metastatic liver lesions have variable vascularity, they also evaluated the angiographic tumour vascularity at baseline of all studied lesions, but no significant difference was found for responding lesions (RL) and non-responding lesions (NRL). In this study, the use of an additional lower b-value of 100–150 s/mm^2 to obtain information on tissue perfusion effects certainly would have been beneficial [111].

Usefulness of DCE MRI in Clinical Practice

To date, reports of liver perfusion at MRI are limited in number and vary considerably [112]. As described above, T1w DCE-MRI seems a promising method for the detection of cancer [113]. In most cases, only one to a few slices within the whole liver parenchyma have been used to evaluate perfusion parameters. Thanks to new developments in MRI scanning technologies, it is now possible to perform T1w DCE-MRI of the entire liver with high spatial and temporal resolution. The above mentioned 4D THRIVE sequence has already been evaluated for its ability to differentiate benign from malignant (Figure 2) focal liver lesions [89].

Dynamic-contrast enhanced magnetic resonance imaging (DCE MRI) may also be used to study the pathophysiology of tumours [114, 115]. Parameters of interest include microvascular density; vascular permeability; and the extravascular, extracellular space [116]. Notably, malignancy, stage, and prognosis have all been correlated with these enhancement parameters [117-121]. Several studies have shown that successful therapies also result in changes in DCE MRI contrast-enhancement parameters, which may prove to be a more accurate and earlier indication of response [122-125].

In a study by Morgan B et al. [126] patients with advanced colorectal cancers with liver metastases were examined with DCE MRI and these functional perfusion changes were analyzed with relation to clinical effect. MRI scan was performed at baseline (within 1 week before treatment). Further studies were performed on day 2 and at the end of each 28-day cycle (ie, end of cycle 1 (EC1) and end of cycle 2 (EC2)). Patients were imaged between 2 to 9 hours post-dose on these days. Specific (PTK/ZK) treatment in this study was shown to cause a significant reduction in DCE MRI contrast-enhancement parameters (K^{trans}) within 26 to 33 hours of administration of the first dose. The extent of reduction was dose dependent at both day 2 and EC1. There was a statistically significant relationship between reduction in contrast-enhancement and disease response. Thus DCE MRI bidirectional transfer constant (at day 2) appeared to be a strong predictive marker for disease stabilization, thus supporting the use of DCE MRI as a biomarker for early assessment of tumour response in this study.

In a study by Miyazaki K et al. [127], it was shown that it was possible to calculate HPI on a pixel-by-pixel basis by converting the measured T1 signal intensity to quantified gadolinium concentrations. HPI calculation using such a methodology has not been previously reported. The resulting HPI maps could be analysed qualitatively and quantitatively.

Qualitative visual analysis of the HPI maps overlaid on T1-weighted images in patients with metastatic liver disease showed striking increases in relative arterial perfusion around and within hepatic metastases [127]. However, the area of increased peri-tumoural HPI could be larger than the area of T1 peri-tumoural enhancement.

Elevated HPI in liver beyond the tumour boundary determined by anatomical T1-weighted imaging may represent increased hepatic arterial flow in the presence of occult metastases or due to stimulation of angiogenic cytokines by metastases. Another possible mechanism for this appearance may be compression of blood vessels beyond the tumour boundaries. The HPI maps appeared sensitive to vascular perturbations which are not apparent on morphological imaging. HPI maps, therefore, appear to provide additional information about altered hepatic blood flow which may be useful for tumour assessment and could improve our understanding of the process of metastasis development and treatment response [127].

Conclusion

Although the primary modalities for liver imaging are US and CT, recent studies have suggested that MRI is the most sensitive method for detecting (especially) small focal liver lesions. One of the advantages of MRI in liver imaging is the better soft tissue contrast, which reveals better detection and characterization of benign and malignant focal liver lesions. The development of liver-specific MRI contrast agents has further improved the diagnostic yield of MRI in lesion detection and characterization.

Further, two recent developments in MRI sequences for the upper abdomen comprise (unenhanced) diffusion-weighted imaging (DWI) and keyhole-based T1-weighted dynamic contrast-enhanced MRI (4D THRIVE). Unenhanced DWI has been shown to allow an improved detection ($b=10s/mm^2$) of (especially) small (<10mm) focal liver lesions compared with other (more routinely used) MRI sequences and is useful as a road map sequence at the start of each MRI examination of the liver. Also, using higher b-values, the calculation of Apparent Diffusion Coefficient (ADC) value, true diffusion coefficient (D) and the perfusion fraction f can be useful for the characterization of focal liver lesions. Dynamic contrast-enhanced 4D THRIVE enables MRI of the liver with high temporal and spatial resolution with full liver coverage. 4D THRIVE improves detection and characterization of focal liver lesions providing multiple arterial and venous phases. The characterization of focal liver lesions using parametric maps seems promising for differentiating benign and malignant focal liver lesions.

Functional imaging techniques (eg. DWI, DCE MRI,...) may aid in determining the biological active dose of a drug. Furthermore, as new targeted therapies may not result in tumour shrinkage and are frequently costly, the ability to detect early treatment effects may help to identify patients who are most likely to benefit. Therefore, functional imaging techniques can be used as a potential biomarker for assessing treatment response in patients with metastatic liver disease.

References

[1] Ferrucci J. Liver tumor imaging. Current concepts. *Radiol. Clin. North Am.* 1994;32:39-54.

[2] Fong Y, Blumgart L, Fortner J, Brennan M. Pancreatic or liver resection for malignancy is safe and effective for the elderly. *Ann. Surg.* 1995;222:426-434.

[3] Ward J. New MR techniques for the detection of liver metastases. *Cancer Imaging* 2006;6:33-42.

[4] Morana G, Grazioli L, Testoni M, Caccia P, Procacci C. Contrast Agents for Hepatic Magnetic Resonance Imaging. *Topics in Magnetic Resonance Imaging* 2002:13:117-150.

[5] Schima W, Kulinna C, Langenberger H, Ba-Ssalamah A. Liver metastases of colorectal cancer: US, CT or MR? *Cancer Imaging* 2005;5:S149-S155.

[6] Lodge I. Modern surgery for liver metastases. *Cancer Imaging* 2000;1:77-79.

[7] Malafosse R, Penna C, Sa Cunha A, Nordlinger B. Surgical management of hepatic metastases from colorectal malignancies. *Ann. Oncol.* 2001;12:887-894.

[8] Miyazaki M, Ito H, Nakagawa K, Ambiru S, Shimizu H, Okuno A, et al. Aggressive surgical resection for hepatic metastases involving the inferior vena cava. *Am. J. Surg.* 1999;177:294-298.

[9] Lodge J, Ammori B, Prasad K, Bellamy M. Ex vivo and in situ resection of inferior vena cava with hepatectomy for colorectal metastases. *Ann. Surg.* 2000;231:471-479.

[10] Jaeck D, Bachellier P, Guiguet M, Boudjema K, Vaillant J, Balladur P, et al. Long-term survival following resection of colorectal hepatic metastases. *Br. J. Surg.* 1997;84:977-980.

[11] Rees M, John T. Current status of surgery in colorectal metastases to the liver. *Hepato-Gastroenterol* 2001;48:341-344.

[12] Scheele J, Stangl R, Altendorf-Hofman A. Hepatic metastases from colorectal cancer: impact of surgical resection on the natural history. *Br. J. Surg.* 1990;77:1241-1246.

[13] Stangl R, Altendorf-Hofman A, Charnely R, Scheele J. Factors influencing the natural history of colorectal liver metastases. *Lancet* 1994;343:1405-1410.

[14] Arai Y, Inaba Y, Takeuchi Y, Ariyoshi Y. Intermittent hepatic arterial infusion of high-dose 5FU on a weekly schedule for liver metastases from colorectal cancer. *Cancer Chemother Pharmacol.* 1997;40:526–530.

[15] Kuszyk B, Bluemke D, Urban B, Choti M, Hruban R, Sitzmann J, et al. Portal-phase contrast-enhanced helical CT for the detection of malignant hepatic tumors: sensitivity based on comparison with intra-operative and pathologic findings. *AJR Am. J. Roentgenol.* 1996;166:91-95.

[16] Valls C, Lopez E, Guma A, Gil M, Sanchez A, Andia E, et al. Helical CT versus CT arterial portography in the detection of hepatic metastasis of colorectal carcinoma. *AJR Am. J. Roentgenol.* 1998;170:1341-1347.

[17] Ward J, Naik K, Guthrie J, Wilson D, Robinson P. Hepatic lesion detection: comparison of MR imaging after the administration of superparamagnetic iron oxide with dual phase CT by using alternative-free response receiver operating characteristic analysis. *Radiology* 1999;210:459-466.
[18] Valls C, Andia E, Sanchez A, Guma A, Figueras J, Torras J, et al. Hepatic metastases from colorectal cancer: preoperative detection and assessment of resectability with helical CT. *Radiology* 2001;218:55-60.
[19] Furuhata T, Okita K, Tsuruma T, Hata F, Kimura Y, Katsuramaki T, et al. Efficacy of SPIO-MR imaging in the diagnosis of liver metastases from colorectal carcinomas. *Dig. Surg.* 2003;20:321-325.
[20] Wang S, Chiang J, Tsai Y, Lee S, Lin H, Chou Y, et al. Focal hepatic fatty infiltration as a cause of pseudotumors: ultrasonographic patterns and clinical differentiation. *J. Clin. Ultrasound.* 1990;18:401-409.
[21] Janica J, Lebkowska U, Ustymowicz A, Augustynowicz A, Kamocki Z, Werel D, et al. Contrast-enhanced ultrasonography in diagnosing liver metastases. *Med. Sci. Monit.* 2007;13S1:111-115.
[22] Larsen L, Rosenkilde M, Christensen H, Bang N, Bolvig L, Christiansen T, et al. The value of contrast enhanced ultrasonography in detection of liver metastases from colorectal cancer: a prospective double-blinded study. *Eur. J. Radiol.* 2007;62:302-307.
[23] Cosgrove D. Ultrasound contrast agents: an overview. *Eur. J. Radiol.* 2006;60:324-330.
[24] Dietrich C, Kratzer W, Strobe D, Danse E, Fessl R, Bunk A, et al. Assessment of metastatic liver disease in patients with primary extrahepatic tumors by contrast-enhanced sonography versus CT and MRI. *World J. Gastroenterol.* 2006;12:1699-1705.
[25] Li R, Guo Y, Hua X, He Y, Ding J, Guo A, et al. Characterization of focal liver lesions: comparison of pulse-inversion harmonic contrast-enhanced sonography with contrast-enhanced CT. *J. Clin. Ultrasound.* 2007;35:109-117.
[26] Catala V, Nicolau C, Vilana R, Pages M, Bianchi l, Sanchez M, et al. Characterization of focal liver lesions: comparative study of contrast-enhanced ultrasound versus spiral computed tomography. *Eur. Radiol.* 2007;17:1066-1073.
[27] Della Vigna P, Cernigliaro F, Monfardini L, Gandini S, Bellomi M. Contrast-enhanced ultrasonography in the follow-up of patients with hepatic metastases from breast carcinoma. *Radiol. Med.* 2007;112:47-55.
[28] Dai Y, Chen M, Yin S, Yan K, Fan Z, Wu W, et al. Focal liver lesions: can SonoVue-enhanced ultrasound be used to differentiate malignant from benign lesions? *Invest. Radiol.* 2007;42:596-603.
[29] Soye J, Mullan C, Porter S, Beattie H, Barltrop A, Nelson W. The use of contrast-enhanced ultrasound in the characterization of focal liver lesions. *Ulster Med. J.* 2007;76:22-25.
[30] Rappeport E, Loft A. Liver metastases from colorectal cancer: imaging with superparamagnetic iron oxide (SPIO)-enhanced MR imaging, computed tomography and positron emission tomography. *Abdominal. Imaging* 2007;32:624-634.
[31] Silverman P. Liver metastases: imaging considerations for protocol development with multislice CT (MSCT). *Cancer Imaging* 2006;6:175-181.
[32] Bipat S, van Leeuwen M, IJzermans J, Comans E, Planting A, Bossuyt P, et al. Evidence-based guideline on management of colorectal liver metastases in the Netherlands. *Neth J. Med.* 2007;65:5-14.

[33] Carnaghi C, Tronconi MC, Rimassa L, Tondulli L, Zuradelli M, Rodari M, et al. Utility of 18F-FDG PET and contrast-enhanced CT scan in the assessment of residual liver metastasis from colorectal cancer following adjuvant chemotherapy. *Nucl. Med .Rev. Cent East Eur.* 2007;10:12–15.

[34] Lubezky N, Metser U, Geva R, Nakache R, Shmueli E, Klausner JM, et al. The role and limitations of 18-fluoro-2-deoxy-D-glucose positron emission tomography scan and computerized tomography in restaging patients with hepatic colorectal metastases following neoadjuvant chemotherapy: comparison with operative and pathological findings. *J. Gastrointest Surg.* 2007;11:472–478.

[35] Angliviel B, Benoist S, Penna C, El Hajjam M, Chagnon S, Julie C, et al. Impact of chemotherapy on the accuracy of computed tomography scan for the evaluation of colorectal liver metastases. *Ann. Surg. Oncol.* 2009;16:1247–1253.

[36] Robinson P. The effects of cancer chemotherapy on liver imaging. *Eur. Radiol.* 2009;19:1752–1762.

[37] Benoist S, Brouquet A, Penna C, Julie C, El HM, Chagnon S, Mitry E, et al. Complete response of colorectal liver metastases after chemotherapy: does it mean cure? *J. Clin. Oncol.* 2006;24:3939–3945.

[38] Elias D, Youssef O, Sideris L, Dromain C, Baton O, Boige V, et al. Evolution of missing colorectal liver metastases following inductive chemotherapy and hepatectomy. *J. Surg. Oncol.* 2004;86:4–9.

[39] Boykin K, Zibari G, Lilien D, et al. The use of FDG-positron emission tomography for the evaluation of colorectal metastases of the liver. *Am. J. Surg.* 1999;65:1183-1185.

[40] Delbeke D, Vitola J, Sandler M, et al. Staging recurrent metastatic colorectal carcinoma with PET. *J. Nucl. Med.* 1997;38:1196-1201.

[41] Zhuang H, Sinha P, Pourdehnad M, et al. The role of positron emission tomography with fluorine-18-deoxyglucose in identifying colorectal cancer metastases to liver. *Nucl. Med. Commun.* 2000;21:793-797.

[42] Bipat S, van Leeuwen M, Comans E, Pijl M, Bossuyt P, Zwinderman A, et al. Colorectal liver metastases: CT, MR imaging, and PET for diagnosis--meta-analysis. *Radiology* 2005;237:123-131.

[43] Kinkel K, Lu Y, Both M, et al. Detection of hepatic metastases from cancers of the gastrointestinal tract by using noninvasive imaging methods (US, CT, MR Imaging, PET): a meta-analysis. *Radiology* 2002;224:748-756.

[44] Wiering B, Ruers T, Krabbe P, Dekker H, Oyen W. Comparison of multiphase CT, FDG-PET and intra-operative ultrasound in patients with colorectal liver metastases selected for surgery. *Ann. Surg. Oncol.* 2007;14:818-826.

[45] Shin S, Jeong Y, Min J, Kim H, Chung T, Kang H. Preoperative staging of colorectal cancer: CT vs. integrated FDG PET/CT. *Abdom Imaging* 2008;33:270-277.

[46] Roman C, Martin W, Delbeke D. Incremental value of fusion imaging with integrated PET-CT in oncology. *Clin. Nucl. Med.* 2005;30:470-477.

[47] Morana G, Salviato E, Guarise A. Contrast agents for hepatic MRI. *Cancer Imaging* 2007;7 Spec No A:S24-S27.

[48] Semelka R, Cance W, Marcos H, Mauro M. Liver metastases: comparison of current MR techniques and spiral CT during arterial portography for detection in 20 surgically staged cases. *Radiology* 1999;213:86-91.

[49] Hagspiel K, Neidl K, Eichenberger A, Weder W, Marincek B. Detection of liver metastases: comparison of superparamagnetic iron oxide-enhanced and unenhanced MR imaging at 1.5T with dynamic CT, intraoperative US, and percutaneous US. *Radiology* 1995;196:471-478.

[50] Seneterre E, Taourel P, Bouvier Y, Pradel J, Van Beers B, Daures J, et al. Detection of hepatic metastases : Ferumoxides-enhanced MR imaging versus unenhanced MR imaging and CT during arterial portography. *Radiology* 1996;200:785-792.

[51] Muller R, Vogel K, Neumann K, Hirche H, Barkhausen J, Stoblen F, et al. SPIO-MR imaging versus double-phase spiral CT in detecting malignant lesions of the liver. *Acta Radiol.* 1999;40:628-635.

[52] Lencioni R, Della Pina C, Bruix J, Majno P, Grazioli L, Morana G, et al. Clinical management of hepatic malignancies: ferucarbotran-enhanced magnetic resonance imaging versus contrast-enhanced spiral computed tomography. *Dig. Dis. Sci.* 2005;50:533-537.

[53] Floriani I, Torri V, Rulli E, Garavaglia D, Compagnoni A, Salvolini L, et al. Performance of imaging modalities in diagnosis of liver metastases from colorectal cancer: a systematic review and meta-analysis. *JMRI* 2010;31:19-31.

[54] Kim Y, Lee J, Kim C, Chung G, Kim C, Kim I. Detection of liver metastases: gadobenate dimeglumineenhanced three-dimensional dynamic phases and one-hour delayed phase MR imaging versus superparamagnetic iron oxide-enhanced MR imaging. *Eur. Radiol.* 2005;15:220-228.

[55] Kim M, Kim J, Lim J, Oh Y, Chung J, Choi J, et al. Detection and characterization of focal hepatic lesions: mangafodipir vs. superparamagnetic iron oxide-enhanced magnetic resonance imaging. *JMRI* 2004;20:612-621.

[56] Hamm B, Staks T, Muhler A, et al. Phase I clinical evaluation of Gd-EOB-DTPA as a hepatobiliary MR contrast agent: safety, pharmacokinetics, and MR imaging. *Radiology* 1995;195:785–792.

[57] Vogl T, Kummel S, Hammerstingl R, et al. Liver tumors: comparison of MR imaging with Gd-EOB-DTPA and Gd-DTPA. *Radiology* 1996;200:59–67.

[58] Reimer P, Rummeny E, Shamsi K, et al. Phase II clinical evaluation of Gd-EOB-DTPA: dose, safety aspects, and pulse sequence. *Radiology* 1996;199:177–183.

[59] Zech C, Herrmann K, Reiser M, et al. MR imaging in patients with suspected liver metastases: value of liver-specific contrast agent Gd-EOB-DTPA. *Magn Reson Med. Sci.* 2007;6:43–52.

[60] Le Bihan D, Breton E, Lallemand D, Aubin M, Vignaud J, Laval J. Separation of diffusion and perfusion in intravoxel incoherent motion (IVIM) MR imaging. *Radiology* 1988;168:497-505.

[61] Yamada I, Aung W, Himeno Y, Nakagawa T, Shibuya H. Diffusion coefficients in abdominal organs and hepatic lesions: evaluation with intravoxel incoherent motion echo-planar MR imaging. *Radiology* 1999;210:617-623.

[62] Coenegrachts K, Delanote J, ter Beek L, Haspeslagh M, Bipat S, Stoker J, et al. Evaluation of true diffusion, perfusion factor, and apparent diffusion coefficient in non-necrotic liver metastases and uncomplicated liver hemangiomas using black-blood echo planar imaging. *Eur. J. Radiol.* 2009;69:131-138.

[63] Nagayama M, Watanabe Y, Okumura A, et al. Black-blood T2-weighted SE-EPI imaging of the liver. *Proceedings of the annual meeting of ISMRM 2002* (abstract 1963).

[64] Coenegrachts K, Orlent H, ter Beek L, Haspeslagh M, Bipat S, Stoker J, et al. Improved focal liver lesion detection: Comparison of single-shot spin-echo echo-planar and superparamagnetic iron oxide (SPIO)-enhanced MRI. *JMRI* 2008;27:117-124.

[65] Coenegrachts K, De Geeter F, ter Beek L, Walgraeve N, Bipat S, Stoker J, et al. Comparison of MRI (including SS SE-EPI and SPIO-enhanced MRI) and FDG-PET/CT for the detection of colorectal liver metastases. *Eur. Radiol.* 2009;19:370-379.

[66] Hussain S, De Becker J, Hop W, Dwarkasing R, Wielopolski P. Can a single-shot black-blood T2-weighted spin-echo echo-planar imaging sequence with sensitivity encoding replace the respiratory-triggered turbo spin-echo sequence for the liver? An optimization and feasibility study. *JMRI* 2005;21:219-229.

[67] Nasu K, Kuroki Y, Nawano S, Kuroki S, Tsukamoto T, Yamamoto S, et al. Hepatic metastases: diffusion-weighted sensitivity-encoding versus SPIO-enhanced MR imaging. *Radiology* 2006;239:122-130.

[68] Sun X, Quan X, Huang F, Xu Y. Quantitative evaluation of diffusion-weighted magnetic resonance imaging of focal liver lesions. *World J. Gastroenterol.* 2005;11:6535-6537.

[69] Koh D, Erica S, Collins D, et al. Diffusion coefficients and the perfusion fraction of colorectal hepatic metastases estimated using single-shot echo-planar sensitivity-encoded (SENSE) diffusion-weighted MR imaging. *Proc. Intl. Soc. Mag. Reson Med.* 2004, abstract 908.

[70] Moffat B, Chenevert T, Lawrence T, Meyer C, Johnson T, Dong Q, et al. Functional diffusion map: a noninvasive MRI biomarker for early stratification of clinical brain tumor response. *Proc. Natl. Acad. Sci. USA* 2005;102:5524–5529.

[71] Moffat B, Hall D, Stojanovska J, McConville P, Moody J, Chenevert T, et al. Diffusion imaging for evaluation of tumor therapies in preclinical animal models. *Magma* 2004;17:249–259.

[72] Dudeck O, Zeile M, Pink D, Pech M, Tunn P, Reichardt P, et al. Diffusion-weighted magnetic resonance imaging allows monitoring of anticancer treatment effects in patients with soft-tissue sarcomas. *JMRI* 2008;27:1109–1113.

[73] Cui Y, Zhang X, Sun Y, Tang L, Shen L. Apparent diffusion coefficient: potential imaging biomarker for prediction and early detection of response to chemotherapy in hepatic metastases. *Radiology* 2008;248:894–900.

[74] Thoeny H, De Keyzer F, Chen F, Ni Y, Landuyt W, Verbeken E, et al. Diffusion-weighted MR imaging in monitoring the effect of a vascular targeting agent on rhabdomyosarcoma in rats. *Radiology* 2005;234:756–764.

[75] Thoeny H, De Keyzer F, Vandecaveye V, Chen F, Sun X, Bosmans H, et al. Effect of vascular targeting agent in rat tumor model: dynamic contrast-enhanced versus diffusion-weighted MR imaging. *Radiology* 2005;237:492–499.

[76] Jordan B, Runquist M, Raghunand N, Baker A, Williams R, Kirkpatrick L, et al. Dynamic contrast-enhanced and diffusion MRI show rapid and dramatic changes in tumor microenvironment in response to inhibition of HIF-1alpha using PX-478. *Neoplasia* 2005;7:475–485.

[77] van Rijswijk C, Kunz P, Hogendoorn P, Taminiau A, Doornbos J, Bloem J. Diffusion-weighted MRI in the characterization of soft-tissue tumors. *JMRI* 2002;15:302–307.

[78] Latour L, Svoboda K, Mitra P, Sotak C. Time-dependent diffusion of water in a biological model system. *Proc. Natl. Acad. Sci. USA* 1994;91:1229–1233.

[79] Koh D, Scurr E, Collins D, Kanber B, Norman A, Leach M, Husband J. Predicting response of colorectal hepatic metastasis: value of pretreatment apparent diffusion coefficients. *AJR Am. J. Roentgenol.* 2007;188:1001–1008.

[80] DeVries A, Kremser C, Hein P, Griebel J, Krezcy A, Öfner D, et al. Tumor microcirculation and diffusion predict therapy outcome for primary rectal carcinoma. *Int. J. Radiat. Oncol. Biol. Phys.* 2003; 56:958–965.

[81] Dzik-Jurasz A, Domenig C, George M, Wolber J, Padhani A, Brown G, et al. Diffusion MRI for prediction of response of rectal cancer to chemoradiation. *Lancet* 2002;360:307–308.

[82] Padhani A, Liu G, Koh D, Chenevert T, Thoeny H, Takahara T, et al. Diffusion-weighted magnetic resonance imaging as a cancer biomarker: consensus and recommendations. *Neoplasia* 2009;11:102–125.

[83] Low R. Abdominal MRI advances in the detection of liver tumours and characterization. *The Lancet Oncology* 2007;8:525-535.

[84] Rofsky N, Lee V, Laub G, Pollack M, Krinsky G, Thomasson D, et al. Abdominal MR imaging with a volumetric interpolated breath-hold examination. *Radiology* 1999;212:876-884.

[85] Bonaldi V, Bret P, Reinhold C, Atri M. Helical CT of the liver: value of an early hepatic arterial phase. *Radiology* 1995;197:357-363.

[86] Lee V, Lavelle M, Rofsky N, Laub G, Thomasson D, Krinsky G, et al. Hepatic MR Imaging with a Dynamic Contrast-Enhanced Isotropic Volumetric Interpolated Breath-hold Examination: Feasibility, Reproducibility, and Technical Quality. *Radiology* 2000;215:365-372.

[87] Beck G, De Becker J, Jones A, von Falkenhausen M, Willinek W, Gieseke J. A Contrast-Enhanced Timing Robust Acquisition order with a Preparation of the Longitudinal Signal component, CENTRA Plus, for 3D Contrast Enhanced Abdominal Imaging. *JMRI* 2008;27:1461–1467.

[88] Beck G, Herigault G, Glantenay A, Coenegrachts K, Denolin V. Ultra-fast time resolved contrast enhanced abdominal imaging using an elliptical centric fat suppressed 3D profile sharing acquisition technique, SENSE and partial Fourier *Proc. Intl. Soc. Mag. Reson. Med.* 2008;16:2622.

[89] Coenegrachts K, Ghekiere J, Denolin V, Beck G, Hérigault G, Haspeslagh M, et al. Perfusion maps of the whole liver based on high temporal and spatial resolution contrast-enhanced MRI (4D THRIVE): Feasibility and initial results in focal liver lesions. *Eur. J. Radiol.* 2010;74:529-535.

[90] Padhani A. MRI for assessing antivascular cancer treatments. *BJR* 2003;76:60-80.

[91] Wang L, Van den Bos I, Hussain S, Pattynama P, Vogel M, Krestin G. Post-processing of dynamic gadolinium-enhanced magnetic resonance imaging exams of the liver: explanation and potential clinical applications for color-coded qualitative and quantitative analysis. *Acta Radiol.* 2008;49:6-18.

[92] Aronen H, Gazit I, Louis D, et al. Cerebral blood volume maps of gliomas: comparison with tumor grade and histologic findings. *Radiology* 1994;191:41-51.

[93] Parker G, Suckling J, Tanner S, et al. Probing tumor microvascularity by measurement, analysis and display of contrast agent uptake kinetics. *JMRI* 1997;7:564-574.

[94] Gribbestad I, Nilsen G, Fjosne H, Kvinnsland S, Haugen O, Rinck P. Comparative signal intensity measurements in dynamic gadolinium-enhanced MR mammography. *JMRI* 1994;4:477-480.

[95] Wernecke K, Rummeny E, Bongartz G, Vassallo P, Kivelitz D, Wiesmann W, et al. Detection of hepatic masses in patients with carcinoma: Comparative sensitivities of sonography, CT, and MR imaging. *AJR Am. J. Roentgenol.* 1991;157:731-739.

[96] Schulz W, Borchard F. The size of the liver metastases in a low metastatic count. A quantitative study of postmortem livers. *Rofo Fortschr Geb Rontgenstr Neuen Bildgeb Verfahr* 1992;156:320-324.

[97] Imam K, Bluemke D. MR imaging in the evaluation of hepatic metastases. *Magn Reson Imaging Clin. N. Am.* 2000;8:741-756.

[98] Outwater E, Tomaszewski J, Daly J, Kressel H. Hepatic colorectal metastases: Correlation of MR imaging and pathologic appearance. *Radiology* 1991;180:327-332.

[99] Semelka R, Bagley A, Brown E, Kroeker M. Malignant lesions of the liver identified on TI- but not T2-weighted MR images at 1.5 T. *JMRI* 1994;4:315-318.

[100] Semelka R, Kelekis N. Liver. In: Semelka R, Ascher S, Reinhold C, eds. MRI of the Abdomen and Pelvis. New York: Wiley-Liss, 1997;19-135.

[101] Kim J, Kim M, Suh S, Chung J, Yoo H, Lee J. Characterization of focal hepatic lesions with ferumoxides-enhanced MR imaging: utility of T1-weighted spoiled gradient recalled echo images using different echo times. *JMRI* 2002,15:573-583.

[102] Oudkerk M, van den Heuvel A, Wielopolski P, Schmitz P, Borel Rinkes I, Wiggers T. Hepatic lesions: Detection with ferumoxide-enhanced T1-weighted MR imaging. *Radiology* 1997;203:449-456.

[103] Ichikawa T, Haradome H, Hachiya J et al. Diffusion-weighted MR imaging with a single-shot echoplanar sequence: detection and characterization of focal hepatic lesions. *AJR Am. J. Roentgenol.* 1998;170:397–402.

[104] Naganawa S, Sato C, Nakamura T et al. Diffusion-weighted images of the liver: comparison of tumor detection before and after contrast enhancement with superparamagnetic iron oxide. *JMRI* 2005;21:836–840.

[105] Shimada K, Isoda H, Hirokawa Y, Arizono S, Shibata T, Togashi K. Comparison of gadolinium-EOB-DTPA-enhanced and diffusion-weighted liver MRI for detection of small hepatic metastases. *Eur. Radiol.* 2010;20:2690-2698.

[106] Löwenthal D, Zeile M, Lim W, Wybranski C, Fischbach F, Wieners G, et al. Detection and characterisation of focal liver lesions in colorectal carcinoma patients: comparison of diffusion-weighted and Gd-EOB-DTPA enhanced MR imaging. *Eur. Radiol.* 2011;21:832-840.

[107] Marugami N, Tanaka T, Kitano S, Hirohashi S, Nishiofuku H, Takahashi A, et al. Early Detection of Therapeutic Response to Hepatic Arterial Infusion Chemotherapy of Liver Metastases from Colorectal Cancer Using Diffusion-Weighted MR Imaging. *Cardiovasc. Intervent. Radiol.* 2009;32:638-646.

[108] Higano S, Yun X, Kumabe T, et al. Malignant astrocytic tumors: clinical importance of apparent diffusion coefficient in prediction of grade and prognosis. *Radiology* 2006;241:839–846.

[109] Kremser C, Judmaier W, Hein P, Griebel J, Lukas P, de Vries A. Preliminary results on the influence of chemoradiation on apparent diffusion coefficients of primary rectal carcinoma measured by magnetic resonance imaging. *Strahlenther Onkol.* 2003;179:641–649.

[110] Lee K, Bradley D, Hussain M, Meyer C, Chenevert T, Jacobson J, et al. A feasibility study evaluating the functional diffusion map as a predictive imaging biomarker for detection of treatment response in a patient with metastatic prostate cancer to the bone. *Neoplasia* 2007;9:1003–1011.

[111] Dudeck O, Zeile M, Wybranski C, Schulmeister A, Fischbach F, Pech M, et al. Early prediction of anticancer effects with diffusion-weighted MR imaging in patients with colorectal liver metastases following selective internal radiotherapy. *Eur. Radiol.* 2010; 20:2699-2706.

[112] Pandharipande P, Krinsky G, Rusinek H, Lee V. Perfusion Imaging of the Liver: Current Challenges and Future Goals! *Radiology* 2005;234:661-673.

[113] Evelhoch J. Key Factors in the Acquisition of Contrast Kinetic Data for Oncology. *JMRI* 1999;10:254-259.

[114] Yuh W. An exciting and challenging role for advanced contrast MR imaging. *JMRI* 1999;10:221–222.

[115] Taylor J, Tofts P, Port R, et al. MR imaging of tumors microcirculation: Promise for the new millennium. *JMRI* 1999;10:903–907.

[116] Knopp M, Weiss E, Sinn H, et al. Pathophysiologic basis of contrast enhancement in breast tumors. *JMRI* 1999;10:260–266.

[117] Buadu L, Murakami J, Murayama S, et al. Breast lesions: Correlation of contrast medium enhancement patterns on MR images with histopathologic findings and tumors angiogenesis. *Radiology* 1996;200:639–649.

[118] Hawighorst H, Knapstein P, Weikel W, et al. Angiogenesis of uterine cervical carcinoma: Characterization by pharmacokinetic magnetic resonance parameters and histological microvessel density with correlation to lymphatic involvement. *Cancer Res.* 1997;57:4777–4786.

[119] Hawighorst H, Weikel W, Knapstein P, et al. Angiogenic activity of cervical carcinoma: Assessment by functional magnetic resonance imaging-based parameters and a histomorphological approach in correlation with disease outcome. *Clin. Cancer Res.* 1998;4:2305–2312.

[120] Mayr N, Hawighorst H, Yuh W, et al. MR microcirculation assessment in cervical cancer: Correlations with histomorphological tumors markers and clinical outcome. *JMRI* 1999;10:267–276.

[121] Mayr N, Yuh W, Zheng J, et al. Prediction of tumors control in patients with cervical cancer: Analysis of combined volume and dynamic enhancement pattern by MR imaging. *AJR Am. J. Roentgenol.* 1998;170:177–182.

[122] Erlemann R, Sciuk J, Bosse A, et al. Response of osteosarcoma and Ewing sarcoma to preoperative chemotherapy: Assessment with dynamic and static MR imaging and skeletal scintigraphy. *Radiology* 1990;175:791–796.

[123] Fletcher B, Hanna S, Fairclough D, et al. Pediatric musculoskeletal tumors: Use of dynamic, contrast-enhanced MR imaging to monitor response to chemotherapy. *Radiology* 1992;184:243–248.

[124] Reddick W, Taylor J, Fletcher B: Dynamic MR imaging (DEMRI) of microcirculation in bone sarcoma. *JMRI* 1999;10:277–285.

[125] Barentsz J, Berger-Hartog O, Witjes J, et al. Evaluation of chemotherapy in advanced urinary bladder cancer with fast dynamic contrast-enhanced MR imaging. *Radiology* 1998;207:791–797.

[126] Morgan B, Thomas A, Drevs J, Hennig J, Buchert M, Jivan A, et al. Dynamic Contrast-Enhanced Magnetic Resonance Imaging As a Biomarker for the Pharmacological Response of PTK787/ZK 222584, an Inhibitor of the Vascular Endothelial Growth Factor Receptor Tyrosine Kinases, in Patients With Advanced Colorectal Cancer and Liver Metastases: Results From Two Phase I Studies. *J. Clin. Oncol.* 2003;21:3955-3964.

[127] Miyazaki K, Collins D, Walker-Samuel S, Taylor J, Padhani A, Leach M, et al. Quantitative mapping of hepatic perfusion index using MR imaging: a potential reproducible tool for assessing tumour response to treatment with the antiangiogenic compound BIBF 1120, a potent triple angiokinase inhibitor. *Eur. Radiol.* 2008;18:1414-1421.

In: Medical and Biological Frontiers Research Compendium ISBN: 978-1-62417-022-5
Editor: Tsisana Shartava

Chapter 6

Reducing Sodium in Cheese: A Solution for Excess Sodium Intake as a Cause of Hypertension and Heart Diseases

Mamdouh El-Bakry*
Department of Dairy Science and Technology, Faculty of Agriculture,
Cairo University, Giza, Egypt

Abstract

Cheese is a versatile, nutrient-dense dairy food, i.e. a good source of protein, vitamins and minerals particularly calcium and phosphorus, which is an important component in highly consumed convenience foods. However, cheese is perceived as being high in saturated fat, which might contribute to risks of atherosclerosis, and sodium. There is considerable evidence that excess or high sodium intake, which is the case in Western countries, is associated with hypertension and strokes, hence, dietary guidelines recommend that sodium intake be reduced.

This review covers the scientific and technological aspects of the role of sodium in cheese manufacture and functional properties and highlights various strategies for reducing the sodium. The focus is on natural cheese, made from milk by acid and/or rennet-coagulation, and process cheese. This cheese differs from natural cheese in that it is made from natural cheese or casein, which is blended with the necessary emulsifying salts and in the presence of heat, leading to the formation of a homogeneous product with extended shelf-life. Process cheese has numerous end-use applications in processed foods, which counts for ~75% of the dietary sodium in industrialized diets.

The source of sodium in cheese is mainly the added salt (sodium chloride). Salt acts primarily as food preservative and flavor enhancer and also interacts with major components in the cheese and thereby affecting the functionality, e.g. salt increases the protein hydration during manufacture which affects the stability and textural properties. Process cheese contains much higher sodium content, compared to natural cheese, due to

* Department of Dairy Science and Technology, Faculty of Agriculture, Cairo University, Giza, Egypt. E-Mail Address: m.elbakry@um.es, Tel.: +2157857859.

the necessity of using emulsifying salts, such as sodium citrate and phosphate. These salts are crucial for the hydration of the protein, emulsification of fat and the stability of the final product.

Strategies for reducing sodium in cheese are mainly outlined in the reduction of the salt and/or emulsifying salts used and their substitution by the potassium equivalents salts. However, these strategies present many challenges, such as adverse effects on flavor and microbiological stability. In process cheese, a high reduction of emulsifying salts does not allow for the formation of a homogeneous end product. Recent approaches of reducing emulsifying salts used are also discussed, such as utilizing of emulsifiers or protein hydrolyzates in the manufacture of cheese.

A final section in this review is about the future of low sodium cheese manufacture, including suggestions for reducing sodium that has not been systematically investigated in research on various cheese types.

1. Introduction

Although cheese production is a very ancient and traditional craft, it enjoys a consistent and substantial growth rate, with a healthy and positive image. It could be regarded as the original convenience food which may be consumed as the main component of a meal, as a dessert, as a snack, as a condiment, or as a food ingredient. In addition, new varieties continue to be developed, despite the fact that there are 500 types, e.g., Jarlsberg and Araglin (Fox and McSweeney, 2004).

Cheese is a nutritionally valued dairy product that contains a high concentration of essential nutrients relative to its energy content, i.e. cheese contributes ~9% of the protein, 11% of the phosphorus, and 27% of the calcium in the U.S. food supply (O'Brien and O'Connor, 2004). Regarding the vitamin content of the cheese, most cheeses are good sources of vitamin A, as ~85% of its content in milk is retained in the cheese, riboflavin, vitamin B12, and folate (Holland et al., 1989). Cheese fat generally contains ~66% saturated, 30% monounsaturated and 4% polyunsaturated fatty acids. Thus, cheese represents a significant dietary source of both saturated and unsaturated fatty acids.

However, despite these nutritional benefits, cheese is also perceived as being high in fat and sodium. This might discourages some consumers from including cheese in their diets. Evidence exist that high sodium intake can contribute to hypertension, strokes and cardiovascular diseases, particular in the case of salt-susceptible individuals (Cutler, 1999, Johnson et al., 2009, Doyle and Glass, 2010). Adults in Western Societies consume, on average ~5-6g sodium/day, which is much more than the required daily sodium, as the sodium balance in the body can be maintained with a daily intake of less than 2.3g (Taormina, 2010). Salt (sodium chloride), which is mostly the main source of added sodium in cheese, serves several important functions in the cheesemaking process. A wide range of sodium levels are found in cheese due to different amounts of salt added during manufacture.

The objectives is to review the scientific and technological aspects of the role of sodium in cheese manufacture and functional properties, highlights the progress made so far of various strategies for reducing the sodium, and to include a review of recent advances in reducing sodium which has not been sufficiently investigated in research on various cheese types.

2. Sources of Sodium in Cheese

In natural cheese, one of the final steps in the manufacture process is the addition of salt (NaCl). In dry salted cheeses like cheddar, the salt is added directly to the curds just before pressing. In pickled cheeses, the salt is added by submersing the cheese in brine containing about 5 to 10% salt for an appropriate storage time. Salt in some cheeses like Ras cheese is rubbed on the outer surface of the cheese. Salt addition is the major source of sodium in natural cheese. The salt content can vary widely, from 0.5% for cheeses like Emmental to 7% for pickeled cheeses like Domiati (Guinee, 2004).

Process cheese, in broad terms, is defined to be a merge of one or more natural cheeses of different ages and types, emulsifying salts, salt, water, and other dairy and nondairy ingredients like whey proteins, starch, preservatives and flavor enhancers (Guinee et al., 2004). This mixture goes through the necessary continuous thermal and mixing energies, i.e. mixing at ~80°C for several minutes, to produce a homogeneous product. The final product is considered to pasteurised and accordingly has an extended shelf life (Zehren and Nusbaum, 2000). A further advantage of this type of cheese is that wide varieties can be produced due to a multitude of ingredients used in the manufacture. In addition, the manufacture of process cheese allows for the upgrading of defective cheese products if the defects could limit the shelf life but the cheese is still edible (Berger et al., 1989). There are three major sources of the sodium in process cheese. These sources include sodium-based emulsifying salts, natural cheese used as ingredient and salt of ~2% of the cheese weight, contributing to approx. 45, 35 and 20% respectively of the total sodium content (Zehren and Nusbaum, 2000).

3. Role of Sodium in Cheese

3.1. Role of Salt (NaCl)

No matter the way or the amount of the salt added to the cheese, it has been an essential component used to for at least a preservative purpose. Controlling growth of pathogens in foods is essential to public health, particularly for high-risk populations including very young children, pregnant women, the elderly, and people whose immune systems are weakened. Salt also maintains the expected flavor, as consumers expect some degree of saltiness in cheese, and body and texture by controlling the activities of enzymes and microorganisms.

3.1.1. Preservative Action of Salt and its Role in Microbial Safety

The classical methods of food preservation, including salting, fermentation, refrigeration and dehydration, are used to preserve cheese. The preservative action of salt is due to its lowering effect on the water activity (a_w) of the medium and therefore prevent microbial growth, as available water is a critical factor affecting microbial growth on and in foods (Betts, 2007). Salt increases the osmotic pressure of the aqueous phase of foods, causing dehydration of bacterial cells and killing them or at least preventing their growth. The amount of salt in the moisture phase (S/M ratio) of the cheese controls the growth of microorganisms, not the total amount of salt in the food (Guinee, 2004). In addition, during manufacture of natural cheeses, salt affects the syneresis of the cheese curd formed during manufacture resulting in whey expulsion and thus controlling the final moisture of the cheese, which also influences the growth of microorganisms and enzymes.

Table 1 shows the different a_w values and salt content for various types of cheeses. Cheeses have a high aw of 0.95 to 1 and it has been reported that the water activity of young cheese is determined almost entirely by the concentration of NaCl in the aqueous phase (Christian, 2000). In addition to sodium chloride, proteins decrease a_w like reduced a_w of hard cheeses to 0.90-0.92. It is apparent from Table 1 and 2 that the water activity of most cheese varieties is not low enough to prevent the growth of most bacterial pathogens and spoilage microorganisms, but together with a low pH it is quite effective in controlling the microbial growth. Therefore, by inhibiting or retarding the growth and activity of microorganisms, including pathogenic and food-poisoning microorganisms, the safety of cheeses increases.

Table 1. Salt content and water activity (aw) of different cheese types

Cheese	Salt (%)	a_w
Cheese Curd, Whey Cheese	0.0	1.00
Cottage, Quarg Cheese	0.5	0.99
Muenster, Process Cheese	1.0-2.0	0.98
Brie, Camembert	1.0-1.5	0.97
Edam, Havarti	1.5-2.0	0.96
Cheddar, Gorgonzola, Gouda	1.5-2.0	0.95
Mozzarella, Stilton	2.0-2.5	0.94
Danablu, Normana	1.5-2.0	0.93
Parmesan, Zamorano	1.5-2.0	0.92
Provolone, Roquefort	2.5-3.0	0.91
Cabrales, Primost	0-1.0	0.90

Adapted from Zehren and Nusbaum, 2000; Guinee and Fox, 2004.

Table 2. Minimum water activity (aw) required for the growth of different pathogenic and spoilage microorganisms

Microorganisms	Minimum a_w
Aeromonas hydrophila	0.97
Bacillus cereus	0.93
E. coli	0.94
Staph aureus	0.86-0.91
Yersinia enterocolitica	0.96
Vibrio parahaemolyticus	0.94
Shigella spp.	0.96
Clostridium botulinum	0.94-0.97
Campylobacter jejuni	0.99
Salmonella spp.	0.94

Adapted from Guinee and Fox, 2004.

The literature on food safety of cheeses has been recently reviewed (Bishop and Smukowski, 2006), which was especially related to the storage and distribution temperature of the product.

It was recommended that cheeses with ~50% moisture, produced under good manufacturing procedures, with traditional levels of salt, starter culture, pH, and fat be allowed to be distributed at a temperature not exceeding 30°C, if the cheeses contain the necessary content of salt in addition to low pH, which are the main hurdles inherent in maintaining the food safety of these cheeses. Low-fat cheeses have a higher moisture content resulting in a lower S/M ratio, at the same absolute salt content, which negatively affecting the safety and shelf-life especially in the distribution and serving of cheeses.

3.1.2. Flavor and Texture

Saltiness is one of the basic tastes perceived by humans, where sodium is the only edible cations with a taste that is primarily salty. Potassium and calcium contribute to saltiness but they have undesired flavors, which are mostly described as 'metallic' or 'bitter'. Therefore, sodium chloride (table salt) is considered to be the saltiest edible sodium compound. Salt enhances the flavor of cheeses and appears to have a greater impact in low-fat products, as salt is component of the expected taste of the cheese (Johnson et al., 2009; Metzger and Kapoor, 2007). Salt also suppresses or masks bitter flavors.

Salt affects cheese flavor directly and indirectly via its influence on the growth of the microorganisms or starter cultures used, hence, the activities of lipolytic and proteolytic enzymes that produce important characteristic flavor compounds of the cheese type manufacture during the ripening period (Guinee and O'Kennedy, 2007; Johnson et al., 2009). Salt has an impact on the rate and extent of lactose fermentation and thus the final pH obtained in the cheese during the maturation period, where proteolysis and/or lipolysis takes place (Thomas and Pearce, 1985). Proteolysis is necessary for proper flavor and body development. Excessive or insufficient fermentation or proteolysis can lead to defects of both flavor and body of cheese. As an example, cheddar cheese has an intermediate salt content of ~1.5%, which allows for the proteolysis of 95% of the α-casein and 50% of the β-casein, whereas at higher salt content pf above 2%, only 70% of the α-casein and 20% of the β-casein were hydrolysed (Thomas and Pearce, 1985). The high salt content of Roquefort cheese (above 3% salt) is the main aid in selecting growth of the desired mold, *Penicillium roquefortii,* rather than allowing for the growth of salt-sensitive defect-causing microorganisms. In the case of the Parmesan cheese, which is a low-moisture and low a_w cheese, its high salt content of ~2% is the cause of having an extended shelf life of several years. In addition, much of the characteristic fruity flavor of this cheese is due to the action of the microbial lipase. The role and specificity of the lipase enzyme causes the characteristic flavor only at low moisture and low a_w rather than at high moisture and high a_w values (Wolf et al., 2010).

Sodium chloride interacts with other major components in foods thereby affecting the texture of foods. Salt causes changes in cheese proteins that influence cheese texture, protein solubility, and probably protein conformation. For example, salt increases hydration of proteins, which affects the moisture content, and enhances the binding of proteins to each other and to fat. These effects of the salt determine the rheological and textural parameters of the cheese product. In process cheese, during the cooking, moderate concentrations of salt increase the solubilization of casein or para-casein of the natural cheeses used. This will aid in the in the hydration of proteins, which is similar to the effect of the emulsifying salts used (Guinee and O'Kennedy, 2007; Johnson et al., 2009). Further details about the roles of the emulsifying salts used in the manufacture of process cheese will be discussed in the following section.

3.2. Role of Emulsifying Salts in Process Cheese

During the manufacturing of process cheese, the so called emulsifying or melting salts, such as sodium phosphates and citrates, are essentially added. Generally, sodium salts are used as they do not lead to the formation of a much of a precipitate, i.e. crystals which are obvious after the post-manufacture cooling. These salts have two main functions under the mixing and heating applied during the manufacture. First, they increase the pH of the mixture, which is generally about 5.2 to above 6. Second, these salts lower the calcium ion activity to below 0.2 mM by disrupting the calcium–phosphate protein network (Gupta et al., 1984; Caric et al., 1985; Berger et al., 1989). Under these conditions, the protein becomes soluble, i.e. hydration of the protein, and it is able to act as an emulsifier to emulsify and incorporate the fat that could have been added in its free form, e.g. anhydrous milk fat or vegetable oil, due to the exposure of the hydrophilic and hydrophobic sections of the proteins respectively (Ennis et al., 1998; Lee et al., 2003). It was reported that heating and stirring of cheese in the absence of emulsifying salts does not allow for the sufficient protein hydration and also causes considerable coalescence of the fat globules. The quantity of the emulsifying salt required is approximately 10% of the quantity of protein used, which corresponds to a level of 2% to 3% in the final cheese product.

Post-manufacture, the type and concentration of the emulsifying salts used affect various functional properties such as texture and melting properties (Templeton and Sommer, 1936; Meyer, 1973; Gupta et al., 1984; Berger et al., 1989; Zehren and Nusbaum, 2000). Cavalier-Salou and Cheftel (1991) reported increased melting of process cheese with increased citrate ES content (from 0.25 to 3.0%), in comparison to cheese containing phosphate ES at similar concentrations, which could be due to the higher pH (pH = ~6.5) of the former cheese that increased the degree of casein dissociation or solubilization. This casein dissociation in the high pH cheese may have helped in increasing the cheese melting (Savello et al., 1989). In contrast, pyrophosphates and polyphosphates give harder cheese, showing a poor flow on melting (Swenson et al., 2000). From sensory analyses on process cheese, it is generally recognized that sodium citrates impart a 'clean' flavor with no defects such as bitter or acid tastes, while phosphates, especially orthophosphates, may impart off-flavors described as soapy, chemical or salty (Meyer, 1973; Gupta et al., 1984; Caric and Kalab, 1987). In addition, monosodium orthophosphates and pyrophosphates, if used alone as ES, may cause an overacid flavor and bitterness, respectively, if added at a level of 2% or greater (Fox et al., 1996; Zehren and Nusbaum, 2000). Phopshate emulsifying salts are also used as anti-microbial agents providing food safety and extended shelf-life of process cheese (Chambre and Daurelles, 2000; Tanaka et al., 1986).

The general anti-bacterial activity is principally due to the interaction of the phosphates with bacterial proteins and sequestration of calcium, which generally serves as an important cellular cation and cofactor for some microbial enzymes (Stanier et al., 1981). In general microbiology studies, phosphates at concentrations of > 1% showed an anti-microbiological activity against the growth of various *Salmonella* species and many Gram-positive bacteria, including *Staphylococcus aureus, Bacillus subtilis* and *Clostridium* species (Tanaka et al., 1979, 1986; Wagner, 1986; Loessner et al., 1997).

4. Strategies of Sodium Reduction

There are mainly two general approaches to control the amount of sodium chloride (NaCl) in natural cheese. One is simply to restrict the addition of NaCl. The other means is to replace NaCl by its potassium salt (KCl).

4.1. Reducing Sodium Chloride Used in Manufacture

Reducing NaCl content of cheese faces various challenges and complications to cheese manufacturers since salt plays many important roles in cheese, as previously outlined. It is an integral component in cheese, used to maintain shelf-life and contributing to flavor and texture of the final product. Nowadays, many consumers are requesting low-sodium cheeses, as the Western diet has already high sodium content (Taormina, 2010). However, it was reported that that a salt reduction of as little as 25% from typical salt content of cheeses, usually from 1.8% to 1.4% salt, is noticed by consumers and may adversely affect the product acceptability.

As an example of reducing NaCl in natural cheeses, the focus will be on cheddar cheese, which was extensively studied in literature in respect to the salt reduction. In cheddar cheese, Schroeder et al. (1988) investigated the effect of the reduction of sodium chloride, during manufacture and maturation, from 1.44% up to 0.07%. Analysis showed that saltiness was the most important attribute affecting the rating of the overall desirability. The high salt cheeses showed the highest desirability due to the high cheddar intensity flavor and the lack of the unpleasant aftertaste. Similarly, Banks et al. (1993) reported that reduced-fat cheddar cheese at low NaCl content of 1.25% produced a bitter cheese with less cheddar flavor than the one with a higher NaCl content of 1.8% salt. However, the higher salt content produced a firmer cheese. Similar observations were reported by Mistry and Kasperson (1998), who noted a higher firmness when the salt content was increased to 2%. In another study by Rutikowska et al. (2008), cheddar cheeses were manufactured with salt levels ranging from 0.5% to 3.0%. The bacteria of the starter culture and the non-starter lactic acid bacteria substantially survived longer in the case of low salt than in the high salt cheeses with a salt level of above 1.80%. The low-salt cheeses of 0.5% salt had the lowest proteolytic activity resulting in a lower rate of flavor formation and a higher undesired bitterness flavor, which might have been related to the high activity of the non-starter bacteria.

4.2. Replacing Sodium Chloride by Potassium Chloride

Potassium chloride (KCl) is the most chemically similar compound to sodium chloride and accordingly is the most obvious choice for NaCl replacements in cheese products.

Potassium chloride is by far the most popular material used to replace sodium chloride in cheeses. From the nutritional viewpoint, the substitution of NaCl by KCl will give an additional benefit since processed foods, in which cheese is used as an ingredient, is already low in potassium which is known to have a significant effect of reducing the blood pressure and, hence, reducing the risk of cardiovascular diseases (Green et al., 2002). Depending on the usefulness and applications of the cheese, the level of substitution is limited by the bitter undesired taste that might be produced by KCl. At levels up to 50% of sodium substitution the bitterness is well masked by the remaining NaCl (Breslin and Beauchamp, 1997). This replacement of the added sodium chloride with potassium chloride might give the perception of saltiness, without undesired flavors, in mild flavored cheeses. However, this approach may not provide a control of the growth and activity of both desired and undesired microorganisms and thus will make it difficult to achieve the desired characteristic flavors of the different cheese types. In addition, as it was shown by Lindsay et al. (1982), most of the panelists under the study preferred high NaCl cheeses over cheeses with partial substitution of KCl with a ratio of 1:1. In another study by Fitzgerald and Buckley (1985) who evaluated the impact of cheddar cheese produced with different salt substitutes at equivalent concentrations of sodium chloride level of 1.5%. The use potassium chloride produced an unacceptable cheese bitter taste and crumbly texture. However, a mixture of 1:1 ratio of sodium chloride and potassium chloride resulted in a cheese comparable to the cheese containing sodium chloride only.

There are several monovalent salts of chloride investigated as a replacement of sodium chloride, including lithium, ammonium, and choline chloride (Fielding and Locke, 1993). The closest salt to NaCl in its taste is the lithium chloride which does not have any bitterness observed. This salt, however, is considered as toxic as even small amounts are causing nausea as an option for salt replacement. Therefore, potassium chloride remains the best option as a replacement for sodium chloride, the typical table salt, if low sodium cheese manufacture is the main aim.

4.3. Process Cheese

Sodium reduction in process cheese involves the modification and/or reduction of one or all the three ingredients, which were previously mentioned as sodium sources, during process cheese formulations and manufacture. Numerous research efforts have been aimed towards the development of low-sodium natural cheese, which is normally used as an ingredient for process cheese manufacture (Karahadian and Lindsay, 1984; Metzger and Kapoor, 2007). In addition to these efforts, attempts have also been directed towards the development of novel formulations in respect to the utilization of potassium-based emulsifying salts (Gupta et al., 1984; Karahadian and Lindsay, 1984; Henson, 1997; Zehren and Nusbaum, 2000; Metzger and Kapoor, 2007), and flavor enhancers (Karahadian and Lindsay, 1984; Metzger and Kapoor, 2007) without causing an adverse effect on the functional properties of the final process cheese product. Recently, in process imitation cheese, it was possible to lower the sodium content by ~ 20% by just changing the emulsifying salts used in the manufacture (El-Bakry et al., 2011b). The manufacture of this type of cheese was also successful at reduced levels of salt (NaCl), which usually represents approximately 65% of the total sodium content, up to 0% NaCl without adversely affecting the functionalities of the cheese (El-

Bakry et al., 2011a). However, the reduction of sodium in process cheese is still facing a lot of difficulties. First of all, there is lack of information regarding clear systematic strategies for low sodium cheese manufacture, as most research studies were performed at different conditions and with various formulations. Accordingly, despite of these research efforts to develop reduced or low sodium process cheese, there are presently no low-sodium process cheeses that are sold in the marketplace throughout most developed countries (GNPD 2008). Second, the area of food safety and maintaining the microbiological stability, which are important aspects that need to be taken into account when trying to reduce the sodium content in the final product, were not completely solved. There are formulation limitations, i.e. the presence of NaCl and sodium phosphate is necessary for a shelf-stable product (Tanaka et al., 1979, 1986), which did not support any changes towards the production of low sodium cheese. There are no food safety-related challenge studies available to quantify the effectiveness of the replacement of the sodium salts by their potassium one in process cheese (Karahadian and Lindsay, 1984, Zehren and Nusbaum, 2000). Third, there are adverse effects of potassium emulsifying salts on the sensory properties of the cheese, when these salts are substituting the traditionally used sodium-based emulsifying salts. In low sodium process cheese, where the potassium equivalent emulsifying salts were used, an unnatural bitter taste, which becomes more pronounced with storage, and an unpleasant aroma were observed (Karahadian and Lindsay 1984; Zehren and Nusbaum, 2000). These adverse organoleptic properties were more pronounced when citrate emulsifying salts, rather than phosphate emulsifying salts, were replaced by their equivalent potassium equivalents.

5. Recent Approaches to Sodium Reduction in Cheese

The most potential sodium reduction strategy is to adapt the preference of consumers for saltiness by reducing sodium in the food products in small steps. However, this is a time-consuming and unfeasible approach that needs to be widely applied to the industry in order to be effective. Therefore, solutions to reduce the sodium in the food stuff are always investigated with the aim of maintaining the same perceived salt taste intensity at lower sodium levels (Doetsch et al., 2009). Currently applied approaches are resulting in sodium reductions between 20–30%. Further reduction will require new technologies and also research into the physiology of salt taste perception and receptors. For instance, Phan et al. (2008) concluded that sodium release during mastication is mainly influenced by the food moisture content, while saltiness perception is limited by the presence of fat. Therefore, a way to reduce salt in cheese without a negative impact on flavor would be to increase the moisture and decrease the fat. Despite these findings, a balance has to be achieved between the composition and structure to produce cheeses that meet the acceptability of the consumers in terms of salty perception, as well as nutritional recommendations. In this section, a brief overview of the approaches used for high sodium reduction, which are still not widely applied in the cheese industry, is presented.

The use of alternatives to sodium chloride has been reviewed in literature, however these alternatives were not applied, to the authors knowledge, in low sodium cheese manufacture. Arginine amino acid has been most often mentioned as contributing to the salty taste. In some studies very large effects are reported, e.g. more than doubling the saltiness of 4.5 g/l NaCl (Breslin, 2004). In addition, combinations of arginine with aspartame amino acids have been shown a higher salty 'sodium chloride' taste (Angus et al., 2005). Sourness is also known to enhance perceived saltiness (Keast and Breslin, 2003; Hellemann, 1992), as it has been reported that specific acids might give an extra salty flavor. Malate and lactate, usually added as potassium salt, was reported to significantly enhance saltiness at low amounts (Angus et al., 2005; Labruni et al., 2003). However, a limitation for replacing salt with “artificial” salt replacers could be the increasing consumer interest in “natural food" (Searby, 2006). Another important disadvantage for using salt replacers is the costs involved in comparison to salt (NaCl), which is one of the cheapest food ingredients available, e.g. a sodium chloride reduction of ~25% increases costs by up to 30%, depending on the product manufactured.

Process cheeses contain much higher levels of Na than natural cheeses owing to the addition of sodium-based emulsifying salts, as previously discussed. In addition, in general, the salt content of process cheese tends to be more than that of many natural cheeses (Meyer, 1973; Zehren and Nusbaum, 2000). Therefore, there might be greater opportunities and more interest to reduce the total sodium content in these cheese products than in natural cheeses. Attempts have been mainly performed to reduce sodium through the lowering of the sodium emulsifying salts used in the manufacture. Recently, the use of casein hydrolysates has been found to reduce the concentrations of sodium emulsifying salts used for the emulsification and formation of a homogeneous stable product (Kwak et al., 2002). However, the use of such hydrolyzates caused an excessive oiling-off when the cheese product was heated. Another approach may involve the use of traditional emulsifiers such as mono- and diglycerides at various levels, where the cheese functionality was not adversely affected (Lucey 2008; Paulus 2008). In a type of process cheese manufactured in Germany called Kochkäse, its manufacture starts with low-fat ripened quarg cheese, which has a pH of about 4.5 (Walstra et al., 2006). This is followed by yeasts growth and the fermentation of lactic acid, raising the pH to about 5.8. Finally, ~1.5% salt, water or milk and butter are mixed for approximately 10 minutes at 90°C. This product has the ability to form a homogeneous mass and melt without the addition of emulsifying salts, due to the low content of calcium present in the quarg cheese used. This process cheese is consumed as a smooth process cheese spreads, which is considered as a light product, i.e. low in fat.

Conclusion

High sodium intake has been related to diseases, particularly cardiovascular diseases. Accordingly, reducing sodium in food products might have potential health benefits. Processed foods, in which cheese is used as an ingredient, contributes to ~75% of the sodium intake in Western diet. Therefore, it is worthwhile from a nutritional and health perspective to review the strategies and recent advances towards the goal of reducing sodium in the cheese products. Current strategies might only allow for a sodium reduction of ~25%. These strategies include mainly a reduction in the salt (sodium chloride) used or replacing it with its potassium salt in some mild taste cheeses up to a maximum of 50% level of substitution. Therefore, it would be beneficial to consider the recent technologies, outlined above, which were shown in few research work done on cheese as well as sensory tests in order to reduce the salt and other sodium ingredients used in the manufacture of cheese products. For instance, the use of amino acids, which might allow for the same taste like sodium chloride, as an alternative was not extensively studied.

References

[1] Angus, F., Phelps, T., Clegg, S., Narein, C., Ridder den, C. and Kilcast, D. (2005). Salt in processed foods. Leatherhead Food International (No. 00193).

[2] Banks, J.M., Hunter, E.A. and Muir D.D. (1993). Sensory properties of low-fat Cheddar cheese: effect of salt content and adjunct culture. Journal of the Society of Dairy Technoogy, 46, 119–123.

[3] Berger, W., Klostermeyer, H., Merkenich, K. and Uhlmann, G. (1989). *Processed Cheese Manufacture, A JOHA Guide*. BK Ladenburg GmbH., Wurzburg, Germany.

[4] Bishop, J.R. and Smukowski. M. (2006). Storage temperatures necessary to maintain cheese safety. *Food Production Trends*, 26, 714–24.

[5] Breslin, P. A. and Beauchamp, G. K. (1997). Salt enhances flavor by suppressing bitterness. *Nature*, 387-563.

[6] Breslin, P. A. (2004). Chemosensory Challenges for Industry. Philadelphia, US: Monell Chemical Senses Center,

[7] Caric, M., Gantar, M. and Kalab, M. (1985). Effect of emulsifying agents on the microstructure and other characteristics of process cheese – a review. *Food Microstructure*, 4, 297–312.

[8] Caric, M. and Kaláb, M. (1987). Processed cheese products. In: P. F. Fox (Ed), *Cheese: chemistry, physics and microbiology. Vol. 2: Major cheese groups*. London: Elsevier Applied Science.

[9] Cavalier-Salou, C. and Cheftel, J.C. (1991). Emulsifying salts influence on characteristics of cheese analogs from calcium caseinate. *Journal of Food Science,* 56, 1542-1547, 1551.

[10] Chambre, M. and Daurelles, J. (2000). Processed cheese. In Eck . A. and Gillis,J. (Eds), *Cheesemaking from Science to Quality Assurance*, 2nd edition. Lavoisier Publishers, Paris (pp. 641-657).

[11] Christian, J.H. (2000). Drying and reduction of water activity. In The Microbiological Safety and Quality of Food, Lung, B.M. et al (eds). Gaithersburg, Maryland, USA: Aspen Publishers Inc.

[12] Cutler, J. A. (1999). The effects of reducing sodium and increasing potassium intake for control of hypertension and improving health. *Clinical Experimental Hypertension*, 21, 769-783.

[13] Doetsch, M., Busch, J., Batenburg, M., Liem, G., Tareilus, E., Mueller, R. and Meijer, G. (2009). Strategies to Reduce Sodium Consumption: A Food Industry Perspective. *Critical Reviews in Food Science and Nutrition*, 49: 10, 841 – 851.

[14] Doyle, M.E. and Glass, K.A. (2010). Sodium Reduction and Its Effect on Food Safety, Food Quality, and Human Health. *Comprehensive Reviews in Food Science and Food Safety*, 9, 44-56.

[15] El-Bakry, M., Beninati, F., Duggan, E., O'Riordan, E.D. and O'Sullivan, M. (2011a). Reducing Salt in Imitation Cheese: Effects on Manufacture and Functional Properties. *Food Research International*, 44, 589-596.

[16] El-Bakry, M., Duggan, E., O'Riordan, E.D. and O'Sullivan, M. (2011b). Effect of Chelating Salt Type on Casein Hydration and Fat Emulsification during Manufacture and Functionality of Imitation Cheese. *Journal of Food Engineering*, 102, 145-153.

[17] Ennis, M.P., O'Sullivan, M.M. and Mulvihill, D.M. (1998). The hydration behaviour of rennet caseins in calcium chelating salt solution as determined using a rheological approach. *Food Hydrocolloids*, 12, 451-457.

[18] Fielding, S. and Locke, K. W. (1993). Choline-containing compositions as salt substitutes and enhancers and a method of preparation. *Interneuron Pharmaceuticals,* 520-604.

[19] Fitzgerald E. and Buckley J. (1985). Effect of total and partial substitution of sodium chloride on the quality of cheddar cheese. *Journal of Dairy Science*, 68, 3127–3134.

[20] Fox, P.F., O'Connor, T.P., McSweeney, P.L.H., Guinee, T.P., and O'Brien, N.M. (1996). Cheese: Physical, biochemical and nutritional aspects. In Taylor, S.L. (Ed), *Advances in Food and Nutrition Research*, 39, 163-328. London, UK: Academic Press.

[21] Guinee, T.P. (2004). Salting and the role of salt in cheese. *International Journal of Dairy Technology,* 57, 2, 99- 109.

[22] Hellemann, U. (1992). Perceived taste of NaCl and acid mixtures in water and bread. *International Journal of Food Science and Technology*, 27, 201–211.

[23] Fox, P.F. and McSweeney, P. (2004). Cheese: An Overview. In Fox, P.F. et al. (Eds.), *Cheese - Chemistry, Physics and Microbiology Vol. 1* (pp. 1-25). Amsterdam, Netherlands: Academic Press.

[24] GNPD. (2008). Global new product database. Chicago, IL: Mintel Group.

[25] Green D.M., Ropper A.H., Kronmal R.A., Psaty B.M., Burke G.L. (2002). Serum potassium level and dietary potassium intake as risk factors for stroke. *Neurology*, 59, 314-320.

[26] Guinee, T.P. and Fox, P.F. (2004). Salt in Cheese: Physical, Chemical and Biological Aspects. In Fox, P.F. et al. (Eds.), *Cheese - Chemistry, Physics and Microbiology Vol. 1* (pp. 207-259). Amsterdam, Netherlands: Academic Press.

[27] Guinee T.P, Carić M. and Kaláb M. (2004). Pasteurized processed cheese and substitute/imitation cheese products. In: Cheese: Chemistry, Physics and Microbiology, Volume 2. Major cheese groups. London, New York: Elsevier Applied Science.

[28] Gupta S.K., Karahdian C. and Lindsay R.C. (1984). Effect of emulsifier salts on textural and flavor properties of processed cheeses. *Journal of Dairy Science*, 67, 764–78.

[29] Holland, B., Unwin, I.D. andBuss, D.H. (1989). Milk products and eggs. In The Fourth Supplement to McCance and Widdowson's The Composition of Foods, 4th edition. Cambridge, UK: Royal Society of Chemistry/Ministry of Agriculture, Fisheries and Food.

[30] Johnson, M.E., Kapoor, R., McMahon, D.J., McCoy, D.R. and Narasimmon, R.G. (2009). Reduction of Sodium and Fat Levels in Natural and Processed Cheeses: Scientific and Technological Aspects. *Comprehensive Reviews in Food Science and Food Safety*, 8, 252-268.

[31] Henson, L.S. (1997). Reduced sodium content process cheese and method for making it. U.S. patent 5871797A1.
[32] Keast, R.S. and Breslin, P.A. (2003). An overview of taste-taste interactions. *Food Quaityl Preference*, 14, 111–124.
[33] Karahadian, C. and Lindsay, R.C. (1984). Flavor and textural properties of reduced sodium process American cheeses. *Journal of Dairy Science, 61,* 1892-1904.
[34] Kwak, H.S., Choi, S.S., Ahn, J. and Lee, S.W. (2002). Casein hydrolysate fractions act as emulsifiers in process cheese. *Journal of Food Science*, 67,821-825.
[35] Labruni, T., Henry, S., Affolter, M. and Schlichterle-Cerny, H. (2003). Seasoning compositions (EP 1344459).
[36] Lee, S.K., Buwalda, R.J., Euston, S.R., Foegeding, E.A. and McKenna, B. (2003). Changes in the rheology and microstructure of processed cheese during cooking. *LWT-Food Sciend and Technology*, 36, 339–345.
[37] Lindsay R.C., Hargett S.M. and Bush C.S. (1982). Effect of sodium/potassium (1:1) chloride and low sodium chloride concentrations on quality of cheddar cheese. Journal of Dairy Science, 65, 360–370.
[38] Loessner, M.J., Maier, S.K., Schiwek, P. and Scherer, S. (1997). Long-chain polyphosphates inhibit growth of *Clostridium tyrobutyricum* in processed cheese spreads. *Journal of Food Protection*, 60, 493-498.
[39] Lucey, J.A. (2008). Advances in nonfat/lowfat process cheese for melting and ingredient use. *Journal of Dairy Science*, 91, E-Suppl. 1, 153-154.
[40] Metzger, L.E. and Kapoor R. (2007). Novel approach for producing with reduced-fat and reduced sodium content. Journal of Dairy Science, 86(Supplement 1), 198.
[41] Meyer, A. (1973). *Processed Cheese Manufacture*. London, UK: Food Trade Press Ltd.
[42] Mistry, V.V. and Kasperson, K.M. (1998). Influence of salt on the quality of reduced fat Cheddar cheese. Journal of Dairy Science 81, 1214–1221.
[43] O'Brien, N.M. and O'Connor, T.P. (2004). Nutritional aspects of cheese. . In Fox, P.F. et al. (Eds.), *Cheese - Chemistry, Physics and Microbiology Vol. 1* (pp. 572-583). Amsterdam, Netherlands: Academic Press.
[44] Paulus, K. (2008). New mozzarella breaks low fat impasse. Wisconsin Center for Dairy Research. *Dairy Pipeline*, 2, 1-6.
[45] Phan VA, Yven C, Lawrence G, Chabanet C, Reparet JM and Salles, C. (2008). In vivo sodium release related to salty perception during eating model cheeses of different textures. *International Dairy Journal*, 18, 956-963.
[46] Rutikowska A, Kilcawley K.N., Doolan I., Alonso-Gomez M., Beresford T.P. and Wilkinson M.G. (2008). Influence of sodium chloride on the quality of cheddar cheese. IDF symposium: 5th IDF symposium on cheese ripening, March 9-13, 2008, Berne, Switzerland.
[47] Savello, P.A., Ernstrom, C.A. and Kalab, M. (1989). Microstructure and meltability of model process cheese made with rennet and acid casein. *Journal of Dairy Science*, 72, 1-11.
[48] Schroeder, C.L., Bodyfeh, E.W., Wyatt, C.J. and McDaniel, M.R. (1988). Reduction of sodium chloride in cheddar cheese: effect on sensory, microbiological, and chemical properties. *Journal of Dairy Science*, 71, 2010-2020.
[49] Searby, L. (2006). Pass the salt. *International Food Ingredients*, 2-3.

[50] Stanier, R.Y., Adelberg, E.A. and Ingraham, J.L. (1981). General Microbiology, 4th edition, The Macmillan Press Ltd, London

[51] Swenson, B.J., Wendorff, W.L. and Lindsay, R.C. (2000). Effects of ingredients on the functionality of fat-free process cheese spreads. *Journal of Food Science*, 65, 822-825.

[52] Taormina, P.J.(2010). Implications of Salt and Sodium Reduction on Microbial Food Safety. *Critical Reviews in Food Science and Nutrition*, 50 (3), 209-227.

[53] Tanaka, N., Goepfert, J.M., Traisman, E. and Hoffbeck, W.M. (1979). A challenge of pasteurized process cheese spread with Clostridium botulinum spores. *Journal of Food Protection*, 42, 787-789.

[54] Tanaka, N., Traisman, E., Plantinga, P., Finn, L., Flom, W., Meske, L. and Guggisberg, J. (1986). Evaluation of factors involved in antibotulinal properties of pasteurized process cheese spread. *Journal of Food Protection,* 49, 526-531.

[55] Templeton, H.L. and Sommer, H.H. (1936). Studies on the emulsifying salts used in processed cheese. Journal of Dairy Science, 19, 561-572.

[56] Thomas, T.D. and Pearce, K.N. (1985). Influence of salt on lactose fermentation and proteolysis in Cheddar cheese. *New Zealand Journal of Dairy Technology*, 16, 253-259.

[57] Wagner, M.K. (1986). Phosphates as antibotulinal agents in cured meats, a review. *Journal of Food Protection*. 49, 482-487.

[58] Walstra, P., Wouters, J. and Geurts, T. (2006). Dairy Science and technology, 2nd edition (pp. 739). New York: Francis and Taylor.

[59] Wolf, I.V, Perotti, M.C., Bernal, S.M. and Zalazar, C.A. (2010). Study of the chemical composition, proteolysis, lipolysis and volatile compounds profile of commercial Reggianito Argentino cheese: Characterization of Reggianito Argentino cheese. *Food Research International*, 43, 1204-1211.

[60] Zehren, V.L. and Nusbaum, D.D. (2000). *Process Cheese*. Madison, Wisconsin, USA: Cheese Reporter Publishing, Co, Inc.

In: Medical and Biological Frontiers Research Compendium
Editor: Tsisana Shartava
ISBN: 978-1-62417-022-5

Chapter 7

Interactions between Angiotensin II and PPAR-γ in Cardiac Myofibroblasts

***Laxmansa C. Katwa*[1*] *and Cooduvalli S. Shashikant*[2]**
[1]Department of Physiology, Brody School of Medicine at East Carolina University, Greenville, North Carolina, US
[2]Department of Dairy and Animal Science, College of Agricultural Sciences, The Pennsylvania State University, University Park, PA, US

Abstract

Alterations in Angiotensin II (Ang II) and Peroxisome Proliferator-Activated Receptor-γ (PPAR-γ) affect cardiovascular diseases, diabetes and metabolic disorders, suggesting that these two systems intersect at some common biochemical pathways. Elucidating common cellular signaling factors between these two systems are important for better design of combinatorial drugs for treating patients with these disorders. Inhibitors of Ang II and agonists of PPAR-γ appear to have similar and beneficial effects. Ang II, a pro-fibrotic factor, enhances collagen synthesis and contributes to adverse remodeling in case of hypertensive heart diseases that damage tissue structure and alter cardiac function. In contrast, increased PPAR-γ activity inhibits collagen synthesis, reduces fibrosis and adverse remodeling of the cardiac tissue. Treatments with Ang II blockers or with PPAR-γ agonists improve cardiac function. These effects are evident in cardiac myofibroblasts, which appear at the site of myocardial infarction. Cardiac myofibroblasts are the major cell types involved in tissue repair and remodeling. In this article, we review Ang II and PPAR-γ pathways operative in cardiac myofibroblasts and provide evidence for interactions between these two systems.

* Address for correspondence: Dr. Laxmansa C. Katwa, PhD, Associate Professor, Department of Physiology, Mail Stop 634. The Brody School of Medicine, East Carolina University, 600 Moye Blvd., Greenville, NC 27834. Email: KatwaL@ecu.edu. Tel: 252-744-1906.

Introduction

Cardiac remodeling generally refers to alterations in the structure and architecture of left ventricular heart under pathological conditions [1]. The process is maladaptive as in the case of hypertension, myocardial infarction (MI) and heart failure, which subsequently leads to death. At cellular level, cardiac remodeling is characterized by hypertrophy of cardiac myocytes and excessive production of extracellular matrix proteins (ECM) by cardiac fibroblasts and myofibroblasts. Historically, the role of cardiac myocytes, the muscular compartment of the heart, has been extensively studied both *in vitro* and in animal models. In contrast, the role of cardiac fibroblasts, major non-muscular compartment of the heart, has been appreciated only in recent years [2-5]. Cardiac fibroblasts account for two thirds of the cells in the heart. Until recently, they were considered quiescent, monotonous and uniform cells, but considerable heterogeneity in fibroblast population is now being recognized. Cardiac fibroblasts secrete cytokines, growth factors and ECM proteins. They are mainly responsible for ECM homeostasis, maintenance of structural integrity and physiological environment in which cardiac myocytes function. They provide a mechanical scaffold for cardiomyocytes and coordinate the pump function of the heart. In pathological conditions, cardiac fibroblasts play an important role in regulating cardiac function. In response to injury, cardiac fibroblasts differentiate into a myofibroblast phenotype. Cardiac myofibroblasts acquire smooth muscle cell markers such as α-smooth muscle actin and become contractile [6-8]. They act as both paracrine and autocrine cells, producing growth factors, cytokines, pro-inflammatory and pro-remodeling factors. Cardiac myofibroblasts are proliferative, invasive and possess contractile and motile properties, allowing them to migrate to the site of injury and repair tissue damage. Under normal circumstances, cardiac myofibroblasts undergo apoptosis and disappear from the normal functioning heart. However, under pathological conditions due to continued stress on the heart, they fail to undergo apoptosis, producing excessive collagens and other ECM proteins [3, 5]. Thus, remodeling becomes excessive, maladaptive and causes considerable alterations in the structure and physiology of heart. These changes profoundly influence the function of cardiac myocytes, leading to heart failure and death. Consistent with the central role cardiac fibroblasts play in cardiac remodeling, several classes of drugs, which exert profound effects on cardiac fibroblasts are currently prescribed for treatment of cardiovascular diseases [3]. These include drugs that target Angiotensin II (Ang II) and peroxisome proliferator-activated receptor-γ (PPAR-γ), among others. Our understanding of various biochemical pathways affected by these drug targets largely comes from studies carried out with *in vitro* cultured cardiac fibroblasts and myofibroblasts. In this article, we will summarize recent findings on cross-regulatory interactions between Ang II and PPAR-γ pathways in cardiac fibroblasts and myofibroblasts.

Angiotensin-II (Ang II)

Ang II is the main mediator of the renin-angiotensin-aldosterone system (RAAS) [9, 10]. Ang II is first produced as biologically inactive Angiotensinogen (Ao), which is converted to Ang I by the action of aspertyl or serine proteases. Angiotensin converting enzyme (ACE), a membrane bound ectoenzyme, cleaves Ang I to biologically active Ang II peptide ([11-13]. A second enzyme, ACE2, further cleaves Ang II to a heptapeptide referred to as Ang-(1-7). Ang-(1-7) may antagonize effects of Ang II on cardiac remodeling and thus play a regulatory role. The effect of Ang II and Ang-(1-7) peptides are mediated through specific G-protein coupled receptors (GPCR). Ang II acts through Angiotensin II type 1 (AT1) and type 2 (AT2) receptors; whereas, Ang-(1-7) acts through another GPCR receptor, referred to as Mas, but its biological effects are unclear [14, 15]. Although Ang II, Ang-(1-7) and their receptors have been detected in fibroblasts at the site of fibrosis, most of the effects of RAAS system are mediated by Ang II through the AT1 receptor mediated signaling pathways.

Local RAAS systems are integral to the orderly and sequential nature of the repair process occurring in response to tissue injury [16]. Several lines of evidence suggest a central role for Ang II in the initiation and progression of cardiac remodeling [10, 17]. *De novo* production of Ang II significantly influences the post-infarction remodeling of the heart [9]. Drugs that inhibit RAAS activation have beneficial effects on the remodeling heart [18-19]. Clinical studies have shown that ACE inhibitors and angiotensin II type 1 receptor blockers (ARB's) reduce mortality and morbidity in patients with post-MI dysfunction and heart failure [6-8, 18, 20]. Ang II appears to have multiple, direct cytotoxic effects on myocytes including apoptosis, promoting cell hypertrophy and stimulating myocardial fibrosis [21].

Many of the effects of Ang II on cardiac remodeling are mediated through cardiac fibroblasts and myofibroblasts. Although activated macrophages and endothelial cells also produce Ang II and contribute to the initial process of remodeling, cardiac fibroblasts remain a major target cell type for Ang II mediated biological actions associated with cardiac remodeling [10, 17]. Consistent with this view, the distribution of AT1 receptors is predominant among cardiac fibroblasts compared to other cell types, including cardiomyocytes. The levels of cardiac fibroblast Ang II and AT1 receptors are elevated in post-MI hearts. Myofibroblasts remain the major cells expressing ACE and AT1 receptors in the fibrogenic stage of cardiac repair following MI [22, 23]. Both Ang II and AT1 receptor are expressed in cardiac myofibroblasts isolated from the site of MI [24, 25]. Myofibroblasts associated with the healing of infarct scars show increased production of Ang II and AT1 receptor [24, 26-29]. The levels of ACE are also elevated at the site of MI, co-localized with the myofibroblast population [11, 23, 30, 31].

Ang II influences multiple biochemical pathways in cardiac fibroblasts and myofibroblasts during remodeling (Figure 1). Ang II induces proliferation of myofibroblasts, which in turn participate in collagen synthesis [25, 32-35]. In a rat model of MI, Ang II induced hypertrophy of myofibroblasts at the infarct site. In sham operated control and non-infarct myofibroblasts, mitogenic activity of Ang II treatment was also detected [36]. There are several discrepancies in regards to the proliferative effects of Ang II, but a general consensus is that perhaps some of these effects are secondary due to the induced secretion of other growth factors, including TGF-β1, FGF2 and platelet derived growth factor-AA [10, 37-38].

Ang II induces differentiation of both neonatal and adult cardiac fibroblasts into myofibroblasts by activating TGF-β1 [28, 39-41]. Treatment of cardiac myofibroblasts *in vitro* with Ang II results in rapid accumulation of TGF-β1 mRNA and protein [28, 42-45]. Chronic administration of Ang II induces cardiac expression of TGF-β1 *in vivo* [46-48]. In contrast, blockade of AT1 receptor by antagonists reverses cardiac TGF-β1 expression, cardiac hypertrophy and fibrosis [48-51]. Ang II fails to induce cardiac hypertrophy and fibrosis in mice lacking in functional TGF-β1 [52]. Most of the effects of Ang II on cardiac function are likely mediated through TGF-β1 signaling [41]. Treatment of cardiac fibroblasts with anti-TGF-β1 antibodies reduces Ang II induced collagen I levels [52]. The mechanism by which Ang II induces TGF-β1 expression in cardiac myofibroblasts is not completely understood. However, studies in cardiomyocytes of hypertrophied left ventricle indicate that Ang II regulates TGF-β1 expression at the level of transcription through nuclear activating protein 1(AP1) binding activity [48]. Ang II mediates its effect through AT1 receptor, which in turn activates NAD(P)H oxidase, protein kinase C (PKC), p38 MAP kinase and finally AP1 protein [41, 53].

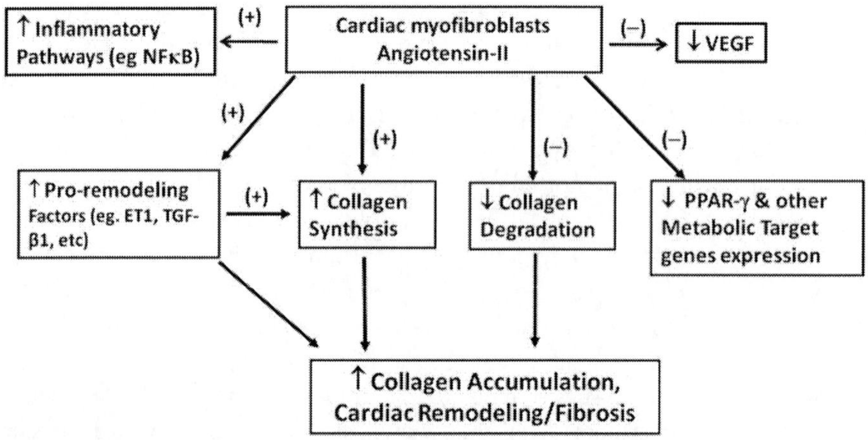

Figure 1. Effect of Ang II on various pathways operative in cardiac myofibroblasts.

Besides inducing TGF-β1, Ang II also induces secretion of other bioactive molecules such as endothelin-1, ET-1 [15, 40, 54, 55], leukemia inhibitory factor, LIF [15], osteopontin [56] vascular endothelial growth factor, VEGF [57], natriuretic peptides [53, 57, 58], and interleukin-6 [60].

Ang II promotes differentiation and proliferation of cardiac fibroblasts. It accelerates pro-fibrotic responses as indicated by increased production of ECM proteins. Ang II treatment increases synthesis of collagens I and II, fibronectin and integrin [15, 36, 42, 61-66]. Ang II is also known to increase the synthesis of tissue inhibitor of metalloproteinase (TIMP) and reduce metalloproteinase (MMP) synthesis thereby inhibiting degradation of ECM proteins (65, 66, 67-69]. Many of these effects are probably indirect and mediated by induction of other pro-remodeling factors, such as ET1 and TFG-β1.

Ang II, also a potent pro-inflammatory agent, influences all stages of the inflammatory response. Through interaction with its AT1 receptor, Ang II activates NADPH oxidase and production of reactive oxygen species. This leads to activation of Ets-1, early growth response 1 and nuclear factor-κB(NF-κB). Some of the inflammatory responses by Ang II are mediated by the caspase-recruitment domain-9 (CARD-9) protein [70]. Ang II also induces known mediators of inflammatory responses such as interferon-γ, INF-γ, and tumor necrosis factor-α, TNF-α [71].

In summary, cardiac myofibroblasts elaborate Ang II mediated multiple signaling pathways at the site of MI. These Ang II induced pathways result in pro-inflammatory and pro-fibrotic effects leading to increased synthesis and accumulation of collagen, a hallmark of fibrosis in MI and resulting heart failure.

PPAR-γ

In recent years, emerging evidence from different experimental systems suggest interactions between a xenobiotic activated transcription factor, peroxisome proliferators-activated receptor, PPAR-γ and various molecules that contribute to the remodeling process. Developing tools and reagents to manipulate PPAR-γ activity may represent a new paradigm in our understanding of cardiac remodeling. PPARs are implicated in the regulation of pathways that interface between intermediate metabolism and inflammation [72]. PPAR-γ plays a critical role in adipocyte differentiation, cellular energy homeostasis, insulin signaling, obesity and inflammation [72-75]. PPAR-γ agonists, such as thiazolidinediones (TZDs) that sensitize cells to insulin are used for their antidiabetic effects in liver, adipose tissue and skeletal muscle [73]. Diabetic patients treated with PPAR-γ agonists also show lower risks for CVD, demonstrating a potential beneficial role for PPAR-γ in modulating cardiac function. Consistent with this hypothesis, treatment with PPAR-γ agonists results in reduced infarct size [76-77], decreased inflammation [74,75], improved vasodialation [76] and decreased left ventricular hypertrophy [78,79]. Thus, PPAR-γ agonists are likely to promote several cellular responses relevant to tissue repair and remodeling.

PPAR-γ agonists could modulate several aspects of cardiac remodeling by affecting the activities of key players, especially in cardiac myofibroblasts (Figure 2). PPAR-γ agonist's show marked influences on collagen synthesis at several levels.

When cultured myofibroblasts are treated with rosiglitazone, a decrease in collagen expression is observed [80]. The molecular mechanism, by which collagen synthesis in cardiac myofibroblasts is reduced, is yet to be elucidated. The effect of PPAR-γ on collagen synthesis could be mediated by decreasing the activities of pro-fibrotic factors including Ang II, ET1, and TGF-β1.

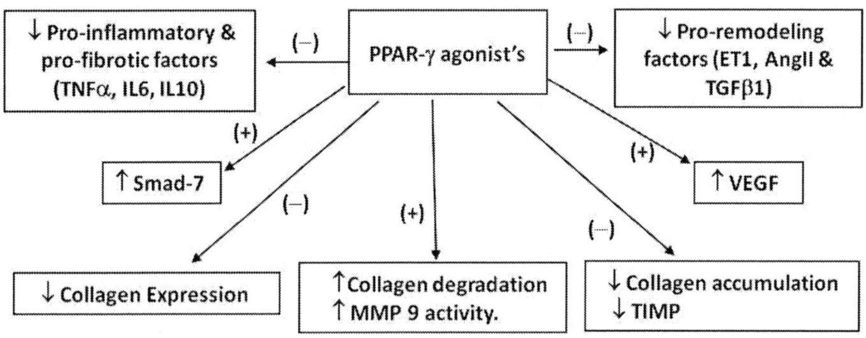

Figure 2. Effect of PPAR-γ agonists on cardiac collagen turn over, pro-angiogenic and pro-fibrotic factors.

When cultured cardiac fibroblasts and myofibroblasts are treated with PPAR-γ agonists such as rosiglitazone or pioglitazone, there is a decrease in both AT1 receptor and the type I collagen expression [80, 81-83]. Rosiglitazone has been shown to significantly attenuate Ang II induced proliferation of cardiac fibroblasts [83]. The mechanism by which PPAR-γ agonists decrease AT1 receptor mediated collagen synthesis is unknown. Ang II and AT1 receptor induce oxidative stress in mouse cardiac fibroblasts. The inhibitory effect of pioglitazone on collagen synthesis is perhaps due to its anti-oxidant effect [82]. In vascular smooth muscle cells, PPAR-γ has been shown to suppress AT1 receptor gene transcription by the inhibition of the Sp1 binding to GC-box related element in the AT1 receptor cis-regulatory/promoter region [84]. Whether a similar mechanism is operative in cardiac myofibroblasts remains to be determined.

Rosiglitazone reduces ET1 expression and collagen synthesis in cultured cardiac myofibroblasts derived from the site of MI (Katwa unpublished observations). The mechanism by which PPAR-γ inhibits ET1 activity in cardiac myofibroblasts remains to be studied. However, in cardiac myocytes, both PPAR-γ overexpression and treatment with rosiglitazone have been shown to inhibit ET1 induced cardiac hypertrophy [85]. Interaction between PPAR-γ and calcineurin/ nuclear factor of activated T cells (NFAT) has been implicated in the inhibition of ET1 activity. PPAR-γ has also been suggested to mediate conjugated linoleic acid mediated inhibition of ET1 activity in reducing cardiac hypertrophy [86]. Treatment of cardiac myofibroblasts with rosiglitazone also results in a decrease in TGF-β1 levels (Katwa, unpublished observations). The effect of rosiglitazone on TGF-β1, however, may not be direct but mediated through its effect on Ang II [6, 80, 83]. The effect of TGF-β1 on collagen synthesis is mediated through the canonical Smad pathway [87]. Smads interact with transcriptional coactivator and histone acetyltransferase, p300, in the regulation of transcriptional activity of collagen promoter [88, 89]. PPAR-γ abrogates Smad-dependent pathways linked to stimulation of collagen synthesis by preventing p300 recruitment and histone H4 hyperacetylation in dermal fibroblasts [88]. In hepatic stellate cells, PPAR-γ inhibits p300 facilitated NF-1 binding to response elements present in the collagen promoter [90]. Although p300 is known to play a role in inflammation as well as cardiac hypertrophy, its role in the regulation of collagen synthesis in cardiac myofibroblasts is yet to be described.

PPAR-γ is known to antagonize TGF-β1stimulated type 1 collagen synthesis in other fibroblast systems by antagonizing the effects of interferon-γ (IFN-γ). PPAR-γ could also increase activities of matrix metalloproteinases, which promote collagen degradation. PPAR-γ agonists appear to cause a decrease in the levels of MMPs in various experimental systems [81, 92, 93]. A similar decrease in the levels of MMPs and TIMPs was observed in cardiac myofibroblasts isolated from site of MI treated with rosiglitazone (Katwa, unpublished observation).

Interactions or Crosstalk between Ang II and PPAR Systems

Both Ang II and PPAR systems are implicated in metabolic syndrome and heart diseases, where they seem to have opposing effects. Increased frequency of left ventricular dysfunction and structural abnormalities are often observed in patients with metabolic syndrome [94-96]. In contrast, animal models of metabolic syndrome often show cardiac fibrosis [94, 97, 98]. Clinical strategies for treating both metabolic syndromes and cardiac failures often employ ACE inhibitors, ARB and PPAR agonists. Although molecular mechanisms that link fibrosis and metabolic syndrome are yet to be elucidated, several studies suggest a link between Ang

II and PPAR systems [70, 80, 94, 99, 100]. Ang II and PPAR-γ mediated pathways intersect and modulate each other's activities in regulating cardiac collagen expression (Figure 3).

In cardiac myofibroblasts, treatment with Ang II leads to decrease in PPAR-γ expression and activity, whereas treatment with ARB (losartan) leads to increase in PPAR-γ expression and activity (Figure 4). In contrast, treatment with PPAR-γ agonist's leads to a decrease in AT1 receptor expression and activities in cardiac myofibroblasts isolated from the site of MI [80].

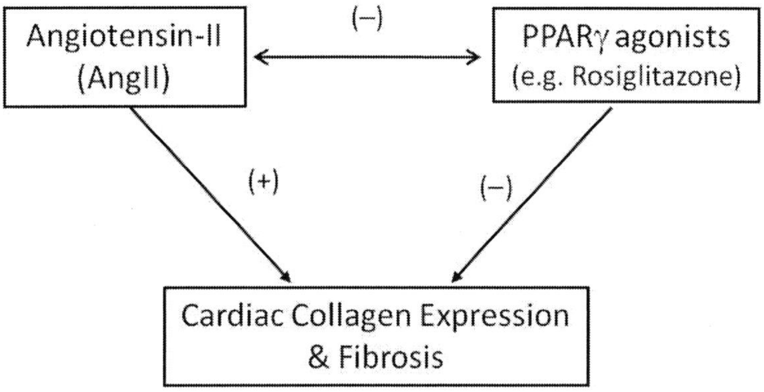

Figure 3. Cross talk between Ang II and PPAR-γ in post-MI cardiac collagen expression and fibrosis.

By mechanisms yet to be elucidated, these interactions affect collagen expression in cardiac myofibroblasts either directly or indirectly. Pro-inflammatory and pro-fibrotic factors could mediate some of the effects of Ang II and PPAR systems. Ang II decreases PPAR-γ expression with a concomitant increase in the expression of pro-inflammatory and pro-fibrotic agents in diabetics with MI and cardiac myofibroblasts [5, 6, 101, 102]. In contrast, PPAR-γ agonists appear to decrease expression of pro-inflammatory and pro-fibrotic agents, including Ang II in cardiac myofibroblasts, and in diabetic heart tissue with MI [80,103, Katwa et al., unpublished data]

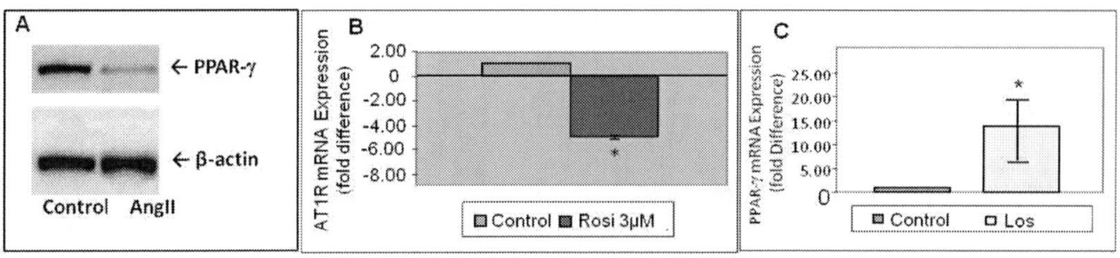

(*p> 0.05).

Figure 4. Cross talk between Ang II and PPAR-γ in cardiac myofibroblasts. Myofibroblasts (passage 4, 90% confluent) were treated in serum free DMEM medium with; (A) Ang II (10^{-7}M) for 24 hours and isolated protein (30μg/well) was analyzed by western blot resulted in the down regulation of PPAR-γ expression. Panel B &C are real-time PCR data of myofibroblasts treated with PPAR-γ agonist Rosiglitazone (3 μM). (B) demonstrates down regulation of AT1 receptor expression by PPAR-γ agonists and (C) results show effects of ARB (Los=Losartan) on myofibroblasts PPAR-γ expression .

Combination of drugs such as PPAR-γ agonists and ARBs have shown beneficial effects in diabetes and CVD by decreasing infarct size and increasing metabolic activities of the cardiac tissue [104, 101,102]. Cardiac myofibroblasts treated with both PPAR-γ agonists and ARBs demonstrated significant decrease in not only collagen expression but also decreased levels of pro-inflammatory and pro-fibrotic agents. Our recent experimental findings on the effects of combination treatment with ARB (e.g. Lasortan) and PPAR-γ agonists (e.g. Rosiglitazone or Pioglitazone) demonstrated an increased PPAR-γ expression and decreased AT1 receptor expression and activity, as well as a significant reduction in collagen expression in cultured rat cardiac myofibroblasts isolated from the site of MI [80].

PPAR-γ agonists have recently been used to treat patients with diabetes and MI. These studies have revealed increased cardiovascular risks and mortality [95, 97, 98, 105]. The clinical relevance of combination therapy of ARBs and PPAR-γ agonists has yet to be determined. Since last decade, the experimental evidence from animal and clinical studies suggest that some of the drugs that interrupt the Ang II system may improve glucose and lipid metabolism and decrease the risk for type 2 diabetes [101,102, 104, 106, 107]. Some of the anti-diabetic properties of ARBs may be mediated by their ability to block adverse effects of Ang II on carbohydrate and lipid metabolism. The beneficial metabolic effects of certain ARBs may go well beyond just simple interruption of the Ang II action, as ARBs have been found to effectively activate PPAR-γ, a well-known target for insulin-sensitizing, antidiabetic drugs [102, 104]. Thus, the identification of ARBs selective PPAR-γ modulating ability suggests new opportunities for developing third-generation ARBs and PPAR-γ activators with enhanced potential for treating hypertension, diabetes and the metabolic syndrome.

Acknowledgments

The authors wish to thank Paul Ferrell and Pranita Katwa for reading the manuscript. This work was supported in part by the National Institutes of Health grant (HL-60047) and East Carolina University Faculty Research Development grant awarded to LCK. CSS is supported by The Pennsylvania State University Experiment Station grant AES 4377.

References

[1] Swynghedauw B. (1999). Molecular mechanisms of myocardial remodeling. *Physiol. Rev.* 79, 215-262.

[2] Brown, R.D., Ambler, S.K., Mitchell, M.D., and Long, C.S. (2005). The cardiac fibroblast: therapeutic target in myocardial remodeling and failure. *Annu. Rev. Pharmacol. Toxicol.*, 45, 657-687.

[3] Porter, K.E., and Turner, N.A. (2009). Cardiac fibroblasts: at the heart of myocardial remodeling. *Pharmacol. Ther.*, 123, 255-278.

[4] Baum, J., and Duffy, H.S. (2011). Fibroblasts and myofibroblasts: what are we talking about? *J. Cardiovasc. Pharmacol.* 57, 376-379.

[5] Katwa, L.C., and Shashikant, C.S. (2011). Cardiac remodeling and fibrosis: Role of myofibroblasts. In: N.A. Turner (ed), The Cardiac Fibroblasts, 29-52, *Research Signpost*. ISBN: 978-81-308-0435-4.

[6] Campbell, S.E., and Katwa L.C. (1997). Angiotensin II stimulated expression of transforming growth factor-beta1 in cardiac fibroblasts and myofibroblasts. *J. Mol. Cell. Cardiol.*, 29, 1947-1958.

[7] Chintalgattu, V., Harris, G.S., Akula, S.M., and Katwa, L.C. (2007). PPAR-gamma agonists induce the expression of VEGF and its receptors in cultured cardiac myofibroblasts. *Cardiovasc. Res.*, 74, 140-150.

[8] Petrov, V.V., Fagard, R.H., and Lijnen, P.J. (2002). Stimulation of collagen production by transforming growth factor-beta1 during differentiation of cardiac fibroblasts to myofibroblasts. *Hypertension*, 39, 258-263.

[9] Weber, K.T., Sun, Y., and Katwa, L.C. (1997). Myofibroblasts and local angiotensin II in rat cardiac tissue repair. *Int. J. Biochem. Cell Biol.*, 29, 31-42.

[10] Cowling, R.T. and Greenberg, B. (2011). Angiotensin receptors and response to angiotensin peptides in cardiac fibroblasts. In: N.A. Turner (ed), The Cardiac Fibroblasts,173-195, *Research Signpost*. ISBN: 978-81-308-0435-4.

[11] Katwa, L.C., Ratajska, A., Cleutjens, J.P., Sun, Y., Zhou, G., Lee, S.J., Weber, K.T. (1995). Angiotensin converting enzyme and kininase-II-like activities in cultured valvular interstitial cells of the rat heart. *Cardiovasc. Res.*, 29, 57-64.

[12] Katwa, L.C., Tyagi, S.C., Campbell, S.E., Lee, S.J., Cicila, G.T., Weber, K.T. (1996). Valvular interstitial cells express angiotensinogen and cathepsin D, and generate angiotensin peptides. *Int. J. Biochem. Cell Biol.*, 28, 807-821.

[13] Katwa, L.C., Sun, Y., Campbell, S.E., Tyagi, S.C., Dhalla, A.K., Kandala, J.C., Weber, K.T. (1998). Pouch tissue and angiotensin peptide generation. *J. Mol. Cell. Cardiol.*, 30, 1401-1413.

[14] Santos, R.A.S., Silva, A.C.S.E., Maric, C., Silva, D.M.R., Machado, R.P., de Buhr, I., Heringer-Walther, S., Pinheiro, S.V.B., Lopes, M.T., Bader, M., Randy T. Cowling and Barry Greenberg Mendes, E.P., Lemos, V.S., Campagnole-Santos, M.J., Schultheiss, H.P., Speth, R., and Walther, T. (2003). Angiotensin-(1-7) is an endogenous ligand for the G protein-coupled receptor Mas. *Proc. Natl. Acad. Sci. USA.*, 100, 8258-8263.

[15] Iwata, M., Cowling, R.T., Gurantz, D., Moore, C., Zhang, S., Yuan, J.X., and Greenberg, B.H. (2005). Angiotensin-(1-7) binds to specific receptors on cardiac fibroblasts to initiate antifibrotic and antitrophic effects. *Am. J. Physiol Heart Circ. Physiol,* 289, H2356-H2363.

[16] Lijnen, P.J., Petrov, V.V. (2003). Role of intracardiac renin-angiotensin-aldosterone system in extracellular matrix remodeling. *Methods Find Exp. Clin. Pharmacol.*, 25, 541–64.

[17] Sun, Y., (2010). Intracardiac renin-angiotensin system and myocardial repair/remodeling following infarction. *J. Mol. Cell Cardiol.*, 48, 483–489.

[18] Pfeffer, M.A., Lamas, G.A., Vaughan, D.E., Parisi, A.F., and Braunwald, E. (1988). Effect of captopril on progressive ventricular dilatation after anterior myocardial infarction. *N. Engl. J. Med.*, 319, 80-86.

[19] Greenberg, B., Quinones, M.A., Koilpillai, C., Limacher, M., Shindler, D., Benedict, C., and Shelton, B. (1995). Effects of long-term enalapril therapy on cardiac structure

and function in patients with left ventricular dysfunction. Results of the SOLVD echocardiography substudy. *Circulation*, 91, 2573-2581.

[20] Gabbiani, G., Hirschel, B.J., Ryan, G.B., Statkov, P.R., and Majno, G. (1972). Granulation tissue as a contractile organ. A study of structure and function. *J. Exp. Med.* 135, 719-734.

[21] Gajarsa, J.J., Kloner, R.A. (2011). Left ventricular remodeling in the post-infarction heart: a review of cellular, molecular mechanisms, and therapeutic modalities. *Heart Fail Rev.*, 16, 13-21.

[22] Sun, Y., and Weber, K.T. (1996). Angiotensin converting enzyme and myofibroblasts during tissue repair in the rat heart. *J. Mol. Cell. Cardiol.*, 28, 851-858.

[23] Sun, Y., Weber, K.T. (1996). Cells expressing angiotensin II receptors in fibrous tissue of rat heart. *Cardiovasc Res*, 31, 518–525.

[24] Katwa, L.C., Campbell, S.E., Tyagi, S.C., Lee, S.J., Cicila, G.T., Weber, K.T. (1997). Cultured myofibroblasts generate angiotensin peptides de novo. *J. Mol. Cell. Cardiol.*, 29, 1375-1386.

[25] Chintalgattu, V., and Katwa, L.C. (2009). Role of protein kinase C-delta in angiotensin II induced cardiac fibrosis. *Biochem. Biophys. Res. Commun.*, 386, 612-616.

[26] Sun Y, and Weber K.T. (1994). Angiotensin II receptor binding following myocardial infarction in the rat. *Cardiovasc. Res.*, 28, 1623-1628.

[27] Weber, K.T., Sun, Y., Katwa, L.C., Cleutjens, J.P. (1995). Connective tissue: a metabolic entity? *J. Mol. Cell. Cardiol.*, 27,107-120.

[28] Campbell, S.E., and Katwa L.C. (1997). Angiotensin II stimulated expression of transforming growth factor-beta1 in cardiac fibroblasts and myofibroblasts. *J. Mol. Cell. Cardiol.*, 29, 1947-1958.

[29] Sun, Y., and Weber K.T. (2000). Infarct scar: a dynamic tissue. *Cardiovasc. Res.*, 46, 250-256.

[30] Fabris, B., Jackson, B., Kohzuki, M., Perich, R., and Johnston, C.I. (1990). Increased cardiac angiotensin-converting enzyme in rats with chronic heart failure. *Clin. Exp. Pharmacol. Physiol.,* 17, 309-314.

[31] Sun Y, Cleutjens J.P., Diaz-Arias, A.A., and Weber, K.T. (1994). Cardiac angiotensin converting enzyme and myocardial fibrosis in the rat. *Cardiovasc. Res.*, 28, 1423-1432.

[32] Schorb, W., Booz, G.W., Dostal, D.E., Conrad, K.M., Chang, K.C., and Baker, K.M. (1993). Angiotensin II is mitogenic in neonatal rat cardiac fibroblasts. *Circ. Res.,* 72, 1245-1254.

[33] Weber, K.T., Brilla, C.G., Campbell, S.E., Guarda, E., Zhou, G., and Sriram, K. (1993). Myocardial fibrosis: role of angiotensin II and aldosterone. *Basic Res. Cardiol.*, 88 Suppl 1:107-124.

[34] Kim, S., Ohta, K., Hamaguchi, A., Yukimura, T., Miura, K., Iwao, H. (1995). Angiotensin II induces cardiac phenotypic modulation and remodeling in vivo in rats. *Hypertension*, 25, 1252-1259.

[35] Bouzegrhane, F., and Thibault, G. (2002). Is angiotensin II a proliferative factor of cardiac fibroblasts? *Cardiovasc. Res.*, 53, 304-312.

[36] Staufenberger. S., Jacobs, M., Brandstätter, K., Hafner, M., Regitz-Zagrosek, V., Ertl, G., and Schorb, W. (2001). Angiotensin II type 1 receptor regulation and differential trophic effects on rat cardiac myofibroblasts after acute myocardial infarction. *J. Cell. Physiol.,* 187, 326-335.

[37] Simm, A. and Diez, C. (1999). Density dependent expression of PDGF-A modulates the angiotensin II dependent proliferation of rat cardiac fibroblasts. *Basic Res. Cardiol.*, 94, 464-471.

[38] Santiago, J.J., Ma, X., McNaughton, L.J., Nickel, B.E., Bestvater, B.P., Yu, L., Fandrich, R.R., Netticadan, T., Kardami, E. (2011). Preferential accumulation and export of high molecular weight FGF-2 by rat cardiac non-myocytes. *Cardiovasc Res.,* 89, 139-147.

[39] Lee, A.A., Dillmann, W.H., McCulloch, A.D., and Villarreal, F.J. (1995). Angiotensin II stimulates the autocrine production of transforming growth factor-beta 1 in adult rat cardiac fibroblasts. J. Mol.Cell Cardiol., 27, 2347-2357.

[40] Gray, M.O., Long, C.S., Kalinyak, J.E., Li, H.T., and Karliner, J.S. (1998). Angiotensin II stimulates cardiac myocyte hypertrophy via paracrine release of TGF-beta 1 and endothelin-1 from fibroblasts. *Cardiovasc. Res.*, 40, 352-363.

[41] Rosenkranz, S. (2004). TGF-beta1 and angiotensin networking in cardiac remodeling. *Cardiovasc. Res.*, 63, 423-432.

[42] Thibault, G., Lacombe, M.J., Schnapp, L.M., Lacasse, A., Bouzeghrane, F., and Lapalme, G. (2001). Upregulation of alpha(8)beta(1)-integrin in cardiac fibroblast by angiotensin II and transforming growth factor-beta1. *Am. J. Physiol. Cell Physiol.*, 281, C1457-C1467.

[43] Klett, C.P., Palmer, A., Dirig, D.M., Gallagher, A.M., Riosecco-Camacho, N., and Printz, M.P. (1995). Evidence for differences in cultured left ventricular fibroblast populations isolated from spontaneously hypertensive and Wistar-Kyoto rats. *J. Hypertens.*, 13, 1421-1431.

[44] Samuel, C.S., Unemori, E.N., Mookerjee, I., Bathgate, R.A., Layfield, S.L., Mak, J., Tregear, G.W., and Du, X.J. (2004). Relaxin modulates cardiac fibroblast proliferation, differentiation, and collagen production and reverses cardiac fibrosis in vivo. *Endocrinology,* 145, 4125-4133.

[45] Olson, E.R., Naugle, J.E., Zhang, X., Bomser, J.A., and Meszaros, J.G. (2005). Inhibition of cardiac fibroblast proliferation and myofibroblast differentiation by resveratrol. *Am. J. Physiol. Heart Circ. Physiol.*, 288, H1131-H1138.

[46] Crawford, D., Chobanian, A., and Brecher, P. (1994). Angiotensin II induces fibronectin expression associated with cardiac fibrosis in the rat. *Circ. Res.*, 74, 727-739.

[47] Kim, S., Ohta, K., Hamaguchi, A., Omura, T., Yukimura, T., Miura, K., Inada, Y., Ishimura, Y., Chatani, F., and Iwao, H. (1995). Angiotensin II type I receptor antagonist inhibits the gene expression of transforming growth factor-beta 1 and extracellular matrix in cardiac and vascular tissues of hypertensive rats. *J. Pharmacol. Exp. Ther.,* 273, 509-515.

[48] Wenzel, S., Taimor, G., Piper, H.M., and Schlu,¨ter, K.D. (2001). Redox-sensitive intermediates mediate angiotensin II-induced p38 MAP kinase activation, AP-1 binding activity, and TGF-beta expression in adult ventricular cardiomyocytes. *FASEB. J.,* 15, 2291-2293.

[49] Tomita, H., Egashira, K., Ohara, Y., Takemoto, M., Koyanagi, M., Katoh, M., Yamamoto, H., Tamaki, K., Shimokawa, H., and Takeshita, A. (1998). Early induction of transforming growth factor-beta via angiotensin II type 1 receptors contributes to

cardiac fibrosis induced by long-term blockade of nitric oxide synthesis in rats. *Hypertension*, 32, 273-279.

[50] Tokuda, K., Kai, H., Kuwahara, F., Yasukawa, H., Tahara, N., Kudo, H., Takemiya, K., Koga, M., Yamamoto, T., and Imaizumi T. (2004). Pressure-independent effects of angiotensin II on hypertensive myocardial fibrosis. *Hypertension,* 43, 499-503.

[51] Tsutsui, H., Matsushima, S., Kinugawa, S., Ide, T., Inoue, N., Ohta, Y., Yokota, T., Hamaguchi, S., and Sunagawa, K. (2007). Angiotensin II type 1 receptor blocker attenuates myocardial remodeling and preserves diastolic function in diabetic heart. *Hyperten. Res.* 30, 439-449.

[52] Schultz, J.J., Witt, S.A., Glascock, B.J., Nieman, M.L., Reiser, P.J., Nix, S.L., Kimball, T.R., and Doetschman, T. (2002). TGF-beta1 mediates the hypertrophic cardiomyocyte growth induced by angiotensin II. *J. Clin. Invest.*, 109, 787-796.

[53] Wang, S., Wang, X., Yan, J., Xie, X., Fan, F., Zhou, X., Han, L., and Chen, J. (2007). Resveratrol inhibits proliferation of cultured rat cardiac fibroblasts: correlated with NO-cGMP signaling pathway. *Eur. J Pharmacol.*, 567, 26-35.

[54] Fujisaki, H., Ito, H., Hirata, Y., Tanaka, M., Hata, M., Lin, M., Adachi, S., Akimoto, H., Marumo, F., and Hiroe, M. (1995). Natriuretic peptides inhibit angiotensin II-induced proliferation of rat cardiac fibroblasts by blocking endothelin-1 gene expression. *J. Clin. Invest.*, 96, 1059-1065.

[55] Chao, H.H., Chen, J.J., Chen, C.H., Lin, H., Cheng, C.F., Lian, W.S., Chen, Y.L., Juan, S.H., Liu, J.C., Liou, J.Y., Chan, P., and Cheng, T.H. (2005). Inhibition of angiotensin II induced endothelin-1 gene expression by 17-beta-oestradiol in rat cardiac fibroblasts. *Heart*, 91, 664-669.

[56] Ashizawa, N., Graf, K., Do, Y.S., Nunohiro, T., Giachelli, C.M., Meehan, W.P., Tuan, T.L., and Hsueh, W.A. (1996). Osteopontin is produced by rat cardiac fibroblasts and mediates A(II)-induced DNA synthesis and collagen gel contraction. *J. Clin. Invest.*, 98, 2218-2227.

[57] Chintalgattu, V., Katwa, L.C. (2003). Cardiac myofibroblasts: a novel source of vascular endothelial growth factor (VEGF) and its receptors Flt-1 and KDR. *J. Mol. Cell. Cardiol.,* 35, 277-286.

[58] Calderone, A., Bel-Hadj, S., Drapeau, J., El-Helou, V., Gosselin, H., Clement, R., and Villeneuve, L. (2006). Scar myofibroblasts of the infarcted rat heart express natriuretic peptides. *J. Cell. Physiol.*, 207, 165-173.

[59] Makino, N., Sugano, M., Satoh, S., Oyama, J., and Maeda, T. (2006). Peroxisome proliferator-activated receptor-gamma ligands attenuate brain natriuretic peptide production and affect remodeling in cardiac fibroblasts in reoxygenation after hypoxia. *Cell Biochem. Biophys.,* 44, 65-71.

[60] Sano, M., Fukuda, K., Sato, T., Kawaguchi, H., Suematsu, M., Matsuda, S., Koyasu, S., Matsui, H., Yamauchi-Takihara, K., Harada, M., Saito, Y., and Ogawa, S. (2001). ERK and p38 MAPK, but not NF-kappaB, are critically involved in reactive oxygen species-mediated induction of IL-6 by angiotensin II in cardiac fibroblasts. *Circ. Res.*, 89, 661-669.

[61] Villarreal, F.J., Kim, N.N., Ungab, G.D., Printz, M.P., and Dillmann, W.H. (1993). Identification of functional angiotensin II receptors on rat cardiac fibroblasts. *Circulation*, 88, 2849-2861.

[62] Crabos, M., Roth, M., Hahn, A.W., and Erne, P. (1994). Characterization of angiotensin II receptors in cultured adult rat cardiac fibroblasts. Coupling to signaling systems and gene expression. *J. Clin. Invest.*, 93, 2372-2378.

[63] Zhou, G., Kandala, J.C., Tyagi, S.C., Katwa, L.C., and Weber, K.T. (1996). Effects of angiotensin II and aldosterone on collagen gene expression and protein turnover in cardiac fibroblasts. *Mol. Cell Biochem.*, 154, 171-178.

[64] Hafizi, S., Wharton, J., Morgan, K., Allen, S.P., Chester, A.H., Catravas, J.D., Polak, J.M., and Yacoub, M.H. (1998). Expression of functional angiotensin-converting enzyme and AT1 receptors in cultured human cardiac fibroblasts. *Circulation*, 98, 2553-2559.

[65] Lijnen, P.J., Petrov, V.V., and Fagard, R.H. (2001). Angiotensin II-induced stimulation of collagen secretion and production in cardiac fibroblasts is mediated via angiotensin II subtype 1 receptors. *J. Renin Angiotensin Aldosterone Syst.*, 2, 117-122.

[66] Peng, J., Gurantz, D., Tran, V., Cowling, R.T., and Greenberg, B.H. (2002). Tumor necrosis factor-alpha-induced AT1 receptor upregulation enhances angiotensin II-mediated cardiac fibroblast responses that favor fibrosis. *Circ. Res.*, 91, 1119-1126.

[67] Stewart, J.A., Jr., Cashatt, D.O., Borck, A.C., Brown, J.E., and Carver, W.E. (2006). 17beta-estradiol modulation of angiotensin II-stimulated response in cardiac fibroblasts. *J. Mol. Cell. Cardiol.,* 41, 97-107.

[68] Stacy, L.B., Yu, Q., Horak, K., and Larson, D.F. (2007). Effect of angiotensin II on primary cardiac fibroblast matrix metalloproteinase activities. *Perfusion*, 22, 51-55.

[69] Pan, C.H., Wen, C.H., and Lin, C.S. (2008). Interplay of angiotensin II and angiotensin(1-7) in the regulation of matrix metalloproteinases of human cardiocytes. *Exp. Physiol.,* 93, 599-612.

[70] Ren, J., Yang, M., Qi. G., Zheng, J., Jia, L., Cheng, J., Tian, C., Li, H., Lin, X., Du, J. (2011). Proinflammatory protein CARD9 is essential for infiltration of monocytic fibroblast precursors and cardiac fibrosis caused by Angiotensin II infusion. *Am. J. Hypertens.,* 24, 701-707.

[71] Sukumaran, V., Watanabe, K., Veeraveedu, P.T., Gurusamy, N., Ma, M., Thandavarayan, R.A., Lakshmanan, A.P., Yamaguchi, K., Suzuki, K., Kodama, M. (2011). Olmesartan, an AT1 antagonist, attenuates oxidative stress, endoplasmic reticulum stress and cardiac inflammatory mediators in rats with heart failure induced by experimental autoimmune myocarditis. *Int. J. Biol. Sci.*, 7, 154-167.

[72] Bensinger, S.J., Tontonoz, P. (2008). Integration of metabolism and inflammation by lipid-activated nuclear receptors. *Nature,* 454(7203), 470-477.

[73] Lehmann, J.M., Moore, L.B., Smith-Oliver, T.A., Wilkison, W.O., Willson, T.M., Kliewer, S.A. (1995). An antidiabetic thiazolidinedione is a high affinity ligand for peroxisome proliferator-activated receptor gamma (PPAR gamma). *J. Biol. Chem.*, 270, 12953-12956.

[74] Wayman, N.S., Ellis, B.L., and Theimermann, C. (2002). Ligands of the peroxisome proliferator-activated receptor-PPAR-a reduce myocardial infarct size. *Med. Sci. Monit.,* 8, BR243-BR247.

[75] Diep, Q.N., Amiri, F., Benkirane, K., Paradis, P., Schiffrin, E.L. (2004). Long-term effects of the PPAR gamma activator pioglitazone on cardiac inflammation in stroke-prone spontaneously hypertensive rats. *Can. J. Physiol. Pharmacol.*, 82, 976-985.

[76] Tabernero, A., Schoonjans, K., Jesel, L., Carpusca, I., Auwerx, J., Andriantsitohaina, R. (2002). Activation of the peroxisome proliferator-activated receptor alpha protects against myocardial ischaemic injury and improves endothelial vasodilatation. *BMC Pharmacol.,* 2:10, 1-10.

[77] Abdelrahman, M., Sivarajah, A., Thiemermann, C. (2005). Beneficial effects of PPAR-gamma ligands in ischemia-reperfusion injury, inflammation and shock. *Cardiovasc. Res.,* 65, 772-781.

[78] Asakawa, M., Takano, H., Nagai, T., Uozumi, H., Hasegawa, H., Kubota, N., Saito, T., Masuda, Y., Kadowaki, T., Komuro, I. (2002). Peroxisome proliferator-activated receptor gamma plays a critical role in inhibition of cardiac hypertrophy in vitro and in vivo. *Circulation*, 105, 1240-1246.

[79] Sakai, S., Miyauchi, T., Irukayama-Tomobe, Y., Ogata, T., Goto, K., Yamaguchi, I. (2002). Peroxisome proliferator-activated receptor-gamma activators inhibit endothelin-1-related cardiac hypertrophy in rats. *Clin. Sci* (Lond)., 103 Suppl 48, 16S-20S.

[80] Katwa, L.C., and Gould, A.N., (2009). Rosiglitazone treatment downer regulates AT1 receptor and collagen expression in cardiac myofibroblasts. *FASEB J.*, 23, 776.9 (abstract).

[81] Chen, K., Li, D., Zhang, X., Hermonat, P.L., Mehta, J.L. (2004). Anoxia-reoxygenation stimulates collagen type-I and MMP-1 expression in cardiac fibroblasts: modulation by the PPAR-gamma ligand pioglitazone. *J. Cardiovasc. Pharmacol.*, 44, 682-687.

[82] Chen, J., and Mehta, J.L. (2006). Angiotensin II-mediated oxidative stress and procollagen-1 expression in cardiac fibroblasts: blockade by pravastatin and pioglitazone. *Am. J. Physiol. Heart Circ. Physiol.*, 291, H1738-H1745.

[83] Hao, G.H., Niu, X.L., Gao, D.F., Wei, J., Wang, N.P. (2008). Agonists at PPAR-gamma suppress angiotensin II-induced production of plasminogen activator inhibitor-1 and extracellular matrix in rat cardiac fibroblasts. *Br. J. Pharmacol.*, 153, 1409-1419.

[84] Sugawara, A., Takeuchi, K., Uruno, A., Ikeda, Y., Arima, S., Sato, K., Kudo, M., Taniyama, Y., Ito, S. (2001). Differential effects among thiazolidinediones on the transcription of thromboxane receptor and angiotensin II type 1 receptor genes. *Hypertens. Res.*, 24, 229-233.

[85] Bao, Y., Li, R., Jiang, J., Cai, B., Gao, J., Le, K., Zhang, F., Chen, S., Liu, P. (2008). Activation of peroxisome proliferator-activated receptor gamma inhibits endothelin-1-induced cardiac hypertrophy via the calcineurin/NFAT signaling pathway. *Mol. Cell Biochem.,* 317, 189-196.

[86] Alibin, C.P., Kopilas, M.A., Anderson, H.D. (2008). Suppression of cardiac myocyte hypertrophy by conjugated linoleic acid: role of peroxisome proliferator-activated receptors alpha and gamma. *J. Biol. Chem.*, 283, 10707-10715.

[87] Massagué, J., Seoane, J., Wotton, D. (2005). Smad transcription factors. *Genes Dev.*, 19, 2783-2810.

[88] Ghosh, A.K., Bhattacharyya, S., Wei, J., Kim, S., Barak, Y., Mori, Y., Varga, J. (2009). Peroxisome proliferator-activated receptor-gamma abrogates Smad-dependent collagen stimulation by targeting the p300 transcriptional coactivator. *FASEB J.,* 23, 2968-2977.

[89] Ghosh, A.K., Wei, J., Wu, M., Varga, J. (2008). Constitutive Smad signaling and Smad-dependent collagen gene expression in mouse embryonic fibroblasts lacking peroxisome proliferator-activated receptor-gamma. *Biochem. Biophys. Res. Commun.*, 374, 231-236.

[90] Yavrom, S., Chen, L., Xiong, S., Wang, J., Rippe, R.A., Tsukamoto, H. (2005). Peroxisome proliferator-activated receptor gamma suppresses proximal alpha1(I) collagen promoter via inhibition of p300-facilitated NF-I binding to DNA in hepatic stellate cells. *J. Biol. Chem.*, 280, 40650-40659.
[91] Xu, Y., Farmer, S.R., Smith, B.D. (2007). Peroxisome proliferator-activated receptor gamma interacts with CIITA x RFX5 complex to repress type I collagen gene expression. *J. Biol. Chem.*, 282, 26046-26056.
[92] Henderson, B.C., Sen, U., Reynolds, C., Moshal, K.S., Ovechkin, A., Tyagi, N., Kartha, G.K., Rodriguez, W.E., Tyagi, S.C. (2007). Reversal of systemic hypertension-associated cardiac remodeling in chronic pressure overload myocardium by ciglitazone. *Int. J. Biol. Sci.,* 3, 385-392.
[93] Cao, Z., Ye, P., Long, C., Chen, K., Li, X., Wang, H. (2007). Effect of pioglitazone, a peroxisome proliferator-activated receptor gamma agonist, on ischemia-reperfusion injury in rats. *Pharmacology*, 79, 184-192.
[94] Fujita, K., Maeda, N., Sonoda, M., Ohashi, K., Hibuse, T., Nishizawa, H., Nishida, M., Hiuge, A., Kurata, A., Kihara, S., Shimomura, I., Funahashi, T. (2008). Adiponectin protects against angiotensin II-induced cardiac fibrosis through activation of PPAR-alpha. *Arterioscler Thromb Vasc Biol.*, 28, 863-870.
[95] Jain, R., Mullins, C.D., Lee, H., Wong, W. (2011). Use of rosiglitazone and pioglitazone immediately after the cardiovascular risk warnings. *Res. Social Adm. Pharm.*, Jul 5. [Epub ahead of print] PMID: 21733760. doi:10.1016/ j.sapharm. 2010.12.003
[96] Nishio, K., Hosaka, M., Shigemitsu, M., Kobayashi, Y. (2011). Three-year clinical outcome in Type 2 diabetic patients with drug-eluting stents versus bare-metal stents with pioglitazone. *Cardiovasc Revasc. Med.* Jul-Aug;12(4):197-202.
[97] Sarafidis, P.A., Georgianos, P.I., Lasaridis, A.N. (2010). REVIEW: PPAR-γ Agonism for Cardiovascular and Renal Protection. Cardiovasc. Ther., Sep 15. doi:10.1111/j.1755-5922.2010.00222.x. [Epub ahead of print] PubMed PMID: 20840193.
[98] Berthet, S., Olivier, P., Montastruc, J.L., Lapeyre-Mestre, M. (2011). Drug safety of rosiglitazone and pioglitazone in France: a study using the French PharmacoVigilance database. *BMC Clin. Pharmacol.*, May 24;11:5 (http://www.biomedcentral.com/1472-6904/11/5)
[99] Zhang, H., Pi, R., Li, R., Wang, P., Tang, F., Zhou, S., Gao, J., Jiang, J., Chen, S., Liu, P. (2007). PPARbeta/delta activation inhibits angiotensin II-induced collagen type I expression in rat cardiac fibroblasts. *Arch. Biochem. Biophys.*, 460, 25-32.
[100] Maejima, Y., Okada, H., Haraguchi, G., Onai, Y., Kosuge, H., Suzuki, J., Isobe, M. (2011). Telmisartan, a unique ARB, improves left ventricular remodeling of infarcted heart by activating PPAR gamma. *Lab. Invest.*, 91, 932-944.
[101] Goyal, S., Arora, S., Bhatt, T.K., Das, P., Sharma, A., Kumari, S., Arya, D.S. (2010). Modulation of PPAR-gamma by telmisartan protects the heart against myocardial infarction in experimental diabetes. *Chem. Biol. Interact.*, 185, 271-280.
[102] Goyal, S.N., Bharti, S., Bhatia, J., Nag, T.C., Ray, R., Arya, D.S. (2011). Telmisartan, a dual ARB/partial PPAR-γ agonist, protects myocardium from ischaemic reperfusion injury in experimental diabetes. *Diabetes Obes Metab.*, 13, 533-541.

[103] Geng, D.F., Wu, W., Jin, D.M., Wang, J.F., Wu, Y.M. (2006). Effect of peroxisome proliferator-activated receptor gamma ligand. Rosiglitazone on left ventricular remodeling in rats with myocardial infarction. *Int. J. Cardiol.*, 113, 86-91.

[104] Kunz, T.W., and Pravenec, M. (2004). Antidiabetic mechanisms of angiotensin-converting enzyme inhibitors and angiotensin II receptor antagonists: beyond the renin-angiotensin system. *J. Hypertens.*, 22, 2253-2261.

[105] Graham, D.J., Ouellet-Hellstrom, R., MaCurdy, T.E., Ali, F., Sholley, C., Worrall, C., Kelman, J.A. (2010). Risk of acute myocardial infarction, stroke, heart failure, and death in elderly Medicare patients treated with rosiglitazone or pioglitazone. *JAMA.*, 304, 411-418.

[106] Fliegner, D., Westermann, D., Riad, A., Schubert, C., Becher, E., Fielitz, J., Tschöpe, C., Regitz Zagrosek, V. (2007). Up-regulation of PPARgamma in myocardial infarction. *Eur. J. Heart Fail.*, 10, 30-38.

[107] Yamagishi, S., Ueda, S., Matsui, T., Nakamura, K., Okuda, S. (2008). Role of advanced glycation end products (AGEs) and oxidative stress in diabetic retinopathy. *Curr. Pharm. Des.*, 14, 962-968.

In: Medical and Biological Frontiers Research Compendium ISBN: 978-1-62417-022-5
Editor: Tsisana Shartava

Chapter 8

DNA Repair as the Primary Adaptive Function of Sex in Bacteria and Eukaryotes

***Harris Bernstein*[1], *Carol Bernstein*[1] *and Richard E. Michod*[2]**
[1]Department of Cellular and Molecular Medicine, University of Arizona, US
[2]Department of Ecology and Evolutionary Biology, University of Arizona, US

Abstract

The essential feature of sex common to both bacteria and eukaryotes is information exchange (recombination) between two genomic DNA molecules derived from different individuals. In bacteria a naturally occurring sexual process termed transformation is characterized by transfer of DNA from one bacterium to another, followed by recombination between the resident DNA and the incoming DNA. In eukaryotes, the sexual cycle involves recombination between paired DNA molecules (chromosomes) in which the two DNA molecules are derived from two different parents. This process occurs in diploid cells during meiosis, and is followed by formation of haploid gametes. The fusion of gametes from different individuals to generate diploid progeny completes the eukaryotic sexual cycle.

DNA damage appears to be a fundamental problem for life. Here, we present evidence for the view that the enzymatic machinery for carrying out recombination, during transformation in bacteria and meiosis in eukaryotes, is an adaptation for DNA repair. Both bacterial and eukaryotic cells, generally, contain repair enzymes that are adept at removing DNA damages. However there are limits to the capability of cells during ordinary cell divisions to repair their DNA. Damages causing loss of information in both DNA strands (double-strand damages) are particularly difficult to handle since they require information from a second homologous chromosome. A repair process referred to as homologous recombinational repair (HRR) appears designed to carry out repair of such double-strand damages.

Evidence is presented for the hypothesis that sexual processes (i.e. transformation in bacteria and meiosis in eukaryotes) are maintained as evolutionary adaptations to facilitate HRR. In bacteria and microbial eukaryotes the problem of DNA damages is particularly acute during periods of stress, especially oxidative stress. It is during such stressful conditions that sex (which facilitates HRR) tends to occur in these facultatively sexual organisms. In multicellular eukaryotes, meiosis facilitates HRR and appears to be designed to protect against damages to the DNA of gametes, thus minimizing infertility and defective progeny.

Another consequence of recombination during sex is increased genetic variation among progeny. Increased variation appears to have significant consequences at the population level over the long-term and is sometimes considered the primary adaptive function of sex. However, we present evidence that the machinery for sexual recombination is maintained primarily by the strong short-term advantage of passing relatively undamaged DNA from one generation to the next. The genetic variation that is generated appears to be a byproduct of HRR.

Introduction

The adaptive function of sex in bacteria and eukaryotes is widely regarded as a major unsolved problem in biology. However, many investigators in this field consider that understanding the benefit of the exchange of information (recombination) during the sexual process is the key to understanding the adaptive function of sex.

In this chapter, we present evidence from diverse fields (i.e. molecular and cellular biology, microbiology, and ecology and evolutionary biology) bearing on the adaptive function of sex in bacteria and eukaryotes. On the basis of this evidence, particularly recent findings, we propose that DNA repair is the primary adaptive function of sex.

DNA Damage, a Basic Problem for Life

DNA damage appears to be a ubiquitous problem for organisms with a DNA genome. As observed by Haynes (1988), DNA is made up of rather ordinary molecular subunits that are not endowed with any peculiar kind of quantum mechanical stability. He noted that its very "chemical vulgarity" makes DNA vulnerable to all the "chemical horrors" that might befall any such molecule in a warm aqueous medium. These chemical horrors are DNA damages, such as a break in a DNA strand or an adduct molecule added to one of the DNA bases. DNA damages are distinct from mutations. DNA damages are structural and chemical alterations in the DNA, whereas mutations ordinarily involve the normal four bases in new arrangements. Mutations can be replicated when the DNA replicates, in contrast to DNA damages that are altered structures that cannot be replicated.

DNA damages are subject to several different repair processes, but those DNA damages that escape repair can have detrimental consequences. DNA damages may block replication or transcription, leading to cell death. Alternatively, during DNA replication, when a DNA polymerase uses a template DNA strand containing a damaged site, it may bypass the damage and in the process generate a mutation.

In bacteria and eukaryotes, the DNA genome is assaulted both by reactive chemicals naturally present in the intracellular environment and by agents from external sources. A major internal source of DNA damage in both bacteria and eukaryotes is reactive oxygen species (ROS) produced as byproducts of normal aerobic metabolism. For eukaryotes, oxidative reactions appear to be a major source of DNA damage (for review of oxidative damage in humans, see Sedelnikova et al., 2010). It is estimated that about 10,000 oxidative DNA damages occur per cell per day in humans (Ames et al., 1993). In the rat, which has a higher metabolic rate than humans, the number of oxidative DNA damages occurring per cell per day is about 100,000. ROS appear to be an important source of DNA damage in aerobically growing bacteria, as indicated by the finding that 89% of spontaneously occurring base substitution mutations are caused by ROS-induced damages and then inaccurate replication past the damaged bases (Sakai et al., 2006). Most oxidative DNA damages affect only one of the DNA strands, but a fraction, about 1-2%, are double-strand damages such as double-strand breaks (DSBs) (Massie et al., 1972). In humans, it is estimated that the average number of endogenous DNA DSBs per cell occurring at each cell generation is about 50 (Vilenchik and Knudson, 2003). This rate of formation of DSBs likely reflects a natural level of damages, such as may be caused by ROS produced by active metabolism.

There are five major pathways employed in repairing different types of DNA damages. These are base excision repair, nucleotide excision repair, mismatch repair, non-homologous end joining and homologous recombinational repair (HRR) [see Bernstein et al. (2002) for review]). However, only one of these pathways, HRR, can accurately repair double-strand damages, such as double-strand breaks (DSBs). The HRR pathway requires the availability of a second homologous chromosome for recovering the information lost by the first chromosome due to the double-strand damage (Figure 1). As described below, in both haploid and diploid organisms, sex promotes the conditions needed for highly effective HRR of double-strand damages. In diploid organisms sex promotes effective repair without the expression or accumulation of recessive or nearly recessive deleterious mutations.

Bacterial Transformation Is an Adaptive Sexual Process

In haploid organisms, such as bacteria, sex is usually required for the presence in the cell of a second homologous template. Homologous gene transfer followed by recombination (sex) can occur by three recognized processes in bacteria. These processes are (1) bacterial virus (bacteriophage) mediated transduction, (2) plasmid-mediated conjugation and (3) natural bacterial transformation. Bacteriophage mediated transduction of bacterial genes appears to reflect an occasional mistake in assembly of virus particles, rather than an adaptation of the host bacteria. The transfer process is controlled by the bacteriophage's genes rather than by the host's genes. Plasmid-mediated conjugation is controlled by plasmid genes, and is an adaptation for distributing copies of the plasmid from one bacterium to another. Infrequently, during this process, the plasmid may become integrated into the host bacterial chromosome, and subsequently transfer part of the host chromosome to another bacterium. Plasmid mediated transfer of host bacterial DNA also appears to generally be an accidental process, rather than a bacterial adaptation.

Natural bacterial transformation involves the transfer of DNA from one bacterium to another through the surrounding medium. In contrast to the first two processes, transformation is clearly a bacterial adaptation for DNA transfer, since it depends on the expression of numerous bacterial genes whose products appear to be specifically designed to carry out this process (Chen and Dubnau, 2004). Transformation is a complex, energy requiring, developmental process. In order for a bacterium to bind, take up and recombine exogenous DNA into its chromosome, it must enter a special physiological state referred to as competence. In *Bacillus subtilis*, expression of about 40 genes is required for development of competence (Solomon and Grossman, 1996). Ordinarily, but with rare exceptions, the DNA integrated into the host bacterial chromosome is from another bacterium of the same species, and thus is homologous to the resident chromosome. The amount of DNA transferred during a transformation event can be a substantial portion of the bacterial chromosome. In *B. subtilis* the transferred DNA can be as large as a third to the whole chromosome (Akamatsu and Taguchi, 2001; Saito et al., 2006). Transformation appears to be common in the bacterial world, and thus far 67 prokaryote species (in seven different phyla) are known to be naturally competent for transformation (Johnsborg et al., 2007).

Competence Development Is Usually Associated with Stressful Conditions

During logarithmic growth there can be two or more copies of any particular region of the chromosome in a bacterial cell, as cell division and DNA replication are not precisely matched. During this phase, HRR can occur between recently replicated sister chromosome regions. However, once cells approach stationary phase they typically have just one copy of the chromosome and HRR requires input of homologous template from outside the cell by transformation. Therefore it is no surprise that competence for transformation is typically induced by high cell density and/or nutritional limitation, conditions associated with stationary phase. In *Haemophilus influenzae*, transformation occurs most efficiently at the end of exponential growth as the bacteria approach stationary phase (Goodgal and Herriott, 1961). In *Streptococcus mutans*, as well as many other streptococci, development of competence for transformation is associated with high cell density and biofilm formation (Aspiras et al., 2004). In *Bacillus subtilis*, competence is induced toward the end of logarithmic growth, especially under conditions of amino acid limitation (Anagnostopoulos and Spizizen, 1961).

Bacterial Transformation, as an Adaptation for DNA Repair

In this section we review evidence that competence is specifically induced by DNA damaging conditions, and that transformation functions as a DNA repair process employing HRR. The DNA damaging agents mitomycin C (a crosslinking agent) and fluoroquinolone (a topoisomerase inhibitor) induce transformation in *Streptococcus pneumoniae* (Claverys et al., 2006). Transformation in *B. subtilis* is enhanced by ultraviolet light, a DNA-damaging agent (Michod et al., 1988). In *Helicobacter pylori*, ciprofloxacin, which binds DNA gyrase and causes double-strand breaks in DNA, induces expression of competence genes, thus increasing transformation frequency (Dorer et al., 2010). Charpentier et al. (2011) tested 64 toxic molecules to determine which of these induce competence for natural transformation in *Legionella pneumophila*. Of these 64 compounds, only six, all DNA damaging agents, caused strong induction. These agents were mitomycin C (which causes DNA inter-strand crosslinks), norfloxacin, ofloxacin and nalidixic acid [each of which inhibits DNA gyrase leading to DSBs (Albertini et al., 1995)], bicyclomycin [which causes single- and double-strand breaks (Washburn and Gottesman, 2011; Tran et al., 2011)], and hydroxyurea [which induces DNA base oxidation (Sakano et al., 2001)]. Among the toxic molecules that did not induce competence were antibiotics that block cell wall or protein synthesis. UV light, another DNA damaging agent, was also tested and proved to induce competence in *L. pneumophila*. Charpentier et al. (2011) suggested that competence likely evolved as a DNA damage response.

To test whether the adaptive function of transformation is repair of DNA damages, a series of experiments was conducted using *B. subtilis* irradiated by UV light (Hoelzer and Michod, 1991; Michod et al., 1988; Michod and Wojciechowski, 1994; Wojciechowski et al., 1989; and reviewed in Michod et al., 2008). The experimental approach was to administer transforming DNA to cultures grown to competence either before exposing the cells to the DNA damaging effects of UV radiation ("DNA-UV") or after UV radiation ("UV-DNA"). The basic result obtained was that after UV irradiation, survival of those cells that were transformed was greater than survival of the majority of cells in the culture that were not transformed. The enhanced survival of the transformed cells was only observed in the UV-DNA experiments in which the donor DNA was administered after the UV treatment (Michod et al., 1988). These results suggest that the transforming DNA acts to repair DNA damages introduced by UV in the recipient DNA, but is of no benefit for survival when the damages are introduced after transformation is completed. The increase in survival in the UV-DNA experiments occurred even if the transforming DNA was irradiated with UV at levels comparable to that given to the recipient cells (Hoelzer and Michod, 1991). This finding suggested that DNA damages introduced more-or-less at random in the donor DNA did not often correspond to the exact locations of the damages in the recipient DNA, and thus the transforming DNA could provide locally intact template for repair of most recipient DNA damages. In other experiments, H_2O_2, which causes oxidative DNA damage, was used and similar results to that obtained with UV were observed (unpublished results).

The results with *B. subtilis*, described above, are reasonably interpreted in terms of homologous recombinational repair (HRR), a well-established repair process in both bacterial and eukaryotic cells (described in Figure 1, and discussed further, below). HRR is unique among DNA repair processes in that it can accurately repair damages causing loss of information in both DNA strands [double-strand damages, such as double-strand breaks (DSBs) and inter-strand crosslinks]. HRR requires, in addition to the damaged DNA molecule, a second homologous DNA molecule containing an intact sequence corresponding to the damaged sequence in the first DNA molecule, so that information can be exchanged between the two. As already mentioned, *B. subtilis* cells typically become competent in late-log phase, at which time most cells are haploid (presumably because maintaining a second chromosome would be costly under conditions approaching starvation). Haploid, non-replicating cells thus lack a second homolog for HRR. However, homologous template DNA for HRR can be provided by transforming DNA. Thus the association of competence (required for bacterial sex) with haploidy is adaptive in terms of the need for DNA template for use in HRR.

Sex Was Present Early in the Evolution of Eukaryotes

The evidence reviewed in this section indicates that facultative sex was present early in the evolution of eukaryotes. Since the earliest ancestor of eukaryotes had bacterial antecedents, continuity in evolution from bacterial sex to eukaryotic sex is a reasonable possibility. Evidence that eukaryotic meiosis is derived from bacterial transformation was reviewed in Bernstein and Bernstein (2010).

Eukaryotes emerged in evolution more than 1.5 billion years ago. Even though sexual reproduction is widespread among extant eukaryotes, it seemed unlikely, until recently, that sex is a primordial and fundamental characteristic of eukaryotes. The reason for this view was that sexual reproduction appeared to be lacking in early observations on certain human pathogenic single-celled eukaryotes that diverged from early ancestors in the eukaryotic lineage. However, several of these organisms are now known to be capable of, or to recently have had, the capability for meiosis and hence sexual reproduction. As one example, the common intestinal parasite *Giardia intestinalis* had been thought to be a descendant of a lineage that predated the emergence of meiosis and sex. Contradicting this view, *G. intestinalis* was recently found to have a core set of meiotic genes, including five meiosis specific genes (Ramash et al., 2005). More recently, evidence for meiotic recombination, indicative of sexual reproduction, was found in *G. intestinalis* (Cooper et al., 2007). In a second example, parasitic protozoa of the genus *Leishmania*, which cause human diseases, have recently also been shown to have a sexual cycle (Akopyants et al., 2009).

Trichomonas vaginalis, a parasitic unicellular eukaryote is not known to undergo meiosis. However, when Malik et al. (2008) tested for the presence of 29 meiotic genes in *T. vaginalis*, they found 27, including 8 of 9 genes specific to meiosis in model organisms, suggesting that that capability for meiosis may have been present in recent ancestors. Twenty-one of the 27 genes were also present in *G. intestinalis*, indicating that most of these meiotic genes were present in common ancestor of these two species. Because these species are descendants of lineages that are highly divergent among eukaryotes, Malik et al. (2008) suggested that each of these meiotic gens were likely present in a common ancestor of all exkaryotes. Dacks and Roger (1999), based on a phylogenetic analysis, also proposed that facultative sex was present in the common ancestor of eukaryotes. A study of amoebae by Lahr et al. (2011) lent further support to this view. Although amoebae are generally regarded as asexual, these authors presented evidence that most amoeboid lineages are anciently sexual, and that the majority of asexual groups probably arose recently and independently.

The Sexual Cycle in Eukaryotic Microorganisms Occurs under Stressful Conditions

In eukaryotic microorganisms, as in bacteria, sex occurs under stressful conditions. Among extant unicellular or simple multicellular eukaryotes, sex is usually facultative. These organisms generally reproduce asexually under favorable environmental conditions, but reproduce sexually under stressful conditions. Starvation, desiccation, mechanical damage and heat shock are all known to induce sex in these organisms. For instance, the paramecium tetrahymena can be induced to undergo mating (conjugation) by starvation conditions brought about by washing (Elliott and Hayes, 1953). When the unicellular green alga *Chlamydomonas reinhardi* is grown in a medium depleted of a nitrogen source, vegetative cells differentiate into gametes (Sager & Granick, 1954). These gametes can then fuse, form zygotes and undergo meiosis. The haploid fission yeast *Schizosaccharomyces pombe* is a facultatively sexual microorganism that undergoes mating when nutrients become limiting (Davey et al., 1998).

The Sexual Cycle in Unicellular or Simple Multicellular Eukaryotes as a Response to DNA Damaging Conditions

We reviewed evidence, above, that sex was present early in the evolution of eukaryotes, raising the likelihood of continuity in the evolution of bacterial to eukaryotic sex. We also reviewed evidence, above, that bacterial sex (transformation) is an adaptation for repair of DNA damage. In this section we cite evidence that, in simple eukaryotes, sex is induced under conditions of oxidative stress and may be an adaptation for repairing oxidative DNA damage. Thus sex may have been retained through the prokaryotic to eukaryotic evolutionary transition as an adaptation for repairing DNA damage, especially DSBs.

Life depends on a delicate balance of reduction and oxidation reactions. Various metabolic or environmental stress factors can upset this balance, leading to an increase in the cellular levels of reduced and highly reactive molecules, including a series of oxygen-containing compounds collectively termed reactive oxygen species or ROS. At high concentrations, ROS can be damaging to biological systems (i.e., oxidative stress), and cause DNA damage. A variety of adaptive responses have evolved to cope with the DNA-damaging effects of oxidative stress, including cell cycle arrest (CCA, allowing time for DNA repair) and programmed cell death (PCD, allowing for the elimination of damaged cells). It also has been known for some time that stress can trigger the sexual cycle in facultatively sexual species (Williams, 1975). As many forms of stress (temperature, drought, UV, pathogens) trigger an increase in cellular levels of ROS, it is reasonable to expect that the sex-inducing stress in facultatively sexual species might also result in ROS overproduction, and that sex in such species is an additional response to oxidative stress and its consequences such as DNA damage.

Oxidative stress causes a variety of DNA damages including modified bases, single-strand breaks and DSBs (Slupphang et al., 2003). To test whether oxidative stress is implicated the induction of sex in the yeast *S. pombe*, Bernstein and Johns (1989) treated late exponential phase *S. pombe* cells with hydrogen peroxide, which produces oxidative stress. This treatment increased the frequency of mating and formation of meiotic spores by 4 to 18-fold. *Phytophthora cinnamoni*, an oomycete fungus, also can be induced to undergo sexual reproduction by exposure to hydrogen peroxide (Reeves and Jackson, 1974). *Volvox carteri*, a simple, haploid, multicellular, facultatively sexual green algae, can be induced to reproduce sexually by heat shock (Kirk and Kirk, 1986). This induction can be inhibited by antioxidants, indicating that oxidative stress mediates the induction of sex by heat shock (Nedelcu and

Michod, 2003). An inhibitor of the mitochondrial electron transport chain that induces oxidative stress also induced sex in *V. carteri* (Nedelcu et al., 2004).

During investigations of the role of ROS in stress-induced sex in the multicellular *V. carteri,* Nedelcu and Michod (2003) noted that the decline in the proportion of sexual progeny with increasing oxidative stress is paralleled by an increase in the proportion of gonidia that arrest and delay cleavage (i.e., the fast successive round of cell divisions that result in formation of the embryo). Many of these arrested gonidia develop into asexual rather than sexual embryos (Nedelcu and Michod, 2003). This pattern suggests the hypothesis that at higher doses of ROS cell-cycle arrest replaces sex as a stress-response. It was also noted that temperatures slightly higher than the one used for inducing sex, increased duration of the heat-stress (3 hours), or the addition of chemicals known to interfere with p53 (a main player in responses to DNA damage – including CCA and PCD in mammals), all result in a PCD-like response in gonidia (Nedelcu, 2006). This relationship between sex and two known responses to DNA damage (CCA and PCD), suggest a connection between sex and DNA damage.

Nedelcu and Michod (2003) and Nedelcu (2006) previously reported three kinds of data suggesting DNA damage is the cause of sex induction by ROS in *V. carteri.* (a) There is a bi-modal response pattern of sex to increasing stress (Nedelcu, 2006) similar to the pattern observed for cellular responses to increasing doses of DNA-damaging H_2O_2. (b) An iron-chelator is effective at reducing the sex response, as is predicted by the DNA damaging effects of the iron-based Fenton reaction (Imlay et al., 1988). (c) The relationship between sex and two known responses to DNA damage, namely, CCA and PCD, imply a connection between sex and DNA damage. Nedelcu (2006) showed in *V. carteri* that sex-inducing stress, when performed in the presence of PFTα (a compound that interferes with p53 activity) triggers PCD in gonidia, which further suggests that DNA damage is involved in sexual induction (Achanta and Huang, 2004; Chlamygenome, 2007). In addition to these data indicating that DNA damage is the basis of ROS' sex-inducing capacity in *V. carteri*, known DNA damaging agents such as glutaraldehyde, formaldehyde and UV have been shown to induce sex in *V. carteri* (Loshon et al., 1999; Zeiger et al., 2005; Starr and Jaenicke, 1988).

The budding yeast *Saccharomyces cerevisiae* divides by mitosis when nutrients are plentiful, but when starved becomes arrested in the G1/G0 phase of the cell cycle. Under this condition oxidative stress increases and DNA DSBs and apurinic/apyrimidinic sites accumulate (Steinboeck et al., 2010). Cells arrested in the G1 phase of the cell cycle undergo meiosis to form haploid spores (Herskowitz, 1988). Since starvation causes oxidative stress and DNA damage in *S. cerevisiae*, the induction of sex by starvation may be mediated by these factors.

Bacterial Transformation and Eukaryotic Meiosis Have Fundamental Similarities

Although transformation in bacteria and meiosis in eukaryotes are complex adaptations encoded by numerous genes, they share their central molecular processes and these processes are carried out by homologous enzymes. Bacterial transformation involves three major steps: (1) the entry of DNA from one "parent" into the cell of another parent; (2) the alignment and genetic recombination between non-sister homologous chromosomes (or parts of chromosomes) that are derived from the different parental bacteria; (3) the recombined chromosome is passed on to progeny bacteria. Meiosis occurs in diploid eukaryotic cells by three steps as well. The key sequential steps in meiosis are (1) pre-meiotic DNA replication of chromosomes that originated from gametes from different parents (chromosomes inherited from the "mother" and the "father"; (2) pairing of non-sister homologs and recombination between them; and (3) two successive cell divisions leading to haploid gametes. When one gamete unites with another gamete (syngamy/fertilization), a diploid progeny is formed. As in transformation, in meiosis the central step (step 2) is the interaction of non-sister homologous chromosomes. This interaction in meiosis, as in transformation, involves the alignment of non-sister homologs followed by genetic recombination. In bacteria and eukaryotes, central to the exchange of genetic information between non-sister homologs is the RecA protein (in bacteria), and its orthologs (e.g. Rad51 and Dmc1) in eukaryotes. In the next section we discuss the key role of the RecA protein in bacterial transformation, and in the section after that we describe the similar central role of RecA orthologs in meiotic recombination.

Role of the RecA Protein in Transformation

In *B. subtilis, S. pneumoniae* and *Neisseria gonorrhoeae* the RecA protein is essential for transformation (Dubnau et al., 1973; Martin et al., 1992; Claverys et al., 2009; Stohl et al., 2011). The RecA protein is induced during development of competence for transformation in *B. subtilis* (Cheo et al., 1992) and *S. pneumoniae* (Mortier-Barriere et al., 1998).

In *B. subtilis*, the RecA protein interacts with several competence proteins to form a multiprotein assembly. This assembly accepts incoming single-stranded DNA (ssDNA) at a cell pole, where the DNA is prepared for recombination with the resident chromosome (Kidane and Graumann, 2005). The incoming ssDNA interacts with the RecA protein to form striking filamentous structures. These filamentous structures emanate from the pole containing the competence machinery and extend into the cytosol. These RecA/ssDNA filamentous threads are considered to represent dynamic nucleofilaments that scan the chromosome for regions of homology. This brings incoming DNA to the corresponding site in the bacterial chromosome where informational exchange occurs (Kidane and Graumann, 2005).

Cox (1991; 1993; 2002) analyzed the molecular interactions of bacterial RecA protein with DNA. This analysis indicated that the RecA protein evolved as the central component of an HRR system for dealing with DNA damage, and that "DNA repair is the most important function of homologous genetic recombination". This conclusion suggests that, in bacterial transformation, the function of RecA is to facilitate repair of damaged DNA. We noted, above, that cells typically become competent in late log phase, when most cells are haploid. Thus the only available source of a second homologous DNA molecule for HRR is from another bacterium. During rapid log phase growth, after DNA replication but before cell division, a bacterial cell may have two homologs present, and thus be able to carry out HRR between sister homologs.

Role of Reca Orthologs in Meiosis of Unicellular Eukaryotes

The HRR machinery appears to be highly conserved. Genes *rad51* and *dmc1* of the unicellular yeasts *S. cerevisiae* and *S. pombe* are orthologs of the bacterial *recA* gene. The *dmc1* gene has also been found in the unicellular eukaryotic microorganisms *Giardia*, *Trypanosoma*, *Leishmania*, *Entamoeba*, and *Plasmodium* (Ramesh et al., 2005). The Rad51 and Dmc1 proteins of yeast interact with ssDNA to form a filamentous intermediate, referred to as a presynaptic filament, that initiates recombination (Sauvageau et al., 2005; San Filippo et al., 2008). This filament is similar to the RecA/ssDNA nucleofilaments formed during bacterial transformation (described above). The Rad51 recombinase acts both during meiosis and mitosis, whereas Dmc1 acts only during meiosis (Bugreev et al., 2011). The tertiary structure of the yeast Dmc1 recombinase is, overall, similar to the bacterial RecA recombinase (Story et al., 1993). Like the bacterial RecA recombinase, the yeast Rad51 recombinase catalyzes ATP-dependent homologous DNA pairing and strand exchange (Sung, 1994). Thus the recombinases Rad51 and Dmc1 that act during meiosis in unicellular eukaryotes appear to be functionally and structurally similar to the RecA bacterial recombinase that acts in transformation. This correspondence suggests continuity in the evolution of the sexual process from bacteria to unicellular eukaryotes.

Role of Reca Orthologs in Meiosis of Complex Multicellular Eukaryotes

The evidence reviewed in this section indicates that orthologs of bacterial RecA play an important role in meiotic recombination in multicellular animals and plants, as they do in unicellular eukaryotes (previous section). Thus there appears to be evolutionary continuity of the central role of recA orthologs in sexual recombination in bacteria, unicellular eukaryotes and multicellular eukaryotes.

As in unicellular eukaryotes, Dmc1 and Rad51 play a key role in HRR during meiosis of complex multicellular eukaryotes. Orthologs of the RecA protein function in meiosis of animals (e.g. nematodes, mice and humans) and of plants (e.g. *Arabidopsis*, rice and lilies). In the nematode *Caenorhabditis elegans*, resistance to X-ray induced DNA damage in meiotic pachytene nuclei depends on the *rad51* gene that is strongly expressed in meiotic cells (Takenami et al., 2000), indicating the repair function of *rad51*. An ortholog of the *recA* gene is expressed at a high level in the testis and ovary of mice, suggesting that this RecA is involved in meiotic recombination (Shinohara et al., 1993). When the mouse *dcm1* gene is mutationally defective, the mice fail to undergo intimate pairing of homologous chromosomes, are unable to complete meiosis and are sterile (Pittman et al., 1998; Yoshida et al., 1998). In humans, Dmc1, the meiosis-specific recombinase, forms nucleoprotein complexes on ssDNA that promote a search for homology and informational exchange, the crucial steps of genetic recombination (Sehorn et al., 2004; Bugreev et al., 2005).

In the plant *Arabidopsis thaliana*, the functions of Rad51 (Li et al., 2004) and Dmc1 (Couteau et al., 1999) are required for meiosis. In the lily, proteins Rad51 and Lim15 (an ortholog of Dmc1) co-localize on meiotic prophase I chromosomes, forming discrete foci (Terasawa et al., 1995). The proteins of these foci are considered to cooperate in the search for, and the pairing of, homologous DNA sequences. In rice, an ortholog of Dmc1 plays a key role in the pairing of homologous chromosomes and is necessary for meiosis (Deng and Wang, 2007).

DNA Damage Increases Meiotic Recombination

Classically, meiotic recombination has been identified and measured by exchange of allelic markers in genetic crosses. When measured in this way, the term "allelic recombination" is often used. A test of whether meiotic allelic recombination reflects the repair process of HRR would be to determine whether allelic recombination increases after exposure to DNA damaging agents. As would be expected if allelic recombination is a reflection of HRR, X-irradiation increases meiotic allelic recombination in *S. cerevisiae* (Kelly et al., 1983) and in the nematode *C. elegans* (Kim and Rose, 1987). In the fruit fly *Drosophila melanogaster,* recombination is increased by UV light (Prudhommeau and Proust, 1973), gamma-rays (Suzuki and Parry, 1964) and mitomycin C (Schewe et al., 1971). Even *D. melanogaster* males, which ordinarily do not display meiotic recombination (Chovnick et al., 1970), can be induced to undergo recombination by X-rays (Hannah-Alava, 1964). That male *D. melanogaster* do not ordinarily undergo recombination, except when exposed to an exogenous DNA damaging agent, is somewhat puzzling. This may reflect a preference for removal of spermatocytes with spontaneous DNA damage by programmed cell death (apoptosis), rather than removal of the DNA damages by HRR; or it may reflect a low level of spontaneous DNA damage requiring HRR during spermatogenesis. In general, these observations show that exposure to DNA damaging agents increase meiotic recombination and are consistent with the view that meiotic recombination is an adaptation for DNA repair.

Crossover and Non-crossover Recombination: Implications for Variation Theories

Recombination involving exchange of genetic information between between non-sister homologs (i.e. homologs originating from different parents) is a near universal feature of meiosis. A double-strand break (DSB) in one of the two DNA homologs is considered to be a general early step in the recombination process (see Figure 1). Succeeding steps lead to the accurate repair of the DSB. When the chromosome arms on opposite sides of a DSB exchange partners during recombination, the event is called a crossover (CO). When the original configuration of the chromosome arms is maintained, the event is referred to as a non-crossover (NCO). CO recombination events produce genetic variation, whereas NCO recombination events have little effect on linkage disequilibrium (the statistical association of genes at different loci). Thus the relative occurrence of CO compared to NCO recombination events provides a test of the plausibility of evolutionary theories of sex based on the assumption that producing genetic variation is the principle function of sex. Variation theories predict that CO recombination should be the preferred product of the complex set of events involved in the recombination process.

Certain fungi are favorable systems for studying the products of individual meiotic events. Tetrad analyses from several species of fungi indicates that about 2/3 of recombination events during meiosis are NCOs [summaries of data from *S. cerevisiae*, *Podospora anserina*, *Sordaria fimicola* and *Sordaria brevicollis* were presented by Whitehouse (1982, Tables 19 and 38)]. In *D. melanogaster*, the ratio of NCOs to COs is about 3:1 (Mehrotra and McKim, 2006). Moens et al. (2002) presented evidence that during meiosis in the mouse there are $\geq$10-fold more DSBs than CO recombinants, and suggested that most DSBs are repaired by NCO recombination. These observations suggest that most recombination events are NCOs. Thus theories for the adaptive function of meiosis and sex that focus exclusively on CO recombination are inadequate to explain most recombination events. This includes theories that attribute the benefit of sex to the generation of genetic diversity.

The Function of NCO Recombination

A succession of molecular models for genetic recombination has been proposed over the years based on information from relevant genetic and biochemical experiments. A model proposed by Szostak et al. (1983), referred to as the Double-Strand Break Repair model, was recognized at the time as providing a good explanation of experimental findings. According to this model, during each recombination event, two Holliday Junctions (see Figure 1) are formed to either side of a DSB, and resolution of these junctions leads to completion of the recombination event. Because of these features, the Double-Strand Break Repair model is also often referred to as the Double-Holliday Junction (DHJ) model (Figure 1). Originally, the DHJ model was thought to explain both CO and NCO types of recombination. Although the DHJ model is still considered to explain how CO recombinants are formed, evidence presented by Allers and Lichten (2001) indicated that NCO recombinants are formed by a different pathway that acts earlier in meiosis.

Several groups (Allers and Lichten, 2001; McMahil et al., 2007; Andersen and Sekelsky, 2010) have reported evidence that NCO recombinants arise during meiosis by an HRR process which they call “Synthesis-Dependent Strand Annealing” or SDSA (Figure 1). In SDSA, an early step is the occurrence of a DSB, as in the DHJ model. This is followed by 5’ to 3’ resections of a single strand on each side of the break.

Next, a single-strand extending from one end of the break invades the homologous chromosome with which it is paired, forming a displacement loop (D-loop). This is followed by continued synthesis of the invading strand using the undamaged complementary strand as a template. Next the invading strand is displaced from its template and anneals with a single strand at the other side of the break. Repair synthesis fills in any remaining gaps. By this process, the information lost in the region of the DSB is accurately restored by copying from the paired intact homolog, without a need for physical exchange of DNA. The process for forming NCO recombinants is one of informational exchange over a small region, rather than physical exchange. By contrast, the process for forming CO recombinants (the DHJ model) does involve physical exchange of DNA segments (Figure 1).

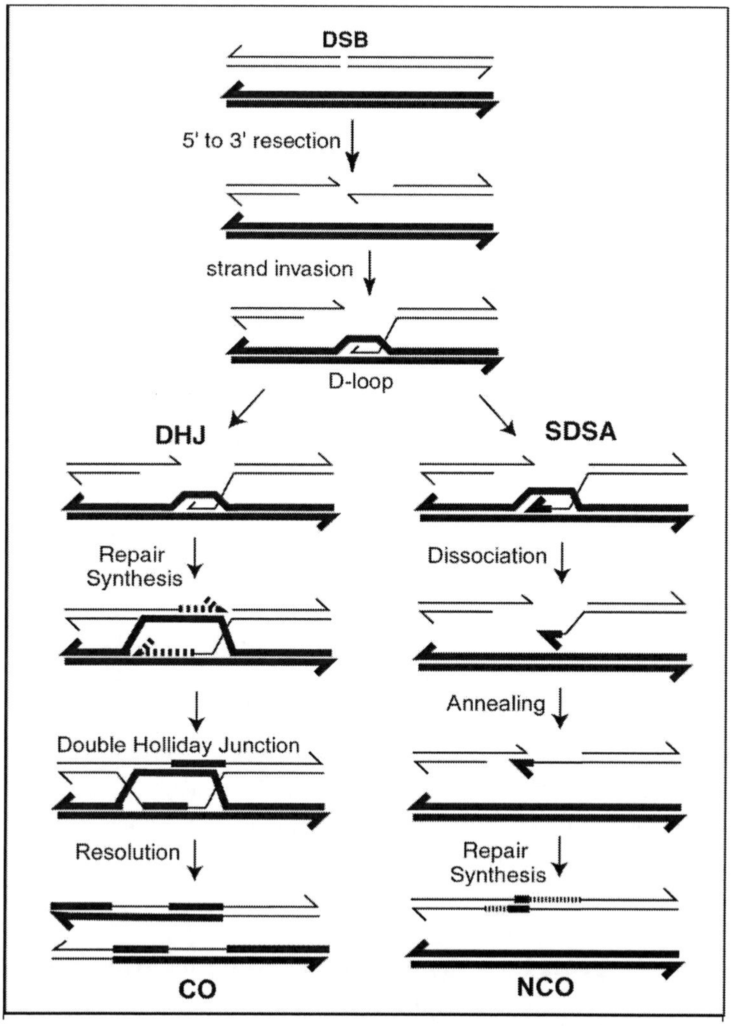

Figure 1. The initiating event in current models of meiotic recombination is formation of a double-strand break (DSB) or gap. This is followed by pairing of the damaged chromosome with a homologous chromosome, and then strand invasion to form a displacement loop (D-loop). Repair of the gap allows restoration of the lost information and can result in a crossover (CO) or non-crossover (NCO) of the flanking regions. CO recombination is considered to arise by the Double Holliday Junction (DHJ) model, shown on the left. NCO recombination is considered to arise mainly by the Synthesis Dependent Strand Annealing (SDSA) model shown on the right. The majority of recombination events during meiosis are likely of the SDSA type.

Although the SDSA model of recombination includes a DSB as an early step, this model may also apply to other types of double-strand damages such as an interstrand-crosslink or single-strand break opposite an altered base in the other strand. In principle, these types of double-strand damage could be converted by nuclease action to a DSB that could then be repaired by SDSA to form a NCO recombination event.

CO and NCO recombination appear to have different functional consequences. The physical exchanges associated with CO recombination appear to be necessary to promote the intimate pairing of homologous chromosomes during meiosis in some organisms. NCO recombination is not thought to have a role in synapsis since there is no physical exchange of

DNA by the SDSA mechanism. Furthermore, CO recombination generates allelic recombination that contributes to genetic diversity among progeny, and this may have long-term benefits. NCO recombination produces relatively little allelic genetic variation. Thus NCO recombination, the most frequent type of recombination during meiosis, appears to be primarily for DNA repair, whereas CO recombination functions in DNA repair, synapsis, and in causing genetic diversity.

Meiotic HRR Is Essential for Fertility and Early Embryonic Survival

One test of the idea that repair of DNA damages during meiosis is adaptively important is to study the effect on fertility of defects in enzymes known to be essential for HRR during mitosis. About 15% of all couples in the US are infertile. An important cause of male infertility is oxidative stress during gametogenesis (Makker et al., 2009). As discussed above, oxidative stress causes DNA damage (Slupphaug et al., 2003). During mouse spermatogenesis, after meiosis is completed and mature sperm are being formed, DNA repair capability declines allowing accumulation of DNA damage in sperm (Marchetti and Wyrobek, 2008). Failure of HRR during meiosis would be expected to exacerbate the problem of DNA damage and increase infertility. Increased DNA damage in the germ line of men is associated with poor semen quality, low fertilization rate, impaired pre-implantation development, increased abortion, and more frequent disease in progeny including childhood cancer (reviewed in Lewis and Aitken, 2005). These authors also commented that the natural causes of this increased DNA damage are unclear, but the principal candidate is oxidative stress.

Table 1. Mutations in genes encoding proteins necessary for HRR cause infertility in humans and/or mice

Species	Gene	Fold-increased expression in testes vs. somatic cells	Infertility in mutant females and /or males	References
Human, Mouse	atm	4×	Females and males in humans and mice are infertile	Galetzka et al., 2007; Barlow et al., 1998
Mouse	brca1	3×	Few surviving male mice are infertile	Galetzka et al., 2007; Cressman et al., 1999
Mouse	mlh1	1.7×	Female and male mice are infertile	Galetzka et al., 2007; Wei et al., 2002

As expected on the hypothesis that meiosis is an adaptation for DNA repair, inherited mutations in human and mouse genes that encode proteins necessary for mitotic HRR are observed to cause infertility (Table 1). This finding indicates that formation of functional gametes depends on HRR. Genes *atm*, *brca1* and *mlh1* are essential for DNA repair during mitosis and are expressed at a higher level during meiosis than mitosis. In summary, it appears that increased damages during meiosis cause infertility, and that HRR of DNA damages during meiosis protects against infertility.

Meiosis is restricted to the cell division preceding gamete formation. This placement of meiosis likely reflects the high cost of producing nonfunctional gametes due to unrepaired DNA damages. A parent provides only one gamete to each progeny, and this gamete must be as free of damage as possible to result in a viable progeny. No other cell in a multicellular organism has as great an influence on reproductive success. Even though DNA repair enzymes involved in HRR are at higher levels during meiosis than during mitosis (Table 1) and thus HRR presumably occurs at a higher level during meiosis, attrition of fertilized eggs and miscarriages are still rather high. Austin (1972) pointed out that about half of fertilized eggs in humans fail to produce surviving embryos, as is generally typical of mammals. Roberts and Lowe (1975) estimated a 78% loss of human conceptions, most of these occurring before the first missed period. Wilcox et al. (1988) concluded that 31% of embryos miscarry after implantation, often before a woman realizes she is pregnant. Although the causes of these malfunctions have not been determined, DNA damage is likely to be an important contributing factor. These observations point to an essential role for DNA repair during meiosis in mammals.

In plants, it is common for fertilized ovules to fail to mature as seeds (Bawa and Webb, 1984). During plant seed dormancy, often associated with unpredictable and stressful environments, DNA damages accumulate (Cheah and Osborne, 1978; Koppen and Verschaeve, 2001; Bray and West, 2005). Thus in plants, as in mammals, DNA damages appear to be a problem for survival, and HRR during meiosis may be necessary for viability of gametes and progeny.

DNA Damages Are Repaired by HRR during Meiosis and Mitosis

In this section, we review findings indicating that DNA damages caused by different exogenous agents are repaired by HRR during mitosis, and that gene products required for mitotic HRR are also required for DNA repair during meiosis. In the next section, we present evidence that during meiosis HRR likely removes a class of DNA damages that cannot be accurately removed during mitosis.

During mitosis, HRR is largely limited to interaction between neighboring sister chromosomes after replication has occurred and before cell division. During mitosis, the frequency of recombination between non-sister homologs is about 1% of that between sister chromosomes (Moynahan and Jasin, 2010). On the other hand, during meiosis, in which there is systematic synapsis between non-sister homologous chromosomes, recombination occurs frequently between these non-sister homologs. Furthermore, while mitotic HRR only rarely leads to CO recombination, meiotic HRR leads to CO far more frequently (Virgin et al.,

2001). This difference may reflect the function of CO recombination in promoting synapsis of non-sister homologs during meiosis, but not during mitosis. In spite of these differences concerning which chromosomes are involved, there appears to be close similarity of the recombination machinery used in meiosis and the HRR machinery used in mitosis. There are many common gene products essential to both processes. The apparent parallels in the machinery of recombination across meiosis and mitosis in eukaryotes, and even extending to the mechanism of transformation in bacteria suggests similarity of function, and this is what we seek to explain through the DNA repair hypothesis of meiosis.

In the yeast *S. cerevisiae*, mutations in a number of genes confer increased sensitivity to radiation and/or genotoxic chemicals, and also cause deficiency in meiotic recombination (Haynes and Kunz, 1981). As an example, studies of *rad52* mutants indicate that the *rad52* gene is necessary for meiotic recombination (Game et al., 1980), and for mitotic recombination (Malone and Esposito, 1980). Mutants defective in *rad52* have increased sensitivity to killing by X-rays, MMS and the crosslinking agent 8-methoxypsoralen-plus-UV light, and in addition have reduced meiotic recombination (Haynes and Kunz, 1981; Henriques and Moustacchi, 1980; Game et al., 1980).

In the nematode *Caenorhabditis elegans*, oocyte nuclei in the pachytene stage of meiosis (the stage in which recombination occurs) are hyper-resistant to X-rays compared to oocytes in diakinesis (a later stage of meiosis) or early embryonic cells after fertilization (Takanami et al., 2000). This pachytene hyper-resistance requires expression of gene *ce-rdh-51*, which is a homolog of yeast *rad51*, a key player in HRR. Furthermore, nuclei in the pachytene stage of meiosis have greater resistance to heavy ion particle irradiation than nuclei in the later diplotene and diakinesis stages and early embryonic cells (Takanami et al., 2003). Resistance during pachytene to heavy ion particle irradiation, like resistance to X-ray irradiation, depends on gene *ce-rdh-51*. This resistance also depends on gene *ce-atl-1*, which is related to gene *atm*, a gene necessary for repair of DSBs by HRR in mammals and for fertility in humans and mice (Table 1). Pachytene nuclei thus appear to effectively repair X-ray and heavy ion-induced DNA damage by meiotic HRR.

In the fruit fly *Drosophila melanogaster*, mutants defective in genes essential to the machinery of recombination (i.e. genes *mei-41*, *mei-9*, *hdm*, *spn* and *brca2*) have increased sensitivity to killing by a variety of DNA damaging agents, compared to wild-type flies. This sensitivity implies a reduced ability of somatic cells to carry out recombinational repair of the DNA damages caused by these agents. These same mutants have reduced recombination during meiosis compared to wild-type flies, indicating that they are deficient in recombination (presumably HRR) during meiosis. Specifically, mutations in the "meiotic genes" *mei-41* and *mei-9* cause increased sensitivity to several DNA damaging agents [X-rays, UV, methylmethane sulfonate (MMS), nitrogen mustard, benzo(s)pyrene and 2-acetyl-aminofluorene], and also have deficient meiotic recombination (Baker et al., 1976; Boyd, 1978; Rasmussen, 1984). Also, *D. melanogaster* mutants defective in genes needed for mitotic HRR (i.e. *hdm*, *DmRad51/spnA* and *brca2*) have increased sensitivity to X-rays and/or MMS, and are also deficient in meiotic recombination (Joyce et al., 2009; Staeva-Viera et al., 2003; Klovstad et al., 2008).

The repair of double-strand damages after γ-irradiation of rat spermatogenic cells was measured in sequential stages of formation of germ cells (Coogan and Rosenblum, 1988). These sequential stages were: spermatagonia and preleptotene spermatocytes, pachytene spermatocytes and spermatid spermatocytes. Pachytene spermatocytes, the meiotic stage in which recombination occurs, showed the greatest repair capability. Thus it appears that a function of meiosis (expressed specifically during the pachytene stage) is to repair double strand damages. The source of DNA damage that most likely provides a natural challenge to gamete formation is reactive (ROS) generated by active metabolism. Fisher and Aitkin (1997) showed that several germ cell stages in mammals, including pachytene spermatocytes, produce levels of ROSs sufficient to cause oxidative stress.

In the plant *A. thaliana*, *rad51* mutants are hypersensitive to the DNA cross-linking agent mitomycin C and are defective in meiotic recombination (Bleuyard and White, 2004; Bleuyard et al., 2005). In maize, mutants defective in orthologs of Rad51 produce embryos that are extremely susceptible to radiation induced DSBs, and are defective in meiosis (Li et al., 2007).

During Meiosis HRR Likely Removes a Class of DNA Damages that Cannot Be Accurately Removed during Mitosis

During meiosis, HRR potentially provides a unique advantage compared to HRR during mitosis. During meiosis, non-sister homologs systematically pair and undergo HRR, whereas during mitosis HRR is largely between sister-homologs and occurs between non-sister homologs in only about 1 in 100 HRR events (Moynahan and Jasin, 2010).

During mitosis, HRR largely involves interaction between the duplicate sister homologs resulting from DNA replication. Consequently, during mitosis, HRR is limited to the portions of the cell cycle in which DNA replication is occurring (S phase) and after DNA replication is complete (G2/M phase) so that a closely adjacent homologous chromosome would be available. Thus double-strand damages occurring during or after DNA replication may be accurately removed by HRR between sister homologs (Tichy et al., 2010). During the portion of the mitotic cell cycle after cell division but prior to DNA replication (G1 phase), double-strand damages, such as DSBs, are ordinarily not repaired by HRR, and are either repaired by an inaccurate process [non-homologous end-joining (NHEJ) that generates mutation] or the DSBs cause cell death. In contrast, during meiosis HRR can likely remove, in an accurate manner, double-strand damages that arise at any stage of the cell cycle because of systematic pairing of non-sister homologs. Cells in the meiotic G1 phase are more resistant to the lethal effects of X-rays than mitotic G1 cells (Kelley et al., 1983). This observation suggests that the types of DNA damage caused by X-rays, which includes DSBs, are more effectively repaired during meiotic G1 than mitotic G1. Thus repair capability in meiosis is likely more effective than during mitosis, since during meiosis HRR proteins are available at an increased level (Table 1) and there is more access to a homolog for the source of needed information to copy.

At each cell division in humans, 30,000 to 50,000 DNA replication origins are activated (Mechali et al., 2010). Consequently, the chromosome is replicated in segments. During meiosis, any segment containing a double-strand damage may fail to complete its replication until the damage is repaired. Such a temporary and limited blockage of replication may result directly from the damage itself or result from signaling by proteins that specifically bind to damaged regions of DNA. Once damage is recognized, HRR can remove the damage during the subsequent prophase I stage of meiosis, when the blocked segment becomes paired with a non-sister homolog. When the damage is removed, replication of the segment can be completed. Hence meiosis provides a means of accurately repairing a class of DNA damages that cannot be accurately repaired during mitosis.

What Are the Consequences of DNA Damages in the Mitotic Divisions Preceding Meiosis in the Germ Line of Multicellular Organisms?

Typically, in multicellular eukaryotes, there are numerous mitotic divisions in the germ line preceding meiosis and the formation of gametes. Double-strand damages occurring during or after DNA replication in the mitotic cells of the germ line can be repaired by HRR involving the two sister-chromosomes.

However, because the non-sister homologs present in a diploid cell ordinarily do not pair and undergo recombination during mitosis, double-strand damages occurring prior to replication are unlikely to be removed by HRR. Consequently when double-strand damages occur before DNA replication during the mitotic divisions in the germ line the result will either be increased mutation or increased apoptotic cell death.

It is likely that the preferred strategy for dealing with pre-replication double-strand damages during the mitotic divisions of the germ line will be apoptosis, since this avoids germ line mutations that could be passed on to progeny. This explanation is suggested by analogy to the behavior of mammalian embryonic stem (ES) cells. These cells use an apoptotic strategy for dealing with DNA damages occurring prior to DNA replication (Tichy et al., 2010). Clonal expansion of ES cells gives rise to all of the mammalian cell types. Since mutations occurring in early embryonic cells are passed on to all clonal descendents, they can be seriously deleterious to the organism as a whole.

Therefore, in ES cells, robust mechanisms are employed for reducing DNA damages and eliminating cells with DNA damage, in order to avoid mutations. Mouse ES cells mainly use high fidelity HRR to repair DSBs, in contrast to differentiated somatic cells that mainly use inaccurate NHEJ (Tichy et al., 2010). In addition, ES cells, upon receiving DNA damage prior to replication (G1 phase) do not undergo cell cycle arrest, but rather undergo apoptosis (Aladjem et al., 1998).

Mouse ES cells have a mutation frequency about 100-fold less than that of isogenic somatic cells (Cervantes et al., 2002). The lower mutation frequency likely reflects, in part, the apoptotic removal of G1 phase cells with DNA damage that would otherwise cause mutation. Thus, increased accuracy likely comes at the cost of somatic selection against cells with unrepaired DNA damages that arose prior to DNA replication. We consider it likely that a similar strategy is used during the mitotic divisions of the germ line preceding meiosis. In this case, the strategy of increased apoptosis in response to damage would substantially reduce transmission of mutations to gametes and progeny.

Crossover Hotspots in Meiosis

A statistical analysis of genetic variation in the human genome has identified about 25,000 hotspots for meiotic CO (Myers et al., 2006). On average, about one cross-over event occurs per 1,300 meioses per hotspot. The nature of hotspots is not well understood. Hotspots may represent sites vulnerable to DNA DSBs and/or DNA sequences that are recognized by a protein that specifically targets the sequence for CO. The number of endogenous DSBs present prior to meiosis is unknown, but Vilenchik and Knudson (2003) have estimated that the average number of endogenous DNA DSBs per somatic cell occurring at each cell generation is about 50, so that a number in this range may apply to pre-meiotic cells. Hochwagen and Marals (2010) have described a DNA-binding protein, PRDM9, which recognizes certain 13-mer sequences characteristic of some hotspots and may determine CO location. In the DHJ model the site of the actual CO (resolution of a Holliday junction) can be distant from the site of the initiating DSB [as indicated by the size of gene conversion tracts during meiosis which are hundreds to thousands of nucleotide pairs long (Judd and Petes, 1988)]. Thus hotspots may occur upstream or downstream of DSBs at sequences that favor Holliday junction resolution.

Evolutionary Forces Maintaining Sex

In this section we present evidence that it is the short-term benefit of DNA repair, rather than the potential long-term benefits of genetic variation, that maintains sex. Explanations for the evolutionary maintenance of sex are often based on the assumption that the main adaptive advantage of sex is the production of genetic variation. This is an active area of research, and a variety of models and reviews have been presented based on this assumption (e.g. Barton and Charlesworth, 1998; Otto and Gerstein, 2006; Agrawal, 2006). However, it has also been noted by Otto and Gerstein (2006) that individuals surviving to reproductive age in a fairly stable environment have genomes that function well in that environment. They ask, why should such individuals risk shuffling their genes with those of another individual? This question and other similar considerations, have led many investigators to doubt that production of genetic diversity is the principal adaptive benefit of sex.

In contrast to the conventional view that sex increases genetic diversity, Heng (2007) and Gorelick and Heng (2011) have reviewed evidence that sex actually decreases most genetic variation. These authors consider that sex acts as a coarse filter, weeding out major genetic changes, such as chromosomal rearrangements, but permitting minor variation, such as changes at the nucleotide or gene level (that often are neutral) to pass through the sexual sieve. Thus they consider that sex acts as a constraint on genomic variation.

It is generally acknowledged that any explanation for the adaptive benefit of sex, to be plausible, must provide benefits that balance the costs of sex. Such costs vary from species to species, depending on the life-style of the organism. However, certain general large costs are widely recognized. These include the "cost of males" (Maynard Smith, 1978; Williams, 1975), the "recombinational load" that is a consequence of the randomization of genetic information during sex and break-up of coadapted gene complexes (Shields, 1982), the cost of finding a mate (Bernstein et al., 1985b), and the cost of sexually transmitted disease

(Michod et al., 2008). These costs apply most strongly to diploid, obligate sexual species. HRR during meiosis, we think, provides an appropriate explanation for the adaptive maintenance of sex (and meiosis), since the benefits are large enough (removal of DNA damages that would otherwise be deleterious/lethal to gametes or progeny) to plausibly balance the large immediate costs of sex.

Furthermore, the explanation that meiosis is an adaptation for repair of DNA damage can be consistently applied to all organisms that undergo meiosis including facultative sexual organisms (as described above), or to species that undergo meiosis but have little or no outcrossing (see below in this section). A number of authors have proposed that the genetic variation produced by sex increases the rate of adaptation (Colegrave et al., 2002; Kaltz and Bell, 2002; Peters and Otto, 2003; Goddard et al., 2005; Cooper et al., 2005; deVisser and Elena, 2007). We consider, however, that genetic variation is a byproduct of HRR and that any long-term benefit of variation would supplement the benefit of DNA repair. We think that, in the short-term, the benefit of variation, by itself, generally would be inadequate to maintain sex in the face of the large costs identified for sex.

Organisms that undergo meiosis, but experience little, or no, outcrossing sex are common in nature. In such cases, recombination produces little, if any, genetic variation among progeny. The budding yeast *S. cerevisiae* appears to outcross very infrequently in nature, although inbreeding sex is frequent. Ruderfer et al. (2006) analyzed the ancestry of natural *S. cerevisiae* strains and concluded that outcrossing occurs about once every 50,000 cell divisions. In contrast, mating between closely related yeast cells is much more common in nature. Mating can happen when haploid yeast cells of opposite mating types, MATa and MATα, contact each other. Ruderfer et al. (2006) and Zeyl and Otto (2007) noted that there are two reasons why mating between closely related *S. cerevisiae* cells is frequent in nature. First, cells of opposite mating type from the same ascus (the sac that holds the cells produced from a single meiosis) are in close proximity. Second, *S. cerevisiae* is capable of homothallism, the ability of haploid cells of one mating type to produce daughter cells of the opposite mating type. Thus, under natural conditions, meiotic events in *S. cerevisiae* that produce little or no recombinational variation are likely far more common than meiotic events that do produce recombinational variation. The relative rarity of outcrossing sex is consistent with the concept that the main adaptive function of meiosis in *S. cerevisiae* is HRR of DNA damages, since this benefit is realized whether meiosis results from inbreeding or outcrossing. If, as is often assumed, the primary adaptive benefit of meiosis is to produce genetic variation, it is difficult to understand how meiosis, a complex process, could be selectively maintained during the 50,000 generations of *S. cerevisiae* in which outcrossing is absent.

Outcrossing sexual reproduction is the most frequent type of reproduction in higher plants. However about 15% of plants undergo meiosis, but are principally self-fertilizing (Bernstein and Bernstein, 1991).

Among vertebrates, one extreme but well studied example of inbreeding is the Mangrove Killifish, *Kryptolebias marmoratus*. This fish occupies brackish water mangrove habitats from Florida to Brazil. It produces eggs and sperm by meiosis and reproduces routinely by self-fertilization. Normally each hermaphroditic individual fertilizes itself when an egg and sperm that are formed by an internal organ unite inside the body of the fish (Sakakura et al., 2006; see Avise, 2008, for review).

The examples reviewed in this section indicate that meiosis often occurs in circumstances that generate little, if any, genetic variation, suggesting that meiosis is maintained by another adaptive benefit, such as the benefit of DNA repair.

Benefits of Outcrossing Sex

The essential feature of sex common to both bacteria and eukaryotes is information exchange between two genomic DNA molecules derived from different individuals. These different individuals (parents) can be closely or distantly related to each other. Above, we discussed some examples of mating between closely related individuals (inbreeding). These examples were discussed to illustrate our argument that meiosis provides a benefit (accurate DNA repair) that is independent of whether significant recombinational variation is also generated. However, meiosis is frequently associated with mating between unrelated or distantly related individuals (outcrossing). We now consider when outcrossing and inbreeding are advantageous.

In predominantly haploid organisms such as bacteria and many unicellular eukaryotes, a simple explanation can be offered for why mating occurs. It serves to create the transient diploid (or partially diploid) state necessary for HRR. It is unclear how frequently outcrossing (vs. inbreeding) occurs in nature in predominantly haploid sexual organisms. In the case of *S. cerevisiae*, as discussed above, evidence indicates that outcrossing is uncommon, whereas mating between related individuals is common (Ruderfer et al., 2006). This is probably also the case for bacteria, where transformation in nature likely most often occurs between clonally related individuals.

Outcrossing sex appears to be preferred in organisms in which diploid cells are the predominant feature of their life cycle. A benefit of diploidy, in contrast to haploidy, is that diploidy allows the masking of recessive deleterious mutations. This masking effect is referred to as "genetic complementation." Once outcrossing is employed because of the benefit of complementation, switching to inbreeding becomes disadvantageous because it leads to expression of the (previously masked) deleterious recessive mutations, resulting in inbreeding depression. This idea has a long history. Charles Darwin (1889), in his book "The Effects of Cross and Self-Fertilization in the Vegetable Kingdom", arrived at clear and definite conclusions concerning the adaptive benefit of outcrossing sex. For example, on page 462 he stated that "the offspring from the union of two distinct individuals, especially if their progenitors have been subjected to very different conditions, have an immense advantage in height, weight, constitutional vigor and fertility over the self-fertilizing offspring from either one of the same parents." He thought that this fact was amply sufficient to account for outcrossing sexual reproduction.

Another possible beneficial consequence proposed for outcrossing is the generation of new genetic variants that may provide a long-term advantage (e.g. Colegrave et al., 2002; Kaltz and Bell, 2002; Peters and Otto, 2003; Goddard et al., 2005; Cooper et al., 2005; deVisser and Elena, 2007).

An analysis of the consequences of genetic complementation indicated that complementation provides a sufficient benefit to maintain outcrossing (Bernstein et al., 1985a; 1987; Michod, 1994). However, recently, more explicit population genetic models have raised some issues concerning this idea. From a population genetics perspective, the basic consequence of outcrossing is to bring populations to Hardy-Weinberg (HW) equilibrium. Consequently, outcrossing can be beneficial under conditions where it is advantageous for a population to go closer to HW equilibrium, and if there is another condition pushing the population away from HW equilibrium, i.e. generating either a deficit or an excess of heterozygotes. Roze and Michod (2010) considered gene conversion to be a potential force pushing away from HW equilibrium, since gene conversion can generate homozygosity. Gene conversion can result from mitotic HRR between non-sister chromosomes. It was concluded that, if deleterious alleles tend to be partially recessive, outcrossing is advantageous in the short-term because it masks deleterious recessive alleles, but disadvantageous in the long-term because purging of deleterious recessive alleles is less efficient. The rate of loss of heterozygosity from gene conversion events during development was a critical parameter in the model determining the outcome of selection on outcrossing. Unfortunately, there is not much data available, but the data reviewed by Roze and Michod (2010) suggests that the loss of heterozygosity may be low which means weak selection for outcrossing.

Aging, Sex and Rejuvenation

Many, if not all, eukaryotes age, yet age-associated changes are not passed on to progeny. Over a century ago, Weismann (1892) commented that among his contemporaries, a widely held view was that the adaptive benefit of sex is rejuvenation (although he did not agree with this view himself). Supporting the rejuvenation concept was the observation that, in some protozoans, vitality declines during the course of successive asexual cell divisions by binary fission, but following sexual interaction (conjugation) vitality is restored. Here we review evidence that lifespan is reset from one generation to the next (rejuvenation) at the time of meiosis, and that this rejuvenation is a consequence, in part, of removal of DNA damages.

The ciliate protozoan *Paramecium tetraurelia* has a diploid micronucleus and a polyploid macronucleus that contains about 800 to 1500 copies of the genome. The micronucleus contains the germline DNA, whereas the macronuclear DNA expresses cellular functions. *P. tetraurelia* is facultatively sexual and can reproduce either by binary fission or by a meiotic process. For *P. tetraurelia* there are two kinds of meiotic process. The first is conjugation, a kind of outcrossing sex. The second is automixis, similar to self-fertilization. In the asexual fission phase, during which cell divisions occur by mitosis rather than meiosis, there is clonal aging, a gradual loss of vitality. An asexual line of clonally aging paramecia will lose vitality and die out after about 200 fissions if it fails to undergo automixis or conjugation.

The cause of clonal aging in *P. tetraurelia* was clarified by transplantation experiments (Aufderheide, 1987). When macronuclei of clonally young paramecia were injected into paramecia of a standard clonal age, the lifespan of the recipient was prolonged. In contrast, transfer of cytoplasm from young paramecia did not prolong the lifespan of the recipient. These experiments suggested that the macronucleus, rather than the cytoplasm, governs clonal aging. Further experiments by Smith-Sonneborn (1979), Holmes and Holmes (1986) and Gilley and Blackburn (1994) showed that, during clonal aging, DNA damage increases dramatically. When clonally aged paramecia are permitted to undergo meiosis, in association with either conjugation or automixis, the progeny are rejuvenated. Furthermore, during these processes, the old macronucleus disintegrates and a new macronucleus is formed by replication of the micronuclear DNA, the DNA that had recently undergone meiosis. There is little, if any, DNA damage in the new macronucleus. These observations suggest that clonal aging is due, in large part, to a progressive increase in DNA damage; and rejuvenation is due to repair of these DNA damages in the micronucleus during meiosis and the reconstitution of the macronucleus by replication of the repaired micronuclear DNA.

In cells of the budding yeast *S. cerevisiae*, mother cells experience replicative aging and death. However, when these cells undergo meiosis and gametogenesis, lifespan is reset (Unal et al., 2011). Gametes (spores) formed by aged cells show the same replicative potential as gametes generated by young cells, and age-associated damage is no longer detectable in the gametes. However in this system, it has not yet been determined if removal of DNA damage during meiosis contributes to the observed rejuvenation.

Parthenogenesis

Parthenogenesis is the development of an individual from an egg without fertilization. In the animal kingdom there are over a million sexual species compared to less than a thousand parthenogenetic species (White, 1973). That is, less than 0.1% of animal species are parthenogenetic, suggesting that parthenogenesis is not a generally successful strategy. The relatively brief evolutionary persistence of most parthenogenic groups is apparent from their lack of high taxonomic rank, and from the low DNA sequence divergence from their nearest sexual relatives

Among vertebrates, some of the most successful and conspicuous animal parthenogens undergo a process called "endomitosis." By this process, there are two sequential pre-meiotic chromosome replications, followed by an apparently normal meiosis resulting in production of diploid eggs (Avise, 2008). The extra chromosome duplication is designated "endomitotic" doubling. Recombination at meiosis in these parthenogens involves pairing between chromosomes derived by replication from the same progenitor chromosome. Unlike meiosis in a sexual species, recombination between non-sister chromosomes is unavailable. One well-studied organism that employs endomitosis is a common type of whiptail lizard (genus *Aspidoscells*) found in the southwestern United States. Other examples of endomitosis have been described among taxa of fish, salamanders, grasshoppers, earthworms, planarians and beetles. Because recombination between non-sister homologous chromosomes is lacking, the maternal genome is passed on intact to daughters. Parthenogenesis by endomitosis might appear to be an ideal strategy, since it provides the benefit of meiotic HRR, while avoiding expression of deleterious recessive alleles. This consideration raises the question of why parthenogenesis, involving endomitosis, does not predominate over sexual reproduction. The answer may be that double-strand damages occurring prior to the first pre-meiotic replication (G1 phase) would be difficult to accurately repair in this form of parthenogenesis. All pairing partners (closely adjacent sister chromosomes) are derived from the same initial chromosome, and if this chromosome had a double-strand damage, there is little opportunity for it to pair with an intact closely neighboring template corresponding to the damaged site. This problem does not occur in ordinary meiosis because systematic pairing and HRR occur between non-sister chromosomes. Thus if double-strand damages are common prior to replication, during the G1 phase of meiosis, parthenogenesis by endomitosis is an unsatisfactory option.

Avise (2008), in reviewing the comparative ecologies of vertebrate parthenogens and sexual reproducers, concluded that some parthenogenetic biotypes can be highly successful in the short or moderate term, but such ecological success does not continue indefinitely, as judged by the fact that no parthenogenetic lineage in vertebrates is demonstrably ancient. This lack of long-term success may reflect the observed reduced fecundity of parthenogens compared to their sexual relatives, in many cases less than 50% (Lynch, 1984).

Another parthenogenetic strategy, employed in plants and invertebrates, is automixis, which involves meiosis followed by fusion of haploid nuclei from the same parent. This is genetically similar to self-fertilization and allows expression of deleterious recessive alleles. Still another common parthenogenetic strategy, especially in plants, is apomixis, an oogenic process that is entirely mitotic, that is, without hints or vestiges of meiosis-type events. An analysis of advantages versus costs of switching from outcrossing sexual reproduction to the various forms of parthenogenesis (endomitosis, automixis and apomixis) led to the conclusion that these alternatives will not generally be favored, except when the costs of outcrossing sex are high (Bernstein et al., 1985a; 1987; 1989). Comparisons of sexual species to related parthenogens, with respect to geographical and ecological correlates, indicate that parthenogens tend to occur where population densities are low (and finding a mate would be very costly) (reviewed in Bernstein et al., 1985b).

Among invertebrates, one exceptional parthenogentic class, the bdelloid rotifers, are thought to have remained asexual for more than 40 million years (Mark Welch and Meselson, 2000). Bdelloid rotifers produce eggs by mitosis, rather than meiosis. Bdelloid rotifers are extraordinarily resistant to ionizing radiation (Gladyshev and Meselson, 2008). This resistance is likely a consequence of an evolutionary adaptation to survive desiccation in temporary pools of water. Desiccation of the rotifers causes considerable DNA breakage, which they can repair. Bdelloid primary oocytes are in the G1 phase of the cell cycle so that sister chromosomes are lacking. MarkWelch et al. (2008) proposed that interaction of non-sister co-linear chromosome pairs provides a mechanism of DNA repair; and that these co-linear chromosome pairs are maintained by natural selection as templates for repair of DSBs caused by frequent desiccation and rehydration. Although lacking sex and meiosis, Bdelloid rotifers appear to retain an essential feature of meiosis, HRR between non-sister homologs.

One can ask why is this not a general strategy for life on earth, and why instead is sex the general strategy with its accompanying costs of outcrossing? We offer the following speculation. Since bdelloid rotifers typically inhabit small transient pools of water, they may often find themselves in pools with no other, or only a few other individuals. Thus finding a mate may often be impossible or very difficult and costly. This condition would tend to select for a parthenogenetic strategy. Furthermore, because bdelloid rotifers are "degenerate tetraploids" (Mark Welch et al., 2008), they may be able to avoid a major cost of producing eggs by mitosis instead of meiosis. If bdelloid cells were only diploid, then recombination between non-sister homologs during the mitotic divisions that produce eggs would generate homozygosity, and hence expression of deleterious recessive alleles. Such a strategy would select against this mode of parthenogenesis and favor a switch to sex. However, because bdelloid rotifers are not diploid, but rather degenerate tetraploids, recombination between non-sister chromosomes leading to homozygosity for one pair of homologs may not ordinarily lead to expression of deleterious recessive mutations due to masking by the second pair of homologs. Thus parthenogenesis in bdelloid rotifers may be a uniquely successful parthenogenetic strategy because of two features specific to the species, a small transient habitat causing a high cost of mating, and degenerate tetraploidy allowing more effective masking of deleterious recessive alleles. This strategy may not be generally advantageous as an alternative to sex because of the costs of maintaining tetraploidy compared to the costs of maintaining diploidy.

Conclusion

DNA damage, particularly oxidative DNA damage, appears to be a ubiquitous problem for organisms. We have summarized evidence bearing on the hypothesis that sex is an adaptation for repairing DNA damage that if unrepaired would cause mutation or inviability. We also reviewed evidence that sex has been maintained by this adaptive benefit throughout evolution in bacteria, simple unicellular eukaryotes and complex multicellular eukaryotes. In bacteria, transformation involves transfer of DNA from one bacterial cell to another and appears to be a primitive form of sex. Since competence for transformation is a complex developmental process dependent on expression of many bacterial genes, it appears to be an adaptation that strongly benefits the bacteria. Development of competence for transformation ordinarily occurs under stressful environmental conditions such as high cell density and nutritional limitation. These are conditions in which DNA damage may be expected. Experiments with several different bacterial transformation systems indicate that transformation is a response to DNA damage, and that it serves to repair DNA by the process of homologous recombinational repair (HRR).

Eukaryotes evolved from bacteria (prokaryotes). As indicated by recent evidence, sexual reproduction was present very early in the evolution of eukaryotes, and sex in eukaryotes likely evolved from ancestral prokaryotic sex. The sexual cycle in eukaryotic microorganisms is facultative and tends to occur under stressful environmental conditions, similar to the conditions that induce sex (competence for transformation) in bacteria. Experiments with a wide variety of different facultatively sexual unicellular or simple multicellular eukaryotes suggest that the sexual cycle is induced by DNA damage. Thus sex may have been retained through the prokaryotic to eukaryotic transition as an adaptation for repairing DNA damage. There are fundamental similarities in the processes employed in bacterial and eukaryotic sex. Both involve the coming together of genomes from two individuals (parents) in a common cytoplasm, the formation of a DNA-RecA (or ortholog) nucleofilament, pairing of homologous regions of the two parental genomes, exchange of information between the genomes (recombination), and passage of the new recombined genomes to progeny.

A characteristic key molecular feature common to recombination in prokaryotes and eukaryotes is the role of the RecA protein and its orthologs in catalyzing the strand invasion step of recombination during transformation and meiosis. RecA protein interacts with DNA to form striking nucleoprotein filaments that scan the partner chromosome for regions of homology. This brings the invading DNA strand to the corresponding site in the partner chromosome where informational exchange occurs. Analysis of the molecular interactions of RecA protein indicates that RecA is the central component of an HRR system for dealing with DNA damage. This basic function of RecA and its orthologs appears to have been maintained through the evolutionary transitions from transformation in bacteria to meiosis in unicellular and simple multicellular eukaryotes, and then to meiosis in higher animals and plants. Experimental exposure of several different eukaryotes to a variety of DNA damaging agents was observed to increase meiotic recombination, consistent with the idea that meiotic recombination is a DNA repair process.

Current molecular models of meiotic recombination assume that an early event is a double-strand break or gap in one of the two pairing chromosomes. The double-strand break may be a direct result of action of a DNA damaging agent, or it may be formed secondarily (e.g. as part of the process of removing another type of damage such as an inter-strand crosslink). During the repair process, two types of recombination event may arise; one in which the chromosome arms flanking the break are exchanged between pairing partners [called a crossover (CO)], and one in which the flanking arms are not exchanged [called a non-crossover (NCO)]. Both the CO and NCO types of recombination are effective repair processes. Evidence indicates that during meiosis the NCO type of recombination is more frequent than the CO type. This observation seems inconsistent with the hypothesis that meiotic recombination is primarily an adaptation for generating genetic diversity, since the NCO type of recombination generates little genetic variation compared to the CO type. The CO and NCO types of recombination arise by different pathways. The CO type arises by a pathway involving two Holliday junctions and the physical exchange of DNA segments. This pathway is referred to as the Double-Holliday Junction (DHJ) pathway. The NCO type arises by a pathway involving transfer of sequence information without physical exchange of DNA. The latter pathway is referred to as the Synthesis Dependent Strand Annealing (SDSA) pathway. The DHJ pathway appears to function during meiosis in three processes: DNA repair, promotion of pairing between non-sister homologous chromosomes, and in causing genetic diversity. The SDSA pathway, the more frequent meiotic pathway, appears to be employed primarily in DNA repair.

Infertility and loss of conceptions appears to be common in animals and plants. Oxidative stress may be an important source of DNA damage during gametogenesis. In humans and mice, mutations in enzymes necessary for recombinational repair cause loss of fertility, suggesting that meiotic HRR is essential for the effective production of functional eggs and sperm. DNA damages caused by a variety of known DNA damaging agents are repaired during mitosis by HRR (between sister homologous chromosomes), and even more effectively during meiosis (by HRR between both sister- and non-sister homologous chromosomes). The HRR processes in meiosis and mitosis seems to be similar in that they employ similar gene products.

During mitosis, double-strand damages can be accurately removed by HRR if they occur after DNA replication when two sister chromosomes are present and adjacent. Because non-sister chromosomes do not ordinarily pair in diploid somatic cells, accurate repair of double-strand damages occurring before replication is not usually possible. However, during meiosis there is systematic pairing of non-sister homologs so that double-strand damages occurring prior to replication may be accurately repaired. Thus a potentially lethal class of DNA damages, that cannot be accurately removed during mitosis, may be accurately removed during meiosis. In multicellular eukaryotes there are typically numerous mitotic cell divisions in the germ line prior to the single meiotic division leading to gamete formation. Double-strand damages occurring subsequent to DNA replication in these mitotic cells can be accurately repaired by HRR between sister-chromosomes. Prior to DNA replication in mitotically dividing cells of the germ line, double-strand damages likely cause programmed cell death (apoptosis). This would avoid the possibility of inaccurate repair of such damages, which would otherwise cause mutations in the germ line that could be passed on to gametes and then to progeny.

The essential characteristic of sex in both bacteria and eukaryotes is recombination associated with mating between different individuals. Mating can be between closely related individuals (inbreeding) or distantly related individuals (outcrossing). Both types of mating provide the benefit of HRR. However, in those eukaryotes whose diploid stage of the life cycle is predominant, as in humans, masking of deleterious recessive mutations also provides a benefit. This benefit, referred to as "genetic complementation" (also "hybrid vigor"), is likely the immediate selective benefit that maintains outcrossing since a switch to inbreeding will cause the expression of the deleterious recessive mutations previously masked (inbreeding depression).

Outcrossing sex also produces genetic variation. This variation may provide long-term benefits to a population, as proposed by numerous investigators. However, in many sexual species, outcrossing (sex between distantly related individuals) is much less frequent than inbreeding (sex between closely related individuals). Such observations suggest that it is not the possible long-term benefits of outcrossing (increased diversity) that generally maintains sex from one generation to the next, but rather the short-term benefit of DNA repair (due to both CO and NCO HRR).

Parthenogenesis is the development of an individual from an unfertilized egg. Parthenogenesis is not a generally successful strategy. It occurs in less than 0.1% of animal species, and parthenogenetic lineages are ordinarily not long-lasting. It appears that parthenogenetic strategies are favored over the sexual strategy when the costs of mating are unusually high, such as under environmental conditions that only allow low population density, when finding a mate is very difficult. Parthenogenetic strategies appear to suffer the disadvantages of inadequate HRR during meiosis or inadequate masking of deleterious recessive mutations. In conclusion, we consider that the preponderance of evidence supports the idea that sex arose as an adaptation for repairing DNA damage and that this has remained the primary adaptive benefit of sex throughout the evolution from bacteria to unicellular eukaryotes, and then to complex multicellular eukaryotes, such as mammals.

Acknowledgments

This work was supported in part by grants NIH 5 R01 CA119087, Arizona Biomedical Research Commission Grant #0803, VA Merit Review Grant 0142 of the Southern Arizona Veterans Affairs Health Care System and NSF DEB-0742383. We also thank Michael Berman for his helpful critical comments on the manuscript.

References

Achanta, G; Huang, P. Role of p53 in sensing oxidative DNA damage in response to reactive oxygen species-generating agents. *Cancer Research*, 2004, 64(17), 6233-6239.

Agrawal, AF. Evolution of sex: why do organisms shuffle their genotypes? *Current Biology*, 2006, 16, R696-R704.

Akamatsu, T; Taguchi, H. Incorporation of the whole chromosomal DNA in protoplast lysates into competent cells of *Bacillus subtilis*. *Bioscience, Biotechnology, and Biochemistry*, 2001, 65(4), 823-829.

Akopyants, NS; Kimblin, N; Secundino, N; Patrick, R; Peters, N; Lawyer, P; Dobson, DE; Beverley, SM; Sacks, DL. Demonstration of genetic exchange during cyclical development of *Leishmania* in the sand fly vector. *Science*, 2009, 324, 265-268.

Aladjem, MI; Spike, BT; Rodewald, LE; Hope, TJ; Klemm, M; Jaenisch, R; Wald, GM. ES cells do not activate p53-dependent stress responses and undergo p53-independent apoptosis in response to DNA damage. *Current Biology*, 1998, 8, 145-155.

Albertini, S; Chetelat, AA; Miller, B; Muster, W; Pujadas, E; Strobel, R; Gocke, E. Genotoxicity of 17 gyrase - and four mammalian topoisomerase II - poisons in prokaryotic and eukaryotic test systems. *Mutagenesis*, 1995, 10(4), 343-351.

Allers, T; Lichten, M. Differential timing and control of noncrossover and crossover recombination during meiosis. *Cell*, 2001, 106, 47-57.

Ames, BN: Shigenaga, MK; Hagen, TM. Oxidants, antioxidants, and degenerative diseases of aging. *Proceedings of the National Academy of Sciences USA*, 1993, 90, 7915-7922.

Anagnostopoulos, C; Spizizen, J. Requirements for transformation in *Bacillus subtilis*, *Journal of Bacteriology*, 1961, 81, 741-746.

Andersen, SL; Sekelsky, J. Meiotic versus mitotic recombination: two different routes for double-strand break repair. *Bioessays*, 2010, 32, 1058-1066.

Aspiras, MB; Ellen, RP; Cvitkovitch, DG. ComX activity of *Streptococcus mutans* growing in biofilms. *FEMS Microbiology Letters*, 2004, 238, 167-174.

Aufderheide, KJ. Clonal aging in *Paramecium tetraurelia*. II. Evidence of functional changes in the macronucleus with age. *Mechanisms of Ageing and Development*, 1987, 37, 265-279.

Avise, JC. Clonality: The genetics, ecology and evolution of sexual abstinence in vertebrate animals. New York, NY: Oxford University Press; 2008.

Austin, CR. Pregnancy losses and birth defects. In: Austin, CR; Short, RV, editors. *Reproduction in Mammals*. Book 2, Chapter 5, London: Cambridge University Press, 1972, 134.

Baker, BS; Boyd, JB; Carpenter, ATC; Green, MM; Nguyen, TD; Ripoll, P; Smith, PD. Genetic controls of meiotic recombination and somatic DNA metabolism in *Drosophila melanogaster*. *Proceedings of the National Academy of Sciences USA*, 1976, 73(11), 4140-4144.

Barlow, C; Liyanage, M; Moens, PB; Tarsounas, M; Nagashima, K; Brown, K; Rottinghaus, S; Jackson, SP; Tagle, D; Ried, T; Wynshaw-Boris, A. Atm deficiency results in severe meiotic disruption as early as leptonema of prophase I. *Development*, 1998, 125, 4007-4017.

Barton, NH; Charlesworth, B. Why sex and recombination? *Science*, 1998, 281, 1986-1990.

Bawa, KS; Webb, CJ. Flower, fruit and seed abortion in tropical forest trees. Implications for the evolution of paternal and maternal reproductive patterns. *American Journal of Botany*, 1984, 71(5), 736-751.

Bernstein, C; Johns,V. Sexual reproduction as a response to H_2O_2 damage in *Schizosaccharomyces pombe*. *Journal of Bacteriology*, 1989, 171(4), 1893-1897.

Bernstein, C; Bernstein, H. *Aging, Sex and DNA Repair*. San Diego: Academic Press, 1991.

Bernstein, C; Bernstein, H; Payne, CM; Garewal, H. DNA repair/pro-apoptotic dual-role proteins in five major DNA repair pathways: fail-safe protection against carcinogenesis. *Mutation Research*, 2002, 571, 145-178.

Bernstein, H; Byerly, HC; Hopf, FA; Michod, RE. Genetic damage, mutation and the evolution of sex. *Science*, 1985a, 229, 1277-1281.

Bernstein, H; Byerly, HC; Hopf, FA; Michod, RE. Sex and the emergence of species. *Journal of Theoretical Biology*, 1985b, 117, 665-690.

Bernstein, H; Hopf, FA; Michod, RE. The molecular basis of the evolution of sex. *Advances in Genetics*, 1987, 24, 323-370.

Bernstein, H; Hopf, FA; Michod, RE. The evolution of sex: DNA repair hypothesis. In: Rasa, AE; Vogel, C; Voland, E., editors. *The Sociobiology of Sexual and Reproductive Strategies*. New York, NY: Chapman and Hall, 1989, 3-18.

Bernstein H; Bernstein, C. Evolutionary origin of recombination during meiosis. *BioScience*, 2010, 60 (7), 498-505.

Bleuyard, JY; White CI. The Arabidopsis homologue of Xrcc3 plays an essential role in meiosis. *The EMBO Journal*, 2004, 23, 439-449.

Bleuyard, JY; Gallego, ME; Savigny, F; White CI. Differing requirements for the Arabidopsis Rad51 paralogs in meiosis and DNA repair. *The Plant Journal*, 2005, 41, 533-545.

Boyd, JB. DNA repair in *Drosophila*. In: Hanawalt, PC; Friedberg, EC; Fox, CF, editors. *DNA Repair Mechanisms*. New York: Academic Press; 1978, 449-452.

Bray, CM; West, CE. DNA repair mechanisms in plants: crucial sensors and effectors for the maintenance of genome integrity. *New Phytology*, 2005, 168(3), 511-528.

Bugreev, DV; Golub, EI; Stasiak,A; Mazin, AV. Activation of human meiosis-specific recombinase Dmc1 by Ca^{2+}. *Journal of Biological Chemistry*, 2005, 280(29) , 26886-26895.

Bugreev, DV; Pezza, RJ; Mazina, OM; Voloshin, ON; Camerini-Otero, RD; Mazin, AV. The resistance of DMC1 D-loops to dissociation may account for the DMC1 requirement in meiosis. *Nature Structural and Molecular Biology*, 2011, 18(1), 56-61.

Cervantes, RB; Stringer, JR; Shao, C; Tischfield, JA; Stambrook, PJ. Embryonic stem cells and somatic cells differ in mutation frequency and type. *Proceedings of the National Academy of Sciences USA*, 2002, 99(6), 3586-3590.

Charpentier, X; Kay, E; Schneider, D; Shuman, HA. Antibiotics and UV radiation induce competence for natural transformation in *Legionella pneumophila*. *Journal of Bacteriology*, 2011, 193 (5), 1114-1121.

Cheah, KSE; Osborne, DJ. DNA lesions occur with loss of viability in embryos of ageing rye seed. *Nature*, 1978, 272, 593-599.

Chen, I; Dubnau, D. DNA uptake during bacterial transformation. *Nature Reviews/Microbiology*, 2004, 2, 241-249.

Cheo, DL; Bayles, KW; Yasbin, RE. Molecular characterization of regulatory elements controlling expression of the *Bacillus subtilis recA*$^{+}$ gene. *Biochimie* 1992, 74, 755-762.

Chlamygenome. Chlamygenome. In http://genome.jgi-psf.org/Chlre3/Chlre3.home.html [electronic mail system]. 2007.

Chovnick, A; Ballantyne GH; Baillie, DL; Holm, DG. Gene conversion in higher organisms: half-tetrad analysis of recombination within the rosy cistron of *Drosophila melanogaster*. *Genetics*, 1970, 66, 315-329.

Claverys, JP; Prudhomme, M; Martin, B. Induction of competence regulons as a general response to stress in gram-positive bacteria. *Annual Review of Microbiology* 2006, 60, 451-475.

Claverys, JP; Martin, B; Polard, P. The genetic transformation machinery: composition, localization and mechanism. *FEMS Microbiology Reviews*, 2009, 33, 643-656.

Colegrave, N; Kaltz, O; Bell, G. The ecology and genetics of fitness in *Chlamydomonas*. VIII. The dynamics of adaptation to novel environments after a single episode of sex. *Evolution*, 2002, 56(1), 14-21.

Coogan, TP; Rosenblum, IY. DNA double-strand damage and repair following γ-irradiation in isolated spermatogenic cells. *Mutation Research*, 1988, 194, 183-191.

Cooper, MA; Adam, RD, Worobey, M; Sterling, CR. Population genetics provides evidence for recombination in *Giardia*. *Current Biology*, 2007, 17, 1984-1988.

Cooper, TF; Lenski, RE; Elena, SP. Parasites and mutational load: an experimental test of a pluralistic theory for the evolution of sex. *Proceedings of the Royal Society B*, 2005, 272, 311-317.

Couteau, F; Belzile, F; Horlow, C; Grandjean, O; Vezon, D; Doutriaux, MP. Random chromosome segregation without meiotic arrest in both male and female meiocytes of a d*mc1* mutant of *Arabidopsis*. *The Plant Cell*, 1999, 11, 1623-1634.

Cox, MM. The RecA protein as a recombinational repair system. *Molecular Microbiology*, 1991, 5(6), 1295-1299.

Cox, MM. Relating biochemistry to biology: How the recombinational repair function of RecA protein is manifested in its molecular properties. *BioEssays*, 1993, 15(9), 617-623.

Cox, MM. The nonmutagenic repair of broken replication forks via recombination. *Mutation Research*, 2002, 510, 107-120.

Cressman, VL; Backlund, DC; Avrutskaya, AV; Leadon, SA; Godfrey, V; Koller, BH. Growth retardation, DNA repair defects, and lack of spermatogenesis in BRCA1-deficient mice. *Molecular and Cellular Biology*, 1999, 19(10), 7061-7075.

Dacks, J; Roger, AJ. The first sexual lineage and the relevance of facultative sex. *Journal of Molecular Evolution*, 1999, 48, 779-783.

Darwin, C. The Effects of Cross and Self Fertilization in the Vegetable Kingdom. New York: D. Appleton and Co; 1889.

Davey, J. Fusion of a fission yeast. *Yeast*, 1998, 14, 1529-1566.

Deng, ZY; Wang,T. *OsDMC1* is required for homologous pairing in *Oryza sativa*. *Plant Molecular Biology*, 2007, 65, 31-42.

DeVisser, JA; Elena, SF. The evolution of sex: empirical insights into the roles of epistasis and drift. *Nature Reviews/Genetics*, 2007, 8, 139-149.

Dorer, MS; Fero, J; Salama, NR. DNA damage triggers genetic exchange in *Helicobacter pylori*. *PloS Pathogens*, 2010, 6(7), 1-10, e1001026.

Dubnau, D; Davidoff-Abelson R; Scher, B; Cirigliano, C. Fate of transforming deoxyribonucleic acid after uptake by competent *Bacillus subtilis*: phenotypic characterization of radiation-sensitive recombination-deficient mutants. *Journal of Bacteriology*, 1973, 114(1), 273-286.

Elliott, AM; Hayes RE. Mating types in tetrahymena. *Biological Bulletin*, 1953, 105, 269-284.

Fisher, HM; Aitken, RJ. Comparative analysis of the ability of precursor germ cells and epididymal spermatozoa to generate reactive oxygen metabolites. *The Journal of Experimental Zoology*, 1997, 277, 390-400.

Galetzka, D; Weis, E; Kohlschmidt, N; Bitz, O; Stein, R; Haaf, T. Expression of somatic DNA repair genes in human testes. *Journal of Cellular Biochemistry*, 2007, 100, 1232-1239.

Game, JC; Zamb, TJ; Braun, RJ; Resnick, M; Roth, RM. The role of radiation (*rad*) genes in meiotic recombination in yeast. *Genetics*, 1980, 94, 51-68.

Gilley, D; Blackburn, EH. Lack of telemere shortening during senescence in *Paramecium*. *Proceedings of the National Academy of Sciences USA*, 1994, 91, 1955-1958.

Gladyshev, E; Meselson, M. Extreme resistance of bdelloid rotifers to ionizing radiation. *Proceedings of the National Academy of Sciences USA*, 105(13), 5139-5144.

Goddard, MR; Godfray, HC; Burt, A. Sex increases the efficacy of natural selection in experimental yeast populations. *Nature*, 2005, 434, 636-640.

Goodgal, SH; Herriott, RM. Studies on transformations of *Hemophilus influenzae*, I: Competence. *Journal of General Physiology* 1961, 44, 1201-1227.

Gorelick, R; Heng, HHQ. Sex reduces genetic variation: A multidisciplinary review. *Evolution*, 2011, 65(4), 1088-1098.

Hannah-Alava, A. The brood pattern of X-ray-induced mutational damage in the germ cells of *Drosophila melanogaster* males. *Mutation Research*, 1964, 1, 414-436.

Haynes, RH. Biological context of DNA repair. In: Friedberg, EC; Hanawalt, PC, editors. *Mechanisms and Consequences of DNA Damage Processing*, New York, Alan R. Liss, 1988, 577-584.

Haynes, RH; Kunz, BA. DNA repair and mutagenesis in yeast. In: Strathern, J; Jones, E; Broach, J, editors. *The Molecular Biology of the Yeast Saccharomyces. Life Cycle and Inheritance*. Cold Spring Harbor, N.Y, Cold Spring Harbor Laboratory, 1981, 371-414.

Heng, HHQ. Elimination of altered karyotypes by sexual reproduction preserves species identity. *Genome*, 2007, 50, 517-524.

Henriques, JAP; Moustacchi, E. Sensitivity to photoaddition of mono- and bifunctional furocoumarins of X-ray sensitive mutants of *Saccharomyces cerevisiae*. *Photochemistry and Photobiology*, 1980, 31, 557-563.

Herskowitz, I. Life cycle of the budding yeast *Saccharomyces cerevisiae*. *Microbiological Reviews*, 1988, 52(4), 536-553.

Hochwagen, A; Marals, GAB. Meiosis: A PRDM9 guide to the hotsposts of recombination. *Current Biology*, 2010, 20(6), R271-R274.

Hoelzer, MA; Michod RE. DNA repair and the evolution of transformation in *Bacillus subtilis*. III. Sex with damaged DNA. *Genetics,* 1991, 128, 215-223.

Holmes, GE; Holmes, NR. Accumulation of DNA damages in aging *Paramecium tetraurelia*. *Molecular and General Genetics*, 1986, 275, 305-315.

Imlay, JA; Chin, SM; Linn, S. Toxic DNA damage by hydrogen peroxide through the Fenton reaction in vivo and in vitro. *Science*, 1988, 240(4852), 640-642.

Johnsborg, O; Eldholm,V; Havarstein, LS. Natural genetic transformation: prevalence, mechanisms and function. *Research in Microbiology*, 2007, 158, 767-778.

Joyce, EF; Tanneti, SN; McKim, KS. Drosophila Hold'em is required for a subset of meiotic crossovers and interacts with the DNA repair endonuclease complex subunits MEI-9 and ERCC1. *Genetics*, 2009, 181, 335-340.

Judd, SR; Petes, TD. Physical lengths of meiotic and mitotic gene conversion tracts in *Saccharomyces cerevisiae*. *Genetics*,1988, 118; 401-410.

Kaltz, O; Bell, G. The ecology and genetics of fitness in *Chlamydomonas*. XII. Repeated sexual episodes increase rates of adaptation to novel environments. *Evolution*, 2002, 56(9), 1743-1753.

Kelly, SL; Merrill, C; Parry, JM. Cyclic variations in sensitivity to X-irradiation during meiosis in *Saccharomyces cerevisiae*. *Molecular and General Genetics*, 1983, 191, 314-318.

Kidane, D; Graumann, PL. Intracellular protein and DNA dynamics in competent *Bacillus subtilis* cells. *Cell*, 2005, 122, 73-84.

Kim, JS; Rose, AM. The effect of gamma radiation on recombination frequency in *Caenorhabditis elegans*. *Genome*, 1987, 29, 457-462.

Kirk, DL; Kirk, MM. Heat shock elicits production of sexual inducer in *Volvox*. *Science*, 1986, 231(4733), 51-54.

Klovstad, M; Abdu, U; Schupbach, T. Drosophila *brca2* is required for mitotic and meiotic DNA repair and efficient activation of the meiotic recombination checkpoint. *PloS Genetics*, 2008, 4(2): e31.doi:10.1371/journal.pgen.0040031.

Koppen, G; Verschaeve, L. The alkaline single-cell gel electrophoresis/comet assay: a way to study DNA repair in radicle cells of germinating *Vicia faba*. *Folia Biol. (Praha)*, 2001, 47(2), 50-54.

Lahr, DJG; Parfrey, LW; Mitchell, EAD; Katz, LA; Lara, E. The chastity of amoebae: re-evaluating evidence for sex in amoeboid organisms. *Proceedings of the Royal Society B Biological Sciences* (published online 23 March 2011) doi: 10.1098/rspb.2011.0289

Lewis, SEM; Aitken, RJ. DNA damage to spermatozoa has impacts on fertilization and pregnancy. *Cell Tissue Research*, 2005, 322, 33-41.

Li, J; Harper, LC; Golubovskaya, I; Wang, CR; Weber, D; Meeley, RB; McElver, J; Bowen, B; Cande, WZ; Schnable, PS. Functional analysis of maize RAD51 in meiosis and double-strand break repair. *Genetics*, 2007, 176,1469-1482.

Li, W; Chen, C; Markmann-Mulisch, U; Timofejeva, L; Schmeizer, E; Ma, H; Reiss, B. The *Arabidopsis AtRAD51* gene is dispensable for vegetative development but required for meiosis. *Proceedings of the National Academy of Sciences USA*, 2004, 101(29), 10596-10601.

Loshon, CA; Genest, PC; Setlow, B; Setlow, P. Formaldehyde kills spores of *Bacillus subtilis* by DNA damage and small, acid-soluble spore proteins of the alpha/beta-type protect spores against this DNA damage. *Journal of Applied Microbiology*, 1999, 87(1), 8-14.

Lynch, M. Destabilizing hybridization, general purpose genotypes and geographic parthenogenesis. *Quarterly Review of Biology*, 1984, 59, 257-290.

Makker, K; Agarwal, A; Sharma, R. Oxidative stress & male infertility. *Indian Journal of Medical Research*, 2009, 129, 357-367.

Malik, SB; Pightling, AW; Stefaniak, LM; Schurko, AM; Logsdon, JM. An expanded inventory of conserved meiotic genes provides evidence for sex in *Trichomonas vaginalis*. *PloS ONE*, 2008, 3(8), 1-13, 2879.

Malone, RE; Esposito, RE. The *RAD52* gene is required for homothallic interconversion of mating types and spontaneous mitotic recombination in yeast. *Proceedings of the National Academy of Sciences USA*, 1980, 77(1), 503-507.

Marchetti, F; Wyrobek, AJ. DNA repair decline during mouse spermiogenesis results in the accumulation of heritable DNA damage. *DNA Repair*, 2008, 7, 572-581.

Mark Welch, D; Meselson, M. Evidence for the evolution of bdelloid rotifers without sexual reproduction or genetic exchange. *Science*, 2000, 288(5469), 1211-1215.

Mark Welch, DB; Mark Welch, JL; Meselson, M. Evidence for degenerate tetraploidy in bdelloid rotifers. *Proceedings of the National Academy of Sciences USA,* 2008, 105(13), 5145-5149.

Martin, B; Ruellan, JM; Angulo, JF; Devoret, R; Claverys, JP. Identification of the *recA* gene of *Streptococcus pneumoniae. Nucleic Acids Research*, 1992, 20(23), 6412.

Massie, HR; Samis, HV; Baird, MB. The kinetics of degradation of DNA and RNA by H_2O_2. *Biochimica et Biophysica Acta*, 1972, 272, 539-548.

Maynard Smith, J. *The evolution of Sex*, London: Cambridge University Press, 1978.

McMahill, MS; Sham, CW; Bishop, DK. Synthesis-dependent strand annealing in meiosis. *PloS Biology*, 2007, 5(11):e299.doi:10.1371/journal.pbio.0050299

Mechali, M. Eukaryotic DNA replication origins: many choices for appropriate answers. *Nature Reviews: Molecular Cell Biology*, 2010, 11, 728-738.

Mehrotra, S; McKim, KS. Temporal analysis of meiotic DNA double-strand break formation and repair in *Drosophila* females. *PloS Genetics*, 2006, 2(11): e200.doi:10.1371/journal. pgen.0020200

Michod, RE; Wojciechowski, MF; Hoelzer, MA. DNA repair and the evolution of transformation in the bacterium *Bacillus subtilis. Genetics,* 1988, 118, 31-39.

Michod, RE; Wojciechowski, MF. DNA repair and the evolution of transformation IV. DNA damage increases transformation. *Journal of Evolutionary Biology*, 1994, 7, 147-175.

Michod, RE. *Eros and Evolution: A Natural Philosophy of Sex*. Reading, MA, Addison-Wesley, 1994.

Michod, RE; Bernstein, H; Nedelcu, AM. Adaptive value of sex in microbial pathogens. *Infection, Genetics and Evolution*, 2008, 8, 267-285.

Moens, PB; Kolas, NK; Tarsounas, M; Marcon, E; Cohen, PE; Spyropoulos, B. The time course and chromosomal localization of recombination-related proteins at meiosis in the mouse are compatible with models that can resolve the early DNA-DNA interactions without reciprocal recombination. *Journal of Cell Science*, 2002, 115, 1611-1622.

Mortier-Barriere, I; de Saizieu, A; Claverys, JP; Martin, B. Competence-specific induction of *RecA* is required for full recombination proficiency during transformation in *Streptococcus pneumoniae. Molecular Microbiology*, 1998, 27(1), 159-170.

Moynahan, ME; Jasin M. Mitotic homologous recombination maintains genomic stability and suppresses tumorigenesis. *Nature Reviews/ Molecular Cell Biology*, 2010, 11, 196-207.

Myers, S; Spencer, CCA; Auton, A; Bottolo, L; Freeman, C; Donnelly, P; McVean, G. The distribution and causes of meiotic recombination in the human genome. *Biochemical Society Transactions*, 2006, 34(4), 526-530.

Nedelcu, AM. Evidence for p53-like-mediated stress responses in green algae. *FEBS Letters*, 2006, 580, 3013-3017.

Nedelcu, AM; Michod, RE. Sex as a response to oxidative stress: The effect of antioxidants on sexual induction in a facultatively sexual lineage. *Proceedings of the Royal Society B*, 2003 (Suppl.), 270, S136-S139.

Nedelcu, AM; Marcu, O; Michod, RE. Sex as a response to oxidative stress: a two-fold increase in cellular reactive oxygen species activates sex genes. *Proceedings of the Royal Society B*, 2004, 271, 1591-1596.

Otto, SP; Gerstein, AC. Why have sex? The population genetics of sex and recombination. *Biochemical Society Transactions*, 2006, 34, 519-522.

Peters, AD; Otto, SP. Liberating genetic variance through sex. *BioEssays*, 2003, 25, 533-537.

Pittman, DL; Cobb, J; Schimenti, KJ; Wilson, LA; Cooper, DM; Brignull, E; Handel, MA; Schimenti, JC. Meiotic prophase arrest with failure of chromosome synapsis in mice deficient for *Dmc1*, a germline-specific *RecA* homolog. *Molecular Cell*, 1998, 1, 697-705.

Prudhommeau, C; Proust, J. UV irradiation of polar cells of *Drosophila melanogaster* embryos. V. A study of the meiotic recombination in females with chromosomes of different structure. *Mutation Research*, 1973, 22, 63-66.

Ramesh, MA; Malik, SB; Logsdon, JM. A phylogenomic inventory of meiotic genes: evidence for sex in *Giardia* and an early eukaryotic origin of meiosis. *Current Biology*, 2005, 15, 185-191.

Rasmusen, A. Effects of DNA-repair-deficient mutants on somatic and germ line mutagenesis in the UZ system of *Drosophila melanogaster*. *Mutation Research*, 1984, 141, 29-33.

Reeves, RJ; Jackson, RM. Stimulation of sexual reproduction in *Phytophthora* by damage. *Journal of General Microbiology*, 1974, 84, 303-310.

Roberts, CJ; Lowe, CR. Where have all the conceptions gone? *Lancet,* 1975, 305(7905), 498-499.

Roze, D; Michod, RE. Deleterious mutations and selection for sex in finite diploid populations. *Genetics*, 2010, 184, 1095-1112.

Ruderfer, DM; Pratt, SC; Seidel, HS; Kruglyak, L. Population genomic analysis of outcrossing and recombination in yeast. *Nature Genetics*, 2006, 38(9), 1077-1081.

Sager, R; Granick, S. Nutritional control of sexuality in *Chlamydomonas reinhardi. Journal of General Physiology*, 1954, 37, 729-742.

Saito, Y; Taguchi, H; Akamatsu, T. Fate of transforming bacterial genome following incorporation into competent cells of *Bacillus subtilis*: A continuous length of incorporated DNA. *Journal of Bioscience and Bioengineering*, 2006, 101(3), 257-262.

Sakai, A; Nakanishi, M; Yoshiyama, K; Maki, H. Impact of reactive oxygen species on spontaneous mutagenesis in *Escherichia coli*. *Genes to Cells*, 2006, 11, 767-778.

Sakakura, Y; Soyano, K; Noakes, DLG; Hagiwara, A. Gonadal morphology in the self-fertilizing mangrove killifish, *Kryptolebias marmoratus*. *Ichthyological Research*, 2006, 53, 427-430.

Sakano, K; Oikawa, S; Hasegawa, K; Kawanishi, S. Hydroxyurea induces site-specific DNA damage via formation of hydrogen peroxide and nitric oxide. *Japanese Journal of Cancer Research*, 2001, 92, 1166-1174.

San Filippo, J; Sung P; Klein H. Mechanism of eukaryotic homologous recombination. *Annual Review of Biochemistry*, 2008, 77, 229-257.

Sauvageau, S; Stasiak, AZ; Banville, I; Ploquin, M; Stasiak, A; Masson, JY. Fission yeast Rad51 and Dmc1, two efficient DNA recombinases forming helical nucleoprotein filaments. *Molecular and Cellular Biology,* 2005, 25, 4377-4387.

Schewe, MJ; Suzuki, DT; Erasmus, U. The genetic effects of mitomycin C in *Drosophila melanogaster*. II. Induced meiotic recombination. *Mutation Research*, 1971, 12, 269-279.

Sedelnikova, OA; Redon, EC; Dickey, JS; Nakamura, AJ; Georgakilas, AG; Bonner, WM. Role of oxidatively induced DNA lesions in human pathogenesis. *Mutation Research/Reviews in Mutation Research*, 2010, 704, 152-159.

Sehorn, MG; Sigurdsson, S; Bussen, W; Unger,VM; Sung, P. Human meiotic recombinase Dmc1 promotes ATP-dependent homologous DNA strand exchange. *Nature*, 2004, 429, 433-437.

Shields, WM. *Philopatry, Inbreeding, and the Evolution of Sex*, Albany, NY: State University of NY Press, 1982.

Shinohara, A; Ogawa, H; Matsuda, Y; Ushio, N; Ikeo, K; Ogawa, T. Cloning of human, mouse and fission yeast recombination genes homologous to *RAD51* and *RecA*. *Nature Genetics*, 1993, 4, 239-243.

Slupphaug, G; Kavli, B; Krokan, HE. The interacting pathways for prevention and repair of oxidative DNA damage. *Mutation Research*, 2003, 531, 231-251.

Smith-Sonneborn, J. DNA repair and longevity assurance in *Paramecium tetraurelia*. *Science*, 1979, 203, 1115-1117.

Solomon, JM; Grossman, AD. Who's competent and when: regulation of natural genetic competence in bacteria. *Trends in Genetics*, 1996, 12(4), 150-155.

Staeva-Vieira, E; Yoo, S; Lehmann, R. An essential role of DmRad51/SpnA in DNA repair and meiotic checkpoint control. *The EMBO Journal*, 2003, 22(21), 5863-5874.

Starr, R; Jaenicke, L. Sexual induction in *Volvox carteri f. nagariensis* by aldehydes. *Sexual Plant Reproduction*, 1988, 1, 28-31.

Steinboeck, F; Hubmann, M; Bogusch, A; Dorninger, P; Lengheimer, T; Heidenreich, E. The relevance of oxidative stress and cytotoxic DNA lesions for spontaneous mutagenesis in non-replicating yeast cells. *Mutation Research*, 2010, 688, 47-52.

Stohl, EA; Gruenig, MC; Cox, MM; Seifert, HS. Purification and characterization of the RecA protein from *Neisseria gonorrhoeae*. PloS ONE, 2011, 6(2), e17101

Story, RM; Bishop, DK; Kleckner, N; Steitz, TA. Structural relationship of bacterial RecA proteins to recombination proteins from bacteriophage T4 and yeast. *Science*, 1993, 259(5103), 1892-1896.

Sung, P. Catalysis of ATP-dependent homologous DNA pairing and strand exchange by yeast RAD51 protein. *Science*, 1994, 265, 1241-1243.

Suzuki, DT; Parry, DM. Crossing over near the centromere of chromosome 3 in *Drosophila melanogaster* females. *Genetics*, 1964, 50, 1427-1432.

Szostak, JW, Orr-Weaver, TL, Rothstein, RJ; Stahl, FW. The double-strand-break repair model for recombination. *Cell*, 1983, 33, 25-35.

Takanami, T; Mori, A; Takahashi, H; Higashitani, A. Hyper-resistance of meiotic cells to radiation due to a strong expression of a single *RecA*-like gene in *Caenorhabditis elegans*. *Nucleic Acids Research*, 2000, 28(21), 4232-4236.

Takanami, T; Zhang, Y; Aoki, H; Abe, T; Yoshida, S; Takahashi, H; Horiuchi, S; Higashitani, A. Efficient repair of DNA damage induced by heavy ion particles in meiotic prophase I nuclei of *Caenorhabditis elegans*. *Journal of Radiation Research*, 2003, 44, 271-276.

Terasawa, M; Shinohara, A; Hotta, Y; Ogawa, H; Ogawa, T. Localization of RecA-like recombination protein on chromosomes of the lily at various meiotic stages. *Genes and Development*, 1995, 9, 925-934.

Tichy, ED; Pillai, R; Deng, L; Liang, L; Tischfield, J; Schwemberger, SJ; Babcock, GF; Stambrook, PJ. Mouse embryonic stem cells, but not somatic cells, predominantly use homologous recombination to repair double-strand breaks. *Stem Cells and Development*, 2010, 19(11), 1699-1711.

Tran, L; van Baarsel, JA; Washburn, RS; Gottesman, ME; Miller, JH. Single-gene deletion mutants of *Escherichia coli* with altered sensitivity to bicyclomycin, an inhibitor of transcription termination factor rho. *Journal of Bacteriology*, 2011, 193(9), 2229-2235.

Unal, E; Kinde, B; Amon, A. Gametogenesis eliminates age-induced cellular damage and resets life span in yeast. *Science*, 2011, 332, 1554-1557.

Vilenchik, MM; Knudson, AG. Endogenous DNA double-strand breaks: Production, fidelity of repair and induction of cancer. *Proceedings of the National Academy of Sciences USA*, 2003, 100(22), 12871-12876.

Virgin, JB; Bailey, JP; Hasteh, F; Neville, J; Cole, A; Tromp, G. Crossing over is rarely associated with mitotic intragenic recombination in *Schizosaccharomyces pombe*. *Genetics*, 2001, 157, 63-77.

Washburn, RS; Gottesman, ME. Transcription termination maintains chromosome integrity. *Proceedings of the National Academy of Sciences USA*, 2011, 108(2), 792-797.

Wei, K, Kucherlapati, R; Edelmann, W. Mouse models for human DNA mismatch-repair gene defects. *TRENDS in Molecular Medicine*, 2002, 8(7), 346-353.

Weismann, A. *Essays upon Heredity and Kindred Biological Problems.* Vol. II. Oxford: Clarendon; 1892, pg. 196.

White, MJD. *Animal Cytology and Evolution*, 3rd edn. London: Cambridge University Press; 1973.

Whitehouse, HLK. *Genetic Recombination.* New York: Wiley; 1982.

Wilcox, AJ; Weinberg, CR; O'Connor, JF; Baird, DD; Schlatterer, JP; Canfield, RE; Armstrong, EG; Nisula, BC. Incidence of early loss of pregnancy. *New England Journal of Medicine*, 1988, 319(4), 189-194.

Williams, GC. *Sex and Evolution.* Princeton, NJ: Princeton University Press; 1975.

Wojciechowski, MF; Hoelzer, MA; Michod, RE. DNA repair and the evolution of transformation in the bacterium *Bacillus subtilis*. II: Role of inducible repair. *Genetics*, 1989, 121, 411-422.

Yoshida, K; Kondoh, G; Matsuda, Y; Habu, T; Nishimune, Y; Morita, T. The mouse *RecA*-like gene *Dmc1* is required for homologous chromosome synapsis during meiosis. *Molecular Cell*, 1998, 1, 707-718.

Zeiger, E; Gollapudi, B; Spencer, P. Genetic toxicity and carcinogenicity studies of glutaraldehyde—a review. *Mutation Research*, 2005, 589(2), 136-151.

Zeyl, CW; Otto, SP. A short history of recombination in yeast. *Trends in Ecology and Evolution*, 2007, 22(5), 223-225.

Reviewed by Dr. Michael Berman, Hematology/Oncology, University of Arizona Cancer Center.

In: Medical and Biological Frontiers Research Compendium ISBN: 978-1-62417-022-5
Editor: Tsisana Shartava

Chapter 9

Paralysis in ALS Patients: An Overview on Assessment and Treatment of Motor Impairment

Paolo Bongioanni
Neurorehabilitation Unit, Neuroscience Department,
University of Pisa, Italy

Abstract

Amyotrophic lateral sclerosis (ALS) is a progressive neurodegenerative disease affecting brain, brainstem and spinal cord motor neurons.

Muscle weakness is a hallmark sign in ALS, occurring in approximately 60% of patients. Early symptoms vary with each individual, but usually include tripping, dropping things, abnormal fatigue of the arms and/or legs, slurred speech, muscle cramps and twitches and/or uncontrollable periods of laughing or crying. There are spinal-onset or bulbar-onset disease forms, according to the first involvement of limbs or speech/swallowing muscles, respectively. With voluntary muscles progressively affected, patients in the later stages of the disease may become totally paralyzed.

In this paper, ALS diagnostic issues, and methods and techniques for assessing severity of motor deficits are discussed. Various treatment options for limb and bulbar palsies are reviewed: in addition to drugs, assistive rehabilitation approaches are presented, from physiotherapy to occupational therapy, from respiratory exercises to swallowing manoeuvres and postures.

Introduction

Amyotrophic lateral sclerosis (ALS), also called *Lou Gehrig's disease*, is a rapidly progressive, invariably fatal neurodegenerative disease that attacks the neurons responsible for controlling voluntary muscles. It belongs to a group of disorders known as *Motor neuron diseases* (*MND*), including *Primary lateral sclerosis*, *Progressive bulbar palsy*, *Progressive muscular atrophy*, *Flail arm syndrome*, *Flail leg syndrome*, and *ALS with multisystemic involvement* (e.g., *ALS-Dementia*). All these syndromes share a common molecular and cellular pathology comprising degeneration of motor neurons (MNs) in cortex, brainstem and/or spinal cord, and the presence of characteristic ubiquitin and TDP-43-immunoreactive intraneuronal inclusions.

ALS is one of the most common neuromuscular disease worldwide: in Western countries, prevalence ranges from 2.7 to 7.4 per 100,000 [Worms, 2001]. In 90 to 95 percent of all patients with ALS (PALS), the disease occurs apparently at random with no clearly associated risk factors (*sporadic ALS*, *sALS*): patients do not have a family history of the disease, and their family members are not considered to be at increased risk for developing ALS. About 5 to 10 percent of all PALS have a family history of ALS (*fALS*). Often there is a Mendelian inheritance and high penetrance, with most cases having a pattern of inheritance that requires only one parent to carry the gene responsible for the disease (autosomal dominant pattern), although autosomal recessive pedigrees have been reported [Mulder et al., 1986; Gros-Louis et al., 2006].

ALS most commonly strikes people between 40 and 60 years of age, but younger and older people also can develop the disease [Haverkamp et al., 1995]. Men are affected more often than women (about 1.5 to 1.0), although more recent data suggest that the gender ratio may be approaching equality [Abhinav et al., 2007; Logroscino et al., 2008; Zoccolella et al., 2008].

The cause of ALS is not known, and it is not clear why ALS strikes some people and not others, but both genetic [Ticozzi et al., 2011] and environmental factors (including excitotoxicity [Rothstein et al., 1992; Steele and McGeer, 2008] and calcium-mediated intracellular damage [Choi, 1988]; oxidative stress [Ferrante et al., 1997], mitochondrial dysfunction [Curti et al., 1996], lack of neurotrophic factors [Henriques et al., 2010] and apoptosis [Cereda et al., 2006]; immune events [Calvo et al., 2010] and neuroinflammation [Wu et al., 2006]; altered axonal flow (probably due to the cytoskeletal damage [Crippa et al., 2010]) and protein aggregation (related also to defective autophagy [Venkatachalam et al., 2008]); exogenous toxicity [Callaghan et al., 2011]) may play a role.

Clinical Signs

In PALS, both the brain upper MNs (UMNs) and the brainstem or spinal cord lower MNs (LMNs) degenerate or die, ceasing to send messages to muscles: unable to function, the muscles gradually weaken, waste away, and twitch, therefore leading to a wide range of disabilities.

Eventually, all muscles under voluntary control are affected, and patients lose their strength and the ability to move their body, but usually maintain control of eye muscles. Only occasionally there are symptoms of bladder dysfunction (such as urgency of micturition), and ALS does not either affect a person's ability to see, smell, taste, hear, or recognize touch; nor impair a person's mind or intelligence (although a small percentage of patients may experience problems with memory or decision-making [Lomen-Hoerth et al., 2003; Ringholz et al., 2005; Raaphorst et al., 2010], and there is growing evidence that some may even develop a form of dementia [Guedj et al., 2007]). Because the disease usually does not affect cognitive abilities, PALS are aware of their progressive loss of function and may become anxious and depressed [Patten et al., 2007].

Approximately 70% of patients with typical ALS have a *spinal form* of the disease: they present with symptoms which may start either distally or proximally in the upper or lower limbs. PALS may have noticed fasciculations (involuntary muscle twitching) or cramps preceding weakness or wasting onset for months, or even years. Rarely, they notice muscle wasting before weakness onset, which may be so subtle that the symptoms are frequently overlooked.

At the beginning weakness is usually asymmetrical (the controlateral limbs being involved sooner or later): body parts affected by early symptoms depend on which muscles in the body are damaged first. Some PALS see the effects of the disease on a hand or arm, as they experience difficulty with simple tasks requiring manual dexterity, such as buttoning a shirt, writing, or turning a key in a lock. In some cases, symptoms initially affect one of the legs, and patients experience awkwardness when walking or running, or they notice that they are tripping or stumbling more often.

Early examination in the course of spinal-onset disease reveals focal muscle atrophy, involving particularly hand, forearm and shoulder muscles in the upper limbs, and proximal thigh or distal foot muscles in the lower limbs. Fasciculations are usually visible in more than one muscle group; spasticity is present in both upper and lower limbs (with clonus and hypertonia). Tendon reflexes are brisk and usually symmetric, including the finger jerks in the upper limbs and positive crossed adductor reflex in the lower limbs, with abnormal spread of tendon reflexes beyond the stimulated muscle group; the Hoffmann's sign may be positive in the upper limbs, and the Babinski's sign in the lower limbs.

Patients with *bulbar-onset* ALS usually present with dysarthria, which arises from either LMN or UMN involvement, leading to slow slurred speech or a nasal quality. They may also develop dysphagia for solid or liquids after noticing speech problems: difficulty in swallowing and chewing impair their ability to eat normally, so that maintaining weight will then become a problem, and the risk of choking increases. Almost all patients with bulbar symptoms develop sialorrhoea with excessive drooling due to difficulty of swallowing saliva and mild UMN-type bilateral facial weakness, which affects the lower part of the face, causing difficulty with lip seal and blowing cheeks. "Pseudobulbar" symptoms, such as emotional lability and excessive yawning, are seen in a significant number of PALS.

The jaw jerk may be brisk, and an UMN type facial weakness affecting the lower half of the face is observed (although often varying degrees of UMN and LMN facial weakness coexist). The gag reflex is preserved and often brisk, whereas the soft palate may be weak. PALS show tongue wasting and fasciculations of the tongue which moves slowly, also due to muscle hypertonia. The other cranial nerves remain intact, although in late stages of the disease patients may very rarely develop a supranuclear gaze palsy or oculomotor palsy [Okuda et al., 1992; Kobayashi et al., 1999].

Bulbar symptoms may develop almost simultaneously with spinal symptoms, and in the vast majority of cases will occur within 1-2 years.

As disease progresses, patients develop the characteristic picture of the combination of UMN (tight and stiff muscles (spasticity) and hyperreflexia, including an overactive gag reflex and Hoffmann's and/or Babinski's signs) and LMN (muscle weakness and atrophy, muscle cramps, and fasciculations) involvement within the same central nervous system (CNS) region, affecting the bulbar, cervical, thoracic and lumbar territories.

About less than 5% of PALS present with respiratory weakness without previous spinal or bulbar signs [Chen et al., 1996; de Carvalho et al., 1996], showing symptoms of respiratory failure or nocturnal hypoventilation, such as dyspnea, orthopnea, disturbed sleep, morning headaches, excessive daytime somnolence, anorexia, decreased concentration, and irritability or mood changes [Polkey et al., 1999]. In later disease stages, when muscles in the diaphragm and chest wall fail, patients eventually lose the ability to breathe on their own and must depend on ventilatory support for survival. Respiratory failure and/or cardiovascular complications are the usual cause of death.

Diagnosis

ALS diagnosis still remains a clinical one supported by neurophysiological evidence: the expert clinician after collection of patient's full medical history and careful neurological examination, in presence of UMN and LMN signs in the same anatomical region(s) with asymmetrical localization, is able to suspect ALS, but he needs a neurophysiological confirmation. On the other hand, suggestive neurophysiological results alone are not adequate for achieving a diagnosis, but must be interpreted in the light of patient's history and clinical findings. Therefore, clinician and neurophysiologist have to rely on each other, since they have the responsibility for the diagnosis of such a dreadful disease. At regular intervals, neurologist usually repeats physical examination to assess whether symptoms (such as muscle weakness and atrophy, hyperreflexia, and spasticity) are getting progressively worse. According to different surveys, the time required to confirm ALS diagnosis from the first signs/symptoms is approximately one year [Chiò and Silani, 2001].

Clinical Criteria

The World Federation of Neurology Research Group on Motor Neuron Diseases have developed the 1994 *El Escorial diagnostic criteria* [Brooks et al., 1994] and the revised 2000 *Airlie House criteria* [Brooks et al., 2000] to aid in diagnosing and classifying patients for research studies and clinical trials. Based on such criteria PALS are classified into "*clinically definite*", "*clinically probable*", "*clinically probable - laboratory supported*" and "*clinically possible*" categories. In the previous 1994 classification, patients with a pure LMN syndrome were classified into the "*clinically suspected*" category, now removed from the revised criteria: however, it is well recognized that several PALS who either have a pure LMN syndrome or early in the disease course do not have obvious UMN signs, will surely develop ALS (or a variant), but they will not fall into the categories of the revised criteria. Such criteria are thus probably more useful for research purposes and treatment trials, rather than daily clinical practice.

A recent rationalization of the El Escorial Criteria during the Awaji Consensus Conference in December 2006 simplifies the criteria [de Carvalho et al., 2008]: the so-called *Awaji-Criteria*, designed for everyday clinical practice, basically recommend that electrophysiological evidence of chronic neurogenic changes should be taken as equivalent to clinical data in the recognition of LMN involvement, and abnormal complex fasciculation potentials should be regarded as equivalent to fibrillation potentials or positive sharp waves.

Neurophysiological Methods

Conventional Electromyography

Electromyography (EMG) findings can support ALS diagnosis, by documenting LMN dysfunction in clinically involved and uninvolved regions, as it has already shown in the first published criteria for ALS electrodiagnosis [Lambert and Mulder, 1957].

EMG-detected LMN involvement should be found in at least 2 of the 4 regions - brainstem (bulbar MNs); and cervical, thoracic, or lumbar spinal cord (anterior horn MNs). It is enough to demonstrate EMG changes in one muscle (e.g. tongue, jaw, or facial muscles), for the brainstem region; either in the paraspinal muscles at or below the T_6 level, or in the abdominal muscles, for the thoracic spinal cord region; in at least 2 muscles innervated by different roots and peripheral nerves, for the cervical and lumbar spinal cord regions [Brooks et al., 2000]. Such revised El-Escorial criteria require evidence of both *active* or *ongoing denervation* (*fibrillation potentials and positive sharp waves*) and *chronic partial denervation* (*large motor unit potentials* of enhanced duration with an increased proportion of polyphasic potentials, often of enhanced amplitude; *reduced interference pattern* with firing rates > 10 Hz - unless there is a significant UMN component, in which case the firing rate may be < 10 Hz; and *unstable motor unit potentials*), although relative proportions may vary from muscle to muscle [Brooks et al., 2000]. Fasciculation potentials are a remarkable sign in ALS, although they can also be seen in normal muscles (*benign fasciculations*) and are not present in all PALS muscles [de Carvalho et al., 2008].

Nerve Conduction Studies

Because ALS symptoms can be similar to those of a wide variety of other, more treatable diseases, appropriate tests must be conducted to exclude the possibility of other clinical conditions. Nerve conduction (NC) techniques are required for detecting or excluding other disorders of peripheral nerve, neuromuscular junction and muscle that confound the diagnosis of ALS. The findings of NC studies (e.g. motor conduction velocity and distal motor latency) in PALS should generally be normal or near normal [de Carvalho and Swash, 2000], unless the compound muscle potential is small [Brooks et al., 2000].

Motor NC studies are also important in excluding *multifocal motor neuropathy*, by the detection of partial conduction block: a marked reduction of proximal amplitude or negative-peak area as compared with the distal ones (over 50%), in short segments (excluding entrapment sites) [de Carvalho et al., 2001]. F-wave studies are particularly useful in assessing proximal conduction, and abnormalities have been reported in PALS: enhanced F-wave latency with normal frequency and increased amplitude, and reduced F-wave velocity with decreased frequency. Prominent UMN features may be associated with an enhanced F-wave frequency [de Carvalho and Swash, 2000].

Sensory NC studies can show abnormalities in case of entrapment syndromes and coexisting peripheral nerve disease [Brooks et al., 2000]. In 10-20% of PALS, a subclinical sensory system involvement has been reported, suggesting an additional polyneuropathy or sensory ganglionopathy [Pugdahl et al., 2007].

Transcranial Magnetic Stimulation

Transcranial magnetic stimulation (TMS) allows a noninvasive evaluation of the corticospinal motor pathways, and detection of UMN lesions in patients without UMN clinical signs. Motor amplitude, central motor conduction time (CMCT), cortical threshold and silent periods can be easily measured using this method [Eisen and Shtybel, 1990]. Electrophysiological features compatible with UMN involvement include [Brooks et al., 2000]: up to a 30% increase in CMCT; and low firing rates of motor unit potentials on maximal effort. Marked CMCT prolongation is seen in fALS patients with D90A SOD1 mutations [Osei-Lah et al., 2004].

Neuroimaging Techniques

The most important use of neuroimaging in ALS diagnosis is to exclude treatable structural lesions (such as spinal cord tumor, a herniated disk in the neck, syringomyelia, or cervical spondylosis) mimicking ALS by producing varying degrees of UMN and LMN signs [Agosta et al., 2010], especially in patients with clinically probable or possible ALS [Brooks et al., 2000].

Magnetic resonance imaging (*MRI*) can be used in detecting corticospinal tract lesions: the most characteristic finding in ALS is corticospinal tract hyperintensity on T_2-weighted, proton density weighted and FLAIR-weighted MRI scans, and it is best visualised in brain, brainstem and, to a less extent, in spinal cord [Goodin et al., 1988; Waragai, 1997]. T_2-weighted MRI may also show hypointensity of the primary motor cortex, usually along the posterior bank of the precentral gyrus, although this is an inconsistent and non-specific finding [Oba et al., 1993].

More advanced structural neuroimaging modalities (such as *magnetic resonance spectroscopy*, *diffusion-weighted imaging*, *diffusion tensor imaging* and *magnetic resonance voxel-based morphometry*) and functional imaging techniques (*single photon emission computerized tomography*, *positron emission tomography* and *functional MRI*) have a limited role in routine clinical practice, but can be useful in understanding ALS pathophysiology *in vivo*, by identifying potential biomarkers of disease progression and detecting changes earlier in the disease course [Lombardo et al., 2009; Turner et al., 2009].

Laboratory Exams

Muscle Biopsy

Biopsy of skeletal muscle (or other tissues) is not required for diagnosis, unless to rule out a mimic syndrome (e.g. affecting muscle). In addition, muscle biopsy may be used to demonstrate LMN dysfunction in a body region when clinical or electrophysiological findings do not support this evidence. Histological findings that are compatible with ALS diagnosis include: scattered hypertrophied muscle fibers; no more than a moderate number of target fibers; fiber-type grouping of no more than mild-to-moderate extent; the presence of few necrotic muscle fibers [Brooks et al., 2000].

Biochemical Assays

Clinician may order tests on blood, urine and/or cerebrospinal fluid (CSF) samples to eliminate the possibility of other diseases, as well as routine laboratory assays. Clinical laboratory tests that may be abnormal in otherwise typical case of ALS include: a) serum muscle enzymes (creatine kinase, transaminases and lactic dehydrogenase); b) serum creatinine; c) chloremia and serum bicarbonate; d) CSF proteins [Brooks et al., 2000].

Moreover, in our experience, oxidative markers and cytokines/growth factors should be assayed overtime, in order to diachronically assess not only the body redox status, but also the dynamic balance among toxic and trophic factors [Bongioanni et al., 2001; 2002_a; 2002_b; 2008].

Functional Assessment

Global Functional Scales

Severity of PALS functional impairment has to be assessed at the first visit and monitored over time.

Evaluation of motor deficit implies an assessment of the resulting deficiency or incapacity and final disability. Many assessments have been proposed for patient's follow-up in order to analyze the state of motor function and their consequences on activities of everyday life [Couratier et al., 2006]. Clinimetric scales must be validated and relatively simple to use, and generate ordinate results allowing statistical analysis. The clinician should be aware of the different scales and their relative utility: knowledge of these scales, their validity, their sensitivity to modification, and their specificity and interpretation pitfalls is a prerequisite to good evaluation in daily practice and in clinical research.

The choice of which scale to use depends on the clinical objective: global scales (*Norris Scale* [Norris et al., 1974], *Appel ALS Rating Scale* [Appel et al., 1987], *ALS Severity Scale* (*ALSSS*) [Hillel et al., 1989], *ALS Functional Rating Scale* (*ALSFRS*) [Cedarbaum and Stambler, 1997]) can be employed to evaluate progression of the disability; other scales (*ALS Health State Scale*, *Global Clinical Impression of Change*) are used to classify patients by homogeneous stage of severity.

The Appel ALS Rating Scale

The total Appel score consists of 5 subscores: bulbar, respiratory, muscle strength, and lower extremity and upper extremity function. Each group is composed of individual tests: a group score of 6 is assigned, if there is no dysfunction and group scores of 30-36 points are assigned for maximal dysfunction. The total Appel ALS score is 30 for healthy subjects and 164 for those with maximal impairment [Appel et al., 1987] The rate of change in the Appel ALS Rating Scale is a significant predictor of survival for PALS [Haverkamp et al., 1995].

The ALS Severity Scale (ALSSS)

The ALS Severity Scale (ALSSS) measures 4 functional domains: a) speech; b) swallowing; c) lower extremity and walking; d) upper extremity, dressing and hygiene. Bulbar score results from speech subscore added to swallowing subscore; spinal score from lower extremity subscore plus the upper extremity subscore. Total score ranges from 4 to 40: the lower the score the more impairment is present. The average estimated reliability coefficient interraters is 0.95. The correlation between the speech rating and objective speech measures is > 0.80. Total score, when combined with measurement of vital capacity, can provide a rapid and accurate assessment of the patient's disease status [Hillel et al., 1989].

ALS Functional Rating Scale

The *ALSFRS* is an instrument, easily administered by a clinician, an allied health professional, or a trained evaluator, for assessing PALS functional status. It is a validated questionnaire-based ordinal score system for measuring physical functions while performing normal daily tasks: it can be used for monitoring diachronically patient's functional changes. The ALSFRS components are grouped into 4 domains encompassing: a) bulbar functions; b) gross motor tasks; c) fine motor tasks, and d) breathing. It consists of 10 items, related to functional activities which are relevant for PALS (speech, salivation, swallowing, handwriting, cutting food and handling utensils, dressing and hygiene, turning in bed and adjusting bed clothes, walking, climbing stairs, and breathing). Each item is rated on a 4 (normal function) to 0 (maximal impairment) scale by the patients and/or caregiver, yielding a maximal score of 40 points [Cedarbaum and Stambler, 1997]. With appropriate training the ALSFRS can be administered with high interrater reliability and test-retest reliability (0.88 for all test items).

ALSFRS results are in close agreement with objective measures of muscle strength and pulmonary function. The ALSFRS may be used as a screening measure for entry into clinical trials, as a surrogate measure of function in situations in which muscle strength cannot be measured directly, or as an adjunct to myometry.

A limit of the ALSFRS as originally designed was that it granted disproportionate weighting to limb and bulbar, as compared to respiratory, dysfunction: authors have then validated a revised version of the ALSFRS, which incorporates additional assessments of dyspnea, orthopnea, and the need for ventilatory support, thus leading to 12 item numerosity (maximal total score: 48/48) [Cedarbaum et al., 1999]. Such a Revised ALSFRS ($ALSFRS_R$) retains the properties of the original scale and shows strong internal consistency and construct validity.

Somatic Muscle Strength Assessment

Besides the abovementioned clinimetric functional global scales, the quantitative assessment of muscle strength (which is a clinically relevant measure of ALS progression) - including the *Manual Muscle Testing* (*MMT*) and the *Maximal Voluntary Isometric Contraction* (*MVIC*) - complete the clinical motor PALS evaluation. Furthermore, the *quantitative EMG* can be regarded as a suitable complement to muscle strength assessment.

Manual Muscle Testing

Muscle strength is measured by a trained evaluator using the British *Medical Research Council* (*MRC*) grading scale in a standardized patient positioning. It was recently demonstrated that if enough muscles are tested, a decline in average grade can be determined early in the disease, and the variability of measurement approximates that of MVIC [Great

Lakes ALS Study Group, 2003]. MMT advantages are speed, expense, and the lack of needed equipment; its disadvantages are low sensitivity to change in muscle strength, the fact that data are ordinal, qualitative and subjective; furthermore, a large number of muscles must be evaluated to reduce variability and improve sensitivity.

Maximal Voluntary Isometric Contraction

The MVIC [Andres et al., 1987] has proven useful as an outcome measure in natural history studies and clinical trials with PALS, and is a valid and reliable measure of disease progression. MVIC can be measured using a hand-held dynamometer or a fixed device with strain gauges. The strength of individual muscle groups is determined quantitatively, and then the scores are normalized and combined into composite scores (called *megascores*). Intrarater and inter-rater reliability have been assessed in a number of clinical trials in ALS: with rigorous training of clinical evaluators, intra- and inter-rater reliability are less than 15% [Hoagland et al., 1997]. The MVIC is a good quantitative measure of the rate of decline of muscle strength, an outcome measure that is highly relevant to the disease. MVIC advantages include good intrarater and inter-rater reliability, sensitivity to small, clinically relevant changes and generation of numerically continuous data which are suitable for parametric statistical analysis. Problems limiting the use of MVIC are: it takes approximately 45 min to perform testing; requires expensive equipment; is not applicable for home visits; and data can not be obtained from very weak muscles.

A faster and portable method uses hand-held dynamometry (HHD) to test isometric strength of multiple muscles, again with standard patient positioning and rigorous training. HHD equipment is inexpensive and takes less than 5 min to complete a test of both upper and lower extremities. It has been directly validated against MVIC in PALS, and shown to change at a similar rate with variability that is only slightly greater than MVIC [Beck et al., 1999]: for both upper and lower extremity muscles, correlations between MVIC and HHD measurements ranged between 0.84 and 0.92, with test-retest variability that was extremely similar as well.

Quantitative Electromyography

Motor unit number estimation (*MUNE*) is a special electrophysiological technique that can provide a quantitative estimate of the number of axons innervating a muscle or group of muscles. MUNE consists of a number of different methods (incremental, multiple point stimulation, spike-triggered averaging, F-wave, and statistical methods), with each having specific advantages and limitations. Despite the lack of a perfect single method for performing MUNE, it may have value in the assessment of progressive motor axon loss in ALS, and may have use as an end-point measure in clinical trials [Bromberg and Brownell, 2008].

Respiratory Muscle Function Assessment

Vital capacity (*VC*), *maximal inspiratory pressure* (*MIP*) and *maximal expiratory pressure* (*MEP*) are the methods most commonly used to evaluate respiratory muscle strength. These measures are widely available, non-invasive and portable.

The *forced vital capacity* (*FVC*) measures volume of air forcefully expired in one breath: usually, the FVC is reported as a percentage of a predicted vital capacity based on subject's height, gender and age. The FVC declines with time in PALS and is a sensitive measure of disease progression. Both the baseline FVC and the rate of decline in FVC are predictive of survival [Varrato et al., 2001].

MIP measures the maximal negative pressure at the mouth after complete exhalation followed by a single sustained maximal inspiratory effort against an occluded airway; whereas MEP is the maximal positive pressure measured at the mouth after inhalation to total lung capacity followed by a maximal expiratory effort against an occluded airway: both MIP and MEP, easy to determine and reproducible, are sensitive early indicators of respiratory muscle weakness.

However, these tests are associated with increased variability in patients with significant bulbar involvement and require maximal respiratory muscle activation [Lyall et al., 2001]: bulbar or facial weakness can prevent the formation of a tight lip-seal around a mouthpiece; vocal cord spasms and excessive saliva and gagging can also interfere with study performance. Other measures of respiratory muscle function that might be more useful in patients with bulbar involvement and as outcome measures include *maximal sniff esophageal*, *transdiaphragmatic*, and *nasal pressures*.

Swallowing Assessment

Proper evaluation of swallowing problems should begin with a detailed history and oropharyngeal examination by the speech therapist. Generic dysphagia scales are reliable indicators of dysphagia in ALS. The bulbar components of the ALS specific scales is sensitive to dysphagia: the bulbar section of the Norris scale [Norris et al., 1974] can be utilised as an independent and reliable indicator of the severity of dysphagia in ALS.

Clinimetric dysphagia assessment has to be supplemented by instrumental evaluation (videofluoroscopy, fiberoptic examination of the swallowing, and oropharyngoesophageal scintigraphy, OPES) [Fattori et al., 2006].

At present, videofluoroscopy is considered the gold standard for assessing dysphagia in PALS; nevertheless, this procedure allows only qualitative visual evaluation of the swallowing act, without providing any quantitative data. On the other hand, OPES not only permits functional evaluation of swallowing, but it is also used to obtain a detailed semiquantitative assessment of the various stages of swallowing, especially data on transit time and retention of the bolus through the mouth, pharynx, and esophagus; moreover, this technique also provides data on the bolus fraction aspirated into the tracheobronchial tract, if present [Fattori et al., 2006]. As for videofluoroscopy, the main limitation of OPES is a low anatomic definition.

In the absence of availability of detailed instrumental swallowing assessment, clinimetric scales (i.e., the Norris and to a lesser degree the ALSFRS bulbar sections) are adequate to follow clinically significant dysphagia in PALS, and can be used as an indicator for dysphagia treatment initiation.

Speech Assessment

Bulbar involvement leads to progressive dysarthria, unintelligibility and anarthria [Tomik and Guiloff, 2010]. It is associated with significant social and psychological problems: significant dysarthria can lead to frustration on the part of the patient when others are unwilling to spend the time to carefully listen. Friends and healthcare workers may tend to "do all the talking" and not listen to the patient; there is a temptation to anticipate answers and finish sentences for the patient.

Yorkston et al. [1993] initially suggested that PALS speaking rate reduction precedes decreases in intelligibility; Ball et al. [2001, 2002] reported that speaking rate on the *Speech Intelligibility Test* (*Sentence Subtest*) [Yorkston et al., 2007] is a relatively good predictor of PALS intelligibility deterioration. This computerized test supports the efficient measurement of speaking rate in clinical settings; it helps patients and their families monitor changes over time, prepare for an *Augmentative and Alternative Communication* (*AAC*) evaluation, and reinforces their understanding of rate and intelligibility. Using this test, speaking rate can be accurately monitored over the telephone if a patient lives at a distance, or is unable to travel [Ball et al., 2005]: it should be noted, anyway, that speech intelligibility could not be objectively assessed over the telephone, as a clinical measure of understandability.

Treatment

Attempts have been undertaken in the past and present and will be undertaken in the future to bring a stop neurodegeneration in PALS: the ideal outcome for the patient would be complete cessation of symptoms and restitution of full muscle strength and motor control.

At the present time, the neurologist's attempts to treat ALS can be organized under the following multiple modalities of treatment: a *pathogenetic therapy* (encompassing drugs and other biological and electrophysiological approaches) – to counteract MN degeneration; and a *symptomatic therapy* (pharmacological and not, including assistive rehabilitation) – to reduce impairments in motor abilities, in particular body movements in activities of daily living, breathing, nutrition, communication, and a variety of related symptoms, such as spasticity, pain, dyspnea, or sialorrhea.

The appropriate implementation of each one of these types of therapy reflects the difficulties that we now have to face in ALS treatment. Differently from an acute, self-limited disease with expected recovery, the choice of appropriate therapeutic options for PALS raises more difficult concerns, since one must take into account many personal and ethical considerations. Several decisions by PALS and their families regarding treatment hinge on their concept of the quality of life that will result from such treatments.

Pathogenetic Treatment

This type of treatment is addressed to counteract the biochemical mechanisms leading to MN degeneration, by employing drugs, cells or an electrophysiological approach.

Neuropharmacological Strategies

Over the years several studies have been performed with different types of drugs, acting on the mechanisms involved in MN degeneration. Potential therapies for ALS are being investigated in animal models: some of this work involves experimental treatments with normal SOD1 and other antioxidants; in addition, neurotrophic factors are being studied for their potential to protect MNs from pathological degeneration. Although no effective cure has yet been found for ALS, investigators are optimistic that these and other basic research studies will eventually lead to treatments for ALS.

In nineties the Food and Drug Administration has approved the first drug treatment for the disease, *Riluzole*: it is believed to reduce damage to MNs by decreasing the release of glutamate. Clinical trials with PALS showed that Riluzole prolongs survival by several months; it also extends the time before a patient needs ventilation support. Nevertheless, it does not reverse the damage already done to MNs, and patients taking the drug must be monitored for liver damage and other possible side effects. However, this first disease-specific therapy offers hope that ALS progression may one day be slowed by new medications or combinations of drugs.

Each mechanism involved in ALS pathogenesis may represent a possible therapeutic approach to counteract MN neurodegeneration. We now focus on some therapeutic clinical trials recruiting PALS or recently concluded, ordered according the pathogenetic mechanism involved.

Excitotoxicity

A pilot study with a noncompetitive modulator of AMPA glutamate receptors, *Talampanel*, showed a slower decline in $ALSFRS_R$ score rate during the 9-month treatment; subsequently, a multinational, multicenter, randomized, double blind, placebo-controlled, parallel-group study to assess the efficacy, tolerability and safety of Talampanel in PALS (ALS-TAL-201) was performed enrolling 550 patients, beginning on September 2008: on May 2010 the pharmaceutical company Teva announced that the results were conclusively negative, since the $ALSFRS_R$ score showed no difference in the progression rate of PALS treated with placebo or either with 2 doses of Talampanel; and side effects were more common in drug-treated participants treated, whereas the dropout rates were very similar in all groups (www.asla.org 2/7/2010).

Given the increase in *excitatory amino acid transporter 2* expression and function documented in transgenic mice overexpressing a mutant SOD1 (mtSOD1) treated with *Ceftriaxone* at symptom onset [Rothstein et al., 2005] and case reports with *cephalosporins* indicating a clinical improvement [Harvey and Martz, 2007], an open label clinical trial with bimonthly drug cycles of Ceftriaxone (2 g/day, for 14 days every two months) was performed: after one-year treatment a significant improvement of antioxidant oxidative stress status was observed, but no clinical improvement [Siciliano et al., 2010]. A wide double blind placebo-controlled clinical trial on about 600 PALS is currently recruiting participants in the United States of America (NCT00349622) [www.clinicaltrial.gov] since July 2006: final data collection for the primary outcome measure (survival and rate of change in $ALSFRS_R$) will be available in June 2012.

Memantine, a low-affinity noncompetitive NMDA receptor antagonist, may be useful in protecting MN from death [Chen and Lipton, 2006]. Recently, the results of a phase II/III, 12-

month, double-blinded, single-centre, randomized clinical trial performed to evaluate the efficacy and safety of Memantine (20 mg/day) in 63 PALS have been reported [de Carvalho et al., 2010]: primary (12-month ALSFRS decline) and secondary (FVC, MMT, visual analogue scale, quality of life, MUNE and neurophysiological index) outcomes were not significantly different between the two groups; Memantine is safe and well tolerated. Actually is ongoing and currently recruiting participants in Canada a "Randomized, double blind, dose-ranging study to determine the effect of Memantine on functional outcomes and motor neuron degeneration in patients with ALS" (NCT00409721).

Oxidative Stress and Apoptosis

Based on several findings of increased oxidative damage in PALS spinal cord and cortex MNs [Ferrante et al., 1997] and imbalance of oxidative stress reported also in CSF [Smith et al., 1998; Ihara et al., 2005], a large variety of antioxidants compounds have been tested in PALS.

Although preclinical studies demonstrated a prolonged survival following treatment with *Coenzyme Q10* [Matthews et al., 1998], an antioxidant, essential mitochondrial cofactor facilitating electron transfer in the respiratory chain, the phase II study in PALS (NCT00243932) showed insufficient promise to warrant Phase III testing [Kaufmann et al., 2009].

After positive results obtained in animal models [Crow et al., 2005], a pilot study with *Manganoporphyrin*, *AEOL 10150*, an antioxidant molecule that catalytically neutralizes superoxide, hydrogen peroxide and peroxynitrite, and inhibits lipid peroxidation [Patel and Day, 1999] showed that single doses of drug, ranging from 3 mg to 30 mg, were tolerated without serious side effects [www.rideforlife.com].

In keeping with maintaining mitochondrial function in ALS, a two-part Phase II randomized, double-blind trial (NCT00647296) with *KNS-760704* including 102 PALS, recently concluded: preliminary results showed that KNS-760704 is safe and well tolerated, and that 300 mg daily may slow the rate of motor function loss [Bozik et al., 2010].

Yoshino and Kimura [2006] investigated the efficacy and safety of *Edaravone*, a free-radical scavenger now widely used for the treatment of acute cerebral infarction for its neuroprotective effect against oxidative damage [Uno et al., 2005], in an open trial design on 20 PALS receiving either 30 mg or 60 mg intravenously once per day. Two weeks of administration were followed by a 2-week observation period: such a 4-week cycle was repeated 6 times. During the 6-month treatment period, the decline in the $ALSFRS_R$ score was significantly less than that in the 6 months prior to Edaravone administration; in almost all patients, CSF 3-nitrotyrosine, a marker for oxidative stress, was markedly reduced to almost undetectable levels at the end of the 6-month treatment period. This study suggested that Edaravone is safe and may delay the progression of functional motor disturbances by reducing oxidative stress in PALS.

Premature apoptosis and/or an aberration in apoptosis regulation is implicated in ALS MN degeneration [Pasinelli et al., 2004]. Transcriptional dysfunction has been implicated in the pathogenesis of many neurodegenerative diseases including ALS [Rouaux et al., 2007]. Therefore, histone deacetylase (HDAC) inhibitors may be promising candidates.

Valproic acid (*VPA*) is a HDAC inhibiting drug [Kanai et al., 2004] that promotes gene transcription and inhibits neuronal cell death by counterbalancing apoptosis, oxidative stress and glutamate toxicity [Morland et al., 2004]. Based on the finding that VPA and other

HDAC inhibitors increased survival in mtSOD1 mice [Sugai et al., 2004], 163 PALS received 1,500 mg VPA or placebo daily ("A randomized, double blind, placebo-controlled sequential clinical trial of sodium valproate in ALS" - NCT00136110): unfortunately, VPA at a dose used in epilepsy did not show a beneficial effect on survival or disease progression in PALS.

In the "Long term extension study of TCH346 and placebo administered once daily in patients with amyotrophic lateral sclerosis" (NCT00230074) conducted on 591 PALS enrolled from 42 sites in Europe and North America, patients received orally once daily for at least 24 weeks either placebo or one of 4 doses (1.0, 2.5, 7.5, or 15 mg) of *TCH346*, an antiapoptotic compound exerting its effects by binding to glyceraldehyde 3-phosphate dehydrogenase (GAPDH) and blocking the apoptotic pathway in which GAPDH is involved. At the end of the study there were no significant differences between placebo and active treatment groups in the mean rate of $ALSFRS_R$ score decline or in the secondary outcome measures (survival, pulmonary function and MMT).

The administration *Minocycline* to PALS in a multicentre, randomized placebo-controlled phase III trial (NCT00047723) produced negative results with $ALSFRS_R$ score deterioration that was faster in the Minocycline group than in the placebo group [Gordon et al., 2007], even if it was reported to prolong survival by 10-22% in transgenic mouse models of ALS [Kriz et al., 2002; Van Den Bosch et al., 2002].

Having shown preclinical studies antioxidant, antiapoptotic and neuroprotective properties of *Tauroursodeoxycholic Acid* (*TUDCA*) in the CNS, in both *in vitro* and *in vivo* models [Castro et al., 2004], a small Italian phase II trial (NCT00877604) involving 20 people with MND is now underway to assess whether the addition of TUDCA to riluzole can slow the disease progression: the trial will run for 12 months and results are expected quite soon.

Neurotrophic Factors

Insulin-like growth factor 1 (*IGF-1*) is a neurotrophic factor that has been tested in a North American and in an European phase III trial, enrolling 266 and 183 PALS, respectively. The two trials showed contrasting results, since IGF-1 either slowed the rate of functional decline by 26% [Lai et al., 1997], or did not produce positive effects [Borasio et al., 1998]. Subsequently, another phase III trial using IGF-1 treatment for 2 years has been performed on 330 PALS, showing that the drug did not produce beneficial effects on MMT, $ALSFRS_R$ or in delaying tracheostomy [Sorenson et al., 2008].

A double blind, randomized, parallel-group study to evaluate safety and tolerability with *VEGF165* administered intracerebroventricularly (NCT00800501) is currently recruiting participants [www.clinicaltrial.gov].

Neuroinflammation

Thalidomide has potent anti-inflammatory properties through the modulation of inflammatory cytokines, such as TNF-α, and appreciably penetrates the CSF [Franks et al., 2004]. Although a pilot study with Thalidomide was interrupted for safety concerns, a non-randomized, open label phase II study was further performed (NCT00140452), showing that the drug can cause side effects without effectively modulating disease progression [Stommel et al., 2009].

Arimoclomol, a molecule able to determine an enhanced production of the heat shock proteins, thus protecting cells from protein aggregation and death [Kieran et al., 2004], determined a prolonged survival of mtSOD1 mice, either if treatment was started in presymptomatic stage [Kieran et al., 2004] or at the onset of symptoms [Kalmar et al., 2008]. After a Phase IIa Arimoclomol trial showed that the drug is safe and well tolerated [Cudkowicz et al., 2008], a phase II/III adaptive, randomized, placebo-controlled clinical trial is still recruiting fALS patients (NCT00706147) [www.clinicaltrial.gov].

Autophagy

Lithium is a drug regulating autophagy: it induces autophagy by inhibiting the intracellular enzyme inositol monophosphatase [Sarkar et al., 2005], whereas glycogen synthase kinase-3β inhibition (at higher drug concentrations) determines a negative regulation of autophagy via the mammalian target of *rapamycin*, *mTOR* [Yang and Guan, 2007]. Lithium-induced autophagy counteracts neurodegeneration [Pasquali et al., 2009] and appears to be neuroprotective for MNs both in organotypic slice cultures of spinal cord [Caldero et al., 2010] and in mtSOD1 mice, where it improves motor function and slows disease progression [Fornai et al., 2008].

A 15-month pilot clinical trial in randomized PALS showed that Lithium and Riluzole co-treatment markedly reduced mortality when compared with matched control patients treated with Riluzole alone [Fornai et al., 2008]. However, inconsistent results have also been reported: in a sibling-matched, gender-balanced, investigator-blinded trial, using a standard mouse model of fALS chronic Lithium treatment showed no benefit [Gill et al., 2009]; another study also found no therapeutic or neuroprotective effects of Lithium in female ALS mice [Pizzasegola et al., 2009].

A randomized, double blind, placebo-controlled trial was conducted on 84 PALS by the Northeast ALS and Canadian ALS Consortia: Lithium did not produce safety concerns, but treatment was interrupted for futility at the first interim analysis (24 weeks), when a 43% improvement did not occur in patients actively treated [Aggarwal et al., 2010].

Neurobiological Strategies

Gene Therapy

Accumulation of altered, misfolded and aggregated proteins in both fALS and sALS seems to be involved in the pathogenesis of the disease. Decreasing levels of these proteins, by downregulating the genes responsible for such accumulations, may represent a therapeutic strategy aimed to ameliorate the disease state. *Antisense oligonucleotides* to SOD1 administered near onset in mtSOD1 rats reduced SOD1 in brain and spinal cord, and significantly slowed disease progression [Smith et al., 2006]. Based on these findings, a clinical trial using Antisense oligonucleotides to SOD1 will start in fALS patients with SOD1 mutations [www.alsa.org].

Stem Cell Therapy

Stem-cell transplantation is an attractive treatment approach for neurological diseases. Previous studies performed in neurodegenerative disease animal models generated optimism about restoring functions or delaying neurodegeneration in human beings: autologous or allogeneic stem cells, undifferentiated or transdifferentiated, might represent a new therapeutic strategy for PALS [Silani et al., 2004]. Although scientifically based clinical trials using stem cells to treat neurodegenerative diseases have already been carried out, unfortunately none of them has achieved a real benefit: nevertheless, such treatments are somewhere offered around the world, often underestimating the potential risks of the procedure [Lau et al., 2008].

We need strict laboratory guidelines based upon well established preclinical studies, and rigorous clinical protocols in order to successfully develop a safe and effective stem cell therapy for neurodegenerative diseases; furthermore, we have to carefully deal with ethical, social and economic implications.

Neurophysiological Strategies

Repetitive Transcranial Magnetic Stimulation

Another approach to modulate glutamatergic circuits of human motor cortex is the *repetitive transcranial magnetic stimulation* (*rTMS*). Such a technique has potential therapeutic effects in several neurological diseases, including ALS [Lefaucheur, 2008]. Repetitive stimulation of the motor cortex was performed for 5 consecutive days every month for 6 consecutive months in 20 PALS participating to a double blind, placebo-controlled clinical trial [Di Lazzaro et al., 2006]: both active and sham patients deteriorated during treatment, with active patients having a modest, but significant, slowing of the deterioration rate. Based on these findings, a double blind, placebo-controlled trial on 20 PALS randomly allocated to blinded real or placebo stimulation was performed, to test the hypothesis that rTMS given as continuous theta burst stimulation, repeated for 5 consecutive days monthly for one year, would affect disease progression: treatment was well tolerated, but there was no significant difference in the $ALSFRS_R$ score between patients' groups [Di Lazzaro et al, 2010].

Symptomatic Treatment

Other treatments are designed to relieve symptoms and improve the quality of life for patients. This supportive care is best provided by multidisciplinary teams of health care professionals such as physicians; pharmacists; physical, occupational, and speech therapists; nutritionists; social workers; and home care and hospice nurses [Bede et al., 2011]. Working with patients and caregivers, these teams can design an individualized plan of medical and physical therapy and provide special equipment aimed at keeping patients as mobile and comfortable as possible.

Pharmacological Strategies

Physicians can prescribe medications to ameliorate fatigue, ease muscle cramps, control spasticity, and reduce excess saliva and phlegm. Drugs also are available to help patients with pain, depression, sleep disturbances, and constipation [Bede et al., 2011].

For an exhaustive review on this topic s. Gordon [2011]; as well as the American Academy of Neurology Practice Parameters [Miller et al., 1999; $2009_{a,b}$] for a meta-analysis of peer-reviewed studies on symptomatic treatment of PALS.

Non Pharmacological Strategies

The primary goal of an effective assistive rehabilitation for PALS is the management of disabilities, symptoms and complications arising from the progressive weakness of limb, trunk, and bulbar muscles [Norris et al., 1985]. Further goals include keeping the patient functioning as independently as possible and maintaining quality of life even into the terminal stage.

The rehabilitation program varies depending on whether the patient has a long clinical course or rapid progression of the disease: in the former case, PALS become able to compensate remarkably well for the motor unit loss and are able to continue with their daily activity for several years [Chen et al., 2008]. The success of the rehabilitation approach depends on the active participation of the patient who should be a full partner in the therapeutic team even during the advanced stages of the disease. It may be difficult for the physician to discuss such a fatal illness: however, a direct approach allows the patient to deal most effectively with the disease and its physical limitations. This also helps in decisions about the intensity of the therapeutic effort [Bede et al., 2011; Gordon, 2011].

The family and other caregivers should be encouraged to participate in the patient's early rehabilitation program: the family role will then likely increase as weakness progresses, requirements for assistive devices change, and new problems arise in the management of activities of daily living.

Physical Exercise

Patients and their families often have questions concerning physical therapy: several may have been exposed to exercise or fitness programs in the past, and others will have known patients who received rehabilitation followed neurological or orthopaedic dysfunction. They might reason that if weakness of a muscle group exists, exercise can strengthen it. It is important for PALS to understand that the cause of his/her weakness is a chronic and progressive loss of MNs that will not be replaced by exercise. The patient must understand that, although there may be temporary improvement in function, other muscle groups will become increasingly involved. However, healthy muscle groups can be strengthened by exercise and used to compensate for the weakness of other muscle groups [Chen et al., 2008].

The question of whether regular exercise is beneficial or not in PALS is still controversial [Francis et al., 1999]. Moderate regular exercise is helpful in the management of many neuromuscular diseases [Lui and Byl, 2009], allowing weak muscles to increase their mitochondrial content and to enhance muscle blood flow and strength.

Some epidemiological studies suggest that vigorous physical activity in the form of heavy labor or competitive athletics increases ALS risk [Chiò et al., 2005]. On the contrary, other studies report earlier disease onset among individuals with a greater amounts of leisure time and reduced physical activity [Veldink et al., 2005] or that physical activity is not a risk factor for developing ALS [Qureshi et al., 2006]: anyway, frequently PALS do not perform any type of physical activity in order to preserve their muscle strength and minimize overwork muscle damage [Longstreth et al., 1991].

Preclinical studies in the transgenic mouse model of ALS have demonstrated beneficial effects of physical activity on motor function. The effects of high and moderate levels of exercise were investigated in mtSOD1 mice [Carreras et al., 2010]: in mtSOD1 mice undergoing moderate exercise, a preservation of motor performance (correlating with higher MN density in the ventral horn of the lumbar spinal cord) was showed.

Investigation of some oxidative stress markers during submaximal incremental exercise at a power level corresponding to the anaerobic lactate threshold in patients), showed an increased production of lactate and lipoperoxides [Siciliano et al., 2002], suggesting that regular aerobic physical activity, rather than anaerobic exercise, may be useful in ALS. Gentle, low-impact aerobic exercise such as walking, swimming, and stationary bicycling can strengthen unaffected muscles, improve cardiovascular health, and help patients fight fatigue and depression. Range of motion and stretching exercises can help prevent painful spasticity and shortening (contracture) of muscles. Physical therapists can recommend exercises that provide these benefits without overworking muscles.

Clinical trials on PALS have suggested that regular physical exercise may be neuroprotective, ameliorating symptoms and improving functionality [Drory et al., 2001; Bello-Haas et al., 2007]. Drory and colleagues [2001] conducted an observational study to determine the effect of moderate regular exercise under professional guidance on motor deficit, disability, fatigue, musculoskeletal pain and perceived quality of life. They randomized 25 PALS to perform either a specific moderate daily exercise program or just their daily physical activity. At 3 months, patients who performed regular exercise showed less deterioration on ALSFRS and Ashworth spasticity scales; at 6 months, there was no significant difference between groups, although a trend towards less deterioration in the treated group on most scales was observed. At 9 and 12 months there were too few patients in each group for statistical evaluation. Their results showed that a regular moderate physical exercise program has a shortlived positive effect on disability in PALS.

Bello-Haas and coworkers [2007] performed a study in which they investigated the effects of resistance exercise on function, fatigue, and quality of life in 27 PALS using ALSFRS, the Fatigue Severity Scale, Short Form-36 (SF-36), FVC and MVIC at baseline and monthly for 6 months. Patients in mild stage of disease were randomly assigned to a resistance exercise group (daily stretching and resistance exercises three times weekly) or to a usual care group (only the daily stretching exercises). Eight of the 13 enrolled resistance exercise patients and 10 of the 14 enrolled usual care patients completed the trial. At 6 months, the resistance exercise group had significantly higher ALSFRS and SF-36 physical function subscale scores and less decline in leg strength, as measured by MVIC. Physical exercise exerts positive effects on healthy MNs, by enhancing dendritic restructuring, protein synthesis, axonal transport and neuromuscular communication [Gardiner et al., 2006; McCrate and Kaspar, 2008].

Physical therapy and special equipment can enhance patients' independence and safety throughout the course of ALS. The role of physical therapy may vary greatly from patient to patient, and it is difficult to evaluate the benefit of therapy in patients whose disease continues to progress: however, the benefits gained, both physical and psychological, are usually worthwhile. Patient function can be improved by the use of supportive appliances and orthotic devices. In many istances, weakness in one area may lead to a loss of balance that impairs function, despite adequate strength in other muscle groups. A device as simple and inexpensive as a soft cervical collar may provide weakened neck muscles with enough support to prevent forward head tilt, resulting in gait imbalance. Use of a support, such as a cane, walker, or brace may greatly improve a patient's ability to ambulate. Many patients deny their problem and refuse to use aids such as a walker: unfortunately, falls secondary to weakness are common, and resulting injuries such as hip fractures can ultimately worsen disability. PALS can be taught to perform various functions using alternative approaches.

Occupational therapists can suggest devices such as ramps, braces, walkers, and wheelchairs that help patients conserve energy and remain mobile. Small investments in the home and work environment can greatly enhance the quality of life. For instance, a patient unable to button clothing can usually use Velcro fasteners. Self-help books, practical manuals from the ALS associations worldwide, and catalogs from vendors dealing in merchandise for the handicapped can all be valuable resources for PALS and their families: simple solutions are often available for difficult problems, and they need only to be considered.

Respiratory Treatment

Most PALS eventually die of complications due to respiratory dysfunction: these problems may arise from weakness of breathing muscles (leading to hypercapnia, hypoxemia and respiratory failure); and from weakness and incoordination of the bulbar muscles (resulting in a weak cough, aspiration and sleep apnea).

The strength of the respiratory muscles should be monitored with pulmonary function studies (s. Functional assessment – Respiratory muscle function assessment): when pulmonary problems are present, they need to be discussed with the patient and his/her family, and alternatives for respiratory management should also be discussed at that time. Once MIP or MEP falls below 25 cmH_2O or the VC is < 1 l, closed attention must be paid to the patient: if the deterioration in respiratory parameters has been relatively slow, and if the patient is asymptomatic, reliable and well supervised, he/she has to be only carefully followed up [Hardiman, 2011].

Respiratory Exercises

Several strategies can be used to improve respiratory muscle strength and decrease respiratory fatigue: the respiratory muscles, while subject to fatigue like other skeletal muscles, are trainable to potentially achieve greater endurance and strength. The opportunity to increase respiratory muscle strength and endurance, and hence to postpone respiratory failure, must be tempered with the possibility that vigorous exercise may itself induce respiratory muscle failure: this might occur in situations where exercise levels require peak inspiratory pressures greater than the critical level for fatigue. Furthermore, the actual stress caused by exercise could theoretically disrupt muscle fibers. The clinician must keep in mind that endurance and strength-building strategies can only work with intact motor units: muscle fibers becoming denervated will be reinnervated by healthy MNs in the early stages of the disease, but eventually the ability of the nervous system to reinnervate can not keep pace with the increasing number of denervated muscle fibers, which are unlikely to respond to any muscle-training exercise [Hardiman, 2011].

Strategies for improving respiratory muscle strength become most important when the normal work of breathing begins to approach a critical threshold; once it is exceeded, the normal act of breathing will lead to fatigue and ventilatory failure. Patients may exceed this work threshold because of other variables, including minor respiratory tract infections which have to be aggressively treated.

Respiratory muscle strength may be maintained or enhanced with inspiratory-resistive training exercises. Home deep-breathing exercises can be repeated frequently and may be more beneficial with an incentive spirometer. Although the exercises may be performed while the patient is in any position, they are best done with the patient in a supine position. While prolonged benefit from training to improve exercise performance should not be expected in PALS, in many cases, anyway, a training program may delay the onset of ventilatory failure, and give an important psychological support from such an active subject's participation in the fight against his/her disease.

Assisted coughing after a deep breath and chest physical therapy for postural drainage are extremely helpful, and the patient's family may be instructed in these maneuvers [Senent et al., 2011].

Mechanical Ventilation

Whereas a normal $PaCO_2$ does not guarantee that rapid deterioration will not occur, an enhanced $PaCO_2$ (> 45 mmHg) suggests the need for mechanical ventilation. Once MIP and MEP drop below 15 cm H_2O, or the $PaCO_2$ rises to even the smallest extent over normal, the initiation of mechanical ventilation is recommended: the decision concerning long-term mechanical ventilation is a complex one and needs to be approached early in the patient's course and re-evaluated at each visit. Respiratory therapists can help caregivers with tasks such as operating and maintaining ventilators.

Intermittent *noninvasive ventilation* (*NIV*) consists in a positive pressure ventilator (delivering two levels of pressure, inspiratory and expiratory: BiPAP) with a tigh-fitting nasal (or orofacial, or facial) mask. At the beginning, BiPAP will be used nightly, to aid breathing during sleep; then, when muscles are no longer able to maintain O_2 and CO_2 levels, this device will has to be used full time. Such a ventilator can help rest fatigued respiratory muscle and, at least in the short term, may be well tolerated by the patient: however, more chronic use often results in skin breakdown and ulcer formation over the bridge of the nose. NIV can postpone the initiation of *invasive ventilation* (*IV*) for several months; prolong life and improve comfort; allow the PALS to experience a limited form of mechanical ventilation while arriving at a decision concerning full IV [Hardiman, 2011].

NIV, however, is less effective than IV in promoting air exchange. Patients must be told that ventilatory devices are not curative and that further deterioration will occur; furthermore, the upper airway will not be protected as it would be with *tracheostomy*.

Swallowing Treatment

Although PALS with bulbar involvement suffer from more severe swallowing problems (such as aspiration), predominantly nonbulbar PALS may also have dysphagia.

Dysphagia in PALS is known to be characterized by impairment of the oral stage of swallowing, with ensuing impact on the next phase of swallowing, the pharyngeal stage. Deficit in the oral stage first results in increased length of the time required to take a meal: with milder abnormalities, the patient may be able to compensate for any swallowing impairment. A predominant deficit in soft palate muscles may result in nasal regurgitation of fluids, although this symptom is often diminished by concomitant deficit in lingual propulsion.

Several problems related to eating can be treated by relatively simple methods.

Dietary content should be changed to foods that are easy for PALS to swallow: in general, soft but firm foods with a smooth texture are easiest to swallow. Patients should be encouraged to experiment with various textures, temperatures, and types of food. Swallowing water and other thin liquids may prove difficult, due to premature spillover into the pharynx; thicker liquids (e.g. fruit nectars, shakes, and commercial food thickeners) may be used. If chewing is a problem, foods requiring less chewing should be replaced and a blender can be used to homogenize food. As dietary content becomes limited, it can be supplemented with commercially available complete liquid diets; if water intake is reduced due to choking, the nutritionist should suggest adding foods that are high in water content.

Swallowing initiation may be improved by chewing ice or thermal stimulation. Neck extensor weakness can often be successfully managed with a cervical collar. Postures and behavioral modifications can correct swallowing difficulties for a variable interval before other therapeutic interventions are necessary. Documentation of aspiration of a particular food warrants initiation of proper swallowing techniques (postural changes and specific exercises) [Logemann, 2008].

As bulbar muscle weakness progresses, symptoms and signs of decompensated swallowing appear. They are dramatic, and include coughing and choking with feeding, aspiration pneumonia, and asphyxia due to a solid bolus obstructing the airway; frequent throat clearing, wet voice, nasal regurgitation, retention of solid food particles in the pharynx, and delayed food passage.

Eventually, the time comes when a decision has to be made concerning the use of a feeding tube. Patients should be clearly informed that modern techniques for feeding tube placement have greatly decreased the discomfort and morbidity associated with the procedure [Spataro et al., 2011].

Sialorrhea Treatment

Patients complain of drooling or difficulty in controlling their saliva: this problem not only is embarrassing, but also can be life-threatening if secretions are aspirated.

Swallowing difficulties may lead to excessive dribbling of saliva in many PALS. Normally, 1-2 ml of saliva are produced each minute: this is usually swallowed without conscious effort. Weakness of neck and facial muscles will cause a patient to tilt the head forward with lips open: instead of saliva running backwards and being swallowed, it runs forward and drips.

Proper positioning, lip-tightening exercises, and a cervical collar may be helpful.

As the problem progresses, pharmacological intervention may be tried with drying agents such as anticholinergics and certain antidepressants (e.g. *amitryptiline*).

Many patients prefer a suction machine to handle oral secretions while avoiding drug side effects. The use of botulinum toxin and radiotherapy of salivary glands have also been proposed [Guidubaldi et al., 2011; Guy et al., 2011].

Speech Treatment

Dysarthric PALS may benefit from working with a *speech therapist.* These health professionals can teach patients adaptive strategies, such as techniques to help them speak louder and more clearly. In early disease stages, patients can be taught to emphasize certain syllables and slow their speech patterns so that others can understand them better: lip and tongue exercises can sometimes help the patient to enunciate words more clearly on a regular basis.

A recent review on ALS communication research [Hanson et al., 2011] concluded that, due to ALS pathophysiology and the intrinsic degenerative nature of disease, speech treatment strategies designed to increase strength or mobility of the oral musculature are not recommended for PALS. Patients or their caregivers, on the contrary, often request oral exercises to improve strength and mobility for speech, as strengthening exercises seem intuitively to them as a way to increase performance: however, such exercise programs should be discouraged, and PALS should be informed that the speaking that they do each day provides a sufficient amount of speech mechanism activity and exercise.

Speech intervention should focus on learning to conserve energy for priority speaking tasks and to rest often to reduce fatigue, instead of increasing effort with speech exercises. PALS speakers should learn to avoid adverse speaking/listening situations by muting the television, inviting people to speak with them in a quiet place rather than in a crowded room, and using voice amplification when speaking in noisy environments to reduce the effort required [Ball et al., 2007; Yorkston et al., 2010].

Writing may be used as a substitute for speech, and devices as simple as paper and pencil, alphabet cards, portable typewriter, and letter boards may be used by patients with adequate hand function. Becoming speech more and more difficult to understand, many PALS supplement their speech by identifying the first letter of each word on an alphabet board (*alphabet supplementation*), or by identifying the topic on a communication board (*topic supplementation*).

As ALS progresses, speech therapists can help patients develop ways for responding to yes-or-no questions with their eyes or by other nonverbal means, and can recommend aids such as speech synthesizers and computer-based communication systems. These methods and devices help patients communicate when they can no longer speak or produce vocal sounds.

It is frequently difficult for PALS speakers, their caregivers and medical personnel to consider AAC strategies when they are still using residual speech to meet daily communication needs. However, their speaking rate should be clinically monitored so that the referral for an AAC intervention is initiated in a timely manner: Ball et al. [2001, 2002] recommend that patients be referred for AAC assessment when their speaking rates reach 125 words/min (normal value: 190 words/min) on the *Speech Intelligibility Test* (*Sentence Subtest*) [Yorkston et al., 2007]. With sufficient education and preparation, PALS and their caregivers are ready to examine their AAC options. Nevertheless, speech deterioration can be so rapid that individuals can be left with limited communication options, if they are not prepared to act in an opportune manner.

Due to the extended use of AAC with deteriorating levels of physical control, it is imperative that recommended technology has adjustable access options to meet the range of motor capability as the disease progresses, that is, PALS should be fitted with AAC technology that supports multiple access methods, such as allowing them to transition from hand access to scanning and/or head/eye-tracking. Many AAC devices now incorporate a variety of access options so that the technology can continue to meet the needs of the user despite a decline in physical capability. The sensitivity of dynamic touch screens can be adjusted to allow for lighter touch. The improved sensitivity of head-tracking technology has allowed many to use this access method with minimal head/neck movement control.

Perhaps the most significant advancement in access technology has occurred with the widespread availability of *eye-tracking systems* to allow cursor control with eye movement to access high-technology AAC devices. As the disease progresses, many PALS require the use of eye-tracking for several reasons. Firstly, eye-tracking is often the least fatiguing movement for AAC access.; eye gaze is natural, and eye muscles generally do not fatigue with use. Compared to other access methods such as switch-activated scanning, eye-tracking is often reported to be the least fatiguing access method by PALS [Gibbons and Beneteau, 2010]. Others have reported that eye-tracking technology requires relatively little effort [Calvo et al., 2008; Harris and Goren, 2009]. Secondly, eye gaze may be the only volitional movement that the individual continues to exhibit over time, particularly in cases where invasive ventilation has been chosen [Ball et al., 2010].

Research is needed to objectively document AAC acceptance and use; further research is also needed to clarify the level of cognitive impairment that tends to interfere with AAC intervention [Iversen et al., 2008].

Conclusion

PALS functional impairments result from a relentlessly progressive muscle weakness, leading ultimately to a widespread body paralysis. Therefore, all movements become more and more difficult up to a complete immobility.

In the late stages of the disease, eventually patients find themselves in a “locked-in” state, totally unable, in the worst cases, to move neck, trunk and limbs; autonomously breath and feed; and speak. Most of them, however, retain their cognitive capabilities, and assist impotent at their functional decay.

Today, much more than in the past, we can give interdisciplinary assistance to those persons and their families who have to face a dreadful condition and cope with many daily problems: motor, respiratory, nutritional and communicational management is indeed getting better now, although it is not enough to fulfil all patients’ demands.

Actively waiting a “world free from ALS”, we keep fighting against the disease together with PALS and their caregivers, by trying to improve our knowledge of pathogenetic mechanisms; develop novel and effective treatments; help suffering persons to maintain their quality of life as high as possible. Besides scientific and clinical achievements, we look forward to building up a more empathic healthcare enriched with humanity and compassion for sick people.

References

[1] Abhinav, K., Stanton, B., Johnston, C., Hardstaff, J., Orrell, R. W., Howard, R., Clarke, J., Sakel, M., Ampong, M. A., Shaw, C. E., Leigh, P. N. and Al-Chalabi, A. (2007). Amyotrophic lateral sclerosis in South-East England: a population-based study. The South- East England register for amyotrophic lateral sclerosis (SEALS Registry). *Neuroepidemiology*, *29*, 44-48.

[2] Aggarwal, S. P., Zinman, L., Simpson, E., McKinley, J., Jackson, K. E., Pinto, H., Kaufman, P., Conwit, R. A., Schoenfeld, D., Shefner, J. and Cudkowicz, M. Northeast and Canadian Amyotrophic Lateral Sclerosis consortia. (2010). Safety and efficacy of lithium in combination with riluzole for treatment of amyotrophic lateral sclerosis: a randomised, double blind, placebo-controlled trial. *Lancet Neurology*, *9*, 481-488.

[3] Agosta, F., Chiò, A., Cosottini, M., De Stefano, M., Falini, A., Mascalchi, M., Rocca, M. A., Silani, V., Tedeschi, G. and Filippi, M. (2010). The present and the future of neuroimaging in amyotrophic lateral sclerosis. *American Journal of Neuroradiology*, *31*, 1769-1777.

[4] Andres, P. L., Thibodeau, L. M., Finison, L. J. and Munsat, T. L. (1987). Quantitative assessment of neuromuscular deficit in ALS. *Neurology Clinics, 5*, 125-141.

[5] Appel, V., Stewart, S., Smith, G. and Appel, S. H. (1987). A rating scale for amyotrophic lateral sclerosis: description and preliminary experience. *Annals of Neurology, 22*, 328-333.

[6] Ball, L. J., Willis, A., Beukelman D. R. and Pattee, G. L. (2001). A protocol for identification of early bulbar signs in amyotrophic lateral sclerosis. *Journal of the Neurological Sciences*, *191*, 1, 43-53.

[7] Ball, L. J., Beukelman, D. R. and Pattee, G. L. (2002). Timing of speech deterioration in people with amyotrophic lateral sclerosis. *Journal of Medical Speech-Language Pathology*, *10*, 231-235.

[8] Ball, L. J., Beukelman, D. R., Ullman, C., Maassen, K. and Pattee, G. L. (2005). Monitoring speaking rate by telephone for persons with amyotrophic lateral sclerosis. *Journal of Medical Speech-Language Pathology*, 13, 233-240.

[9] Ball, L. J., Beukelman, D. R. and Bardach, L. (2007). AAC intervention for ALS. In D. R. Beukelman, K. Garrett and K. Yorkston (Eds.), *Augmentative Communication Strategies for Adults with acute or chronic Medical Conditions* (pp. 287-316). Baltimore, Md, USA: Paul H. Brookes.

[10] Ball, L. J., Nordness, A., Fager, S. K., Kersch, K., Mohr, B., Pattee, G. L. and Beukelman, D. R. (2010). Eye-gaze access of AAC technology for persons with amyotrophic lateral sclerosis. *Journal of Medical Speech-Language Pathology*, *18*, 11-23.

[11] Beck, M., Giess, R., Würffel, W., Magnus, T., Ochs, G. and Toyka, K. V. (1999). Comparison of maximal voluntary isometric contraction and Drachman's hand-held dynamometry in evaluating patients with amyotrophic lateral sclerosis. *Muscle and Nerve*, *22*, 1265-1270.

[12] Bede, P., Oliver, D., Stodart, J., van den Berg, L., Simmons, Z., O Brannagáin, D., Borasio. G. D. and Hardiman, O. (2011). Palliative care in amyotrophic lateral sclerosis: a review of current international guidelines and initiatives. *Journal of Neurology, Neurosurgery and Psychiatry*, *82*, 413-418.

[13] Bello-Haas, V. D., Florence, J. M., Kloos, A. D., Scheirbecker, J., Lopate, G., Hayes, S. M., Pioro, E. P. and Mitsumoto, H. (2007). A randomized controlled trial of resistance exercise in individuals with ALS. *Neurology*, *68*, 2003-2007.

[14] Bongioanni, P., Tararà, M., Metelli, M. R., Carboncini, M. C., Rossi, B. and Pietrini, P. (2001). Cytokine levels in plasma of patients with Amyotrophic Lateral Sclerosis. *Journal of Neurology*, *248(S2)*, 28-29.

[15] Bongioanni, P., Metelli, M. R., Magoni, M., Panicucci, E., Tararà, M., Bozzi, M., Rossi, B. and Pietrini, P. (2002_a). Blood antioxidative markers in sporadic ALS patients. *Biochimica Clinica*, *26*, 294.

[16] Bongioanni, P., Tararà, M., Metelli, M. R., Magoni, M., Chisari, C., Carboncini, M. C., Bonfiglio, L., Pietrini, P. and Rossi, B. (2002_b). Blood levels of growth factors in amyotrophic lateral sclerosis patients. *Amyotrophic Lateral Sclerosis and Other Motor Neuron Disorders*, *3(S2)*, 55-56.

[17] Bongioanni, P., De Tata, V., Martino, L., Metelli, M., Tuccio, M., Manzone, F. and Rossi, B. (2008). Biomarkers of amyotrophic lateral sclerosis in peripheral fluids identified by means of proteomics. *Neurological Sciences*, 29(S), S327.

[18] Borasio, G. D., Robberecht, W., Leigh, P. N., Emile, J., Guiloff, R. J., Jerusalem, F., Silani, V., Vos, P. E., Wokke, J. H. and Dobbins, T. (1998). A placebo-controlled trial of insulin-like growth factor-I in amyotrophic lateral sclerosis. European ALS/IGF-I Study Group. *Neurology*, *51*, 583-586.

[19] Bozik, M. E., Mather, J. L., Kramer, W. G., Gribkoff, V. K. and Ingersoll, E. W. (2010). Safety, Tolerability, and Pharmacokinetics of KNS-760704 (Dexpramipexole) in Healthy Adult Subjects. *Journal of Clinical Pharmacology*, Oct. 19.

[20] Bromberg, M. B. and Brownell, A. A. (2008). Motor unit number estimation in the assessment of performance and function in motor neuron disease. *Physical Medicine and Rehabilitation Clinics of North America*, *19*, 509-532.

[21] Brooks, B. R. (1994). El Escorial World Federation of Neurology criteria for the diagnosis of amyotrophic lateral sclerosis. Subcommittee on Motor Neuron Diseases/Amyotrophic Lateral Sclerosis of the World Federation of Neurology Research Group on Neuromuscular Diseases and the El Escorial "Clinical limits of amyotrophic lateral sclerosis" workshop contributors. *Journal of the Neurological Sciences*, *124 (S)*, 96-107.

[22] Brooks, B. R., Miller, R. G., Swash, M. and Munsat, T. L. (2000). El Escorial revisited: revised criteria for the diagnosis of amyotrophic lateral sclerosis. *Amyotrophic Lateral Sclerosis and Other Motor Neuron Disorders*, *1*, 293-299.

[23] Caldero, J., Brunet, N., Tarabal, O., Piedrafita, L., Hereu, M., Ayala, V. and Esquerda, J. E. (2010). Lithium prevents excitotoxic cell death of motoneurons in organotypic slice cultures of spinal cord. *Neuroscience*, *165*, 1353-1369.

[24] Callaghan, B., Feldman, D., Gruis, K. and Feldman, E. (2011). The association of exposure to lead, mercury, and selenium and the development of amyotrophic lateral sclerosis and the epigenetic implications. *Neurodegenerative Diseases*, *8*, 1-8.

[25] Calvo, A., Chiò, A. and Castellina, E. (2008). Eye tracking impact on quality-of-life of ALS patients. *Proceedings of the Conference on Computers Helping People with Special Needs*, 5101 (*Lecture Notes in Computer Science)*, 70-77.

[26] Calvo, A., Moglia, C., Balma, M. and Chiò, A. (2010). Involvement of immune response in the pathogenesis of amyotrophic lateral sclerosis: a therapeutic opportunity? *CNS Neurological Disorders Drug Targets*, *9*, 325-330.

[27] Carreras, I., Yuruker, S., Aytan, N., Hossain, L., Choi, J. K., Jenkins, B. G., Kowall, N. W. and Dedeoglu, A. (2010). Moderate exercise delays the motor performance decline in a transgenic model of ALS. *Brain Research*, *1313*, 192-201.

[28] Castro, R. E., Sola, S., Ramalho, R. M., Steer, C. J. and Rodrigues, C. M. (2004). The bile acid tauroursodeoxycholic acid modulates phosphorylation and translocation of bad

via phosphatidylinositol 3-kinase in glutamate-induced apoptosis of rat cortical neurons. *Journal of Pharmacology and Experimental Therapeutics*, *311*, 845-852.

[29] Cedarbaum, J. M. and Stambler, N. (1997). Performance of the ALS Functional Rating Scale (ALSFRS) in multicenter clinical trials. *Journal of the Neurological Sciences*, *152(S)*, 1-9.

[30] Cedarbaum, J. M., Stambler, N., Malta, E., Fuller, C., Hilt, D., Thurmond, B. and Nakanishi, A. (1999). The ALSFRS-R: a revised ALS functional rating scale that incorporates assessments of respiratory function. BDNF ALS Study Group (Phase III). *Journal of the Neurological Sciences*, *169*, 13-21.

[31] Cereda, C., Cova, E., Di Poto, C., Galli, A., Mazzini, G., Corato, M. and Ceroni, M. (2006). Effect of nitric oxide on lymphocytes from sporadic amyotrophic lateral sclerosis patients: toxic or protective role? *Neurological Sciences*, *27*, 312-316.

[32] Chen, R., Grand'Maison, F., Strong, M. J., Ramsay, D. A. and Bolton C. F. (1996). Motor neuron disease presenting as acute respiratory failure: a clinical and pathological study. *Journal of Neurology, Neurosurgery and Psychiatry*, *60*, 455-458.

[33] Chen, H. S. and Lipton, S. A. (2006). The chemical biology of clinically tolerated NMDA receptor antagonists. *Journal of Neurochemistry*, *97*, 1611-1626.

[34] Chen, A., Montes, J. and Mitsumoto, H. (2008). The role of exercise in amyotrophic lateral sclerosis. *Physical Medicine and Rehabilitation Clinics of North America*, *19*, 545-57.

[35] Chiò, A. and Silani, V. (2001). Amyotrophic Lateral Sclerosis (ALS) care in Italy: a nationwide study in neurological centers. *Journal of the Neurological Sciences*, *191*, 145-150.

[36] Chiò, A., Benzi, G., Dossena, M., Mutani, R. and Mora, G. (2005). Severely increased risk of amyotrophic lateral sclerosis among Italian professional football players. *Brain*, *128*, 472-476.

[37] Choi, D.W. (1988). Glutamate neurotoxicity and diseases of the nervous system. *Neuron*, *1*, 623-634.

[38] Couratier, P., Torny, F. and Lacoste, M. (2006). [Functional rating scales for amyotrophic lateral sclerosis]. *Revue Neurologie (Paris)*, *162*, 502-507.

[39] Crippa, V., Sau, D., Rusmini, P., Boncoraglio, A., Onesto, E., Bolzoni, E., Galbiati, M., Fontana, E., Marino, M., Carra, S., Bendotti, C., De Biasi, S. and Poletti, A. (2010). The small heat shock protein B8 (HspB8) promotes autophagic removal of misfolded proteins involved in amyotrophic lateral sclerosis (ALS). *Human Molecular Genetics*, *19*, 3440-3456.

[40] Crow, J. P., Calingasan, N. Y., Chen, J., Hill, J. L. and Beal, M. F. (2005). Manganese porphyrin given at symptom onset markedly extends survival of ALS mice. *Annals of Neurology*, *58*, 258-265.

[41] Cudkowicz, M. E., Shefner, J. M., Simpson, E., Grasso, D., Yu, H., Zhang, H., Shui, A., Schoenfeld, D., Brown, R. H. Jr., Wieland, S. and Barber, J. R. Northeast ALS Consortium. (2008). Arimoclomol at dosages up to 300 mg/day is well tolerated and safe in amyotrophic lateral sclerosis. *Muscle and Nerve*, *38*, 837-844.

[42] Curti, D., Malaspina, A., Facchetti, G., Camana, C., Mazzini, L., Tosca, P., Zerbi, F. and Ceroni, M. (1996). Amyotrophic lateral sclerosis: oxidative energy metabolism and calcium homeostasis in peripheral blood lymphocytes. *Neurology*, *47*, 1060-1064.

[43] de Carvalho, M., Matias, T., Coelho, F., Evangelista, T., Pinto, A. and Luis, M. L. (1996). Motor neuron disease presenting with respiratory failure. *Journal of the Neurological Sciences*, *139*, 117-122.

[44] de Carvalho, M. and Swash, M. (2000). Nerve conduction studies in amyotrophic lateral sclerosis. *Muscle and Nerve*, *23*, 344-352.

[45] de Carvalho, M., Johnsen, B. and Fuglsang-Frederiksen, A. (2001). Medical technology assessment. Electrodiagnosis in motor neuron diseases and amyotrophic lateral sclerosis. *Neurophysiologie Clinique*, *31*, 341-348.

[46] de Carvalho, M., Dengler, R., Eisen, A., England, J. D., Kaji, R., Kimura, J., Mills, K., Mitsumoto, H., Nodera, H., Shefner, J. and Swash, M. (2008). Electrodiagnostic criteria for diagnosis of ALS. *Clinical Neurophysiology*, *119*, 497-503.

[47] de Carvalho, M., Pinto, S., Costa, J., Evangelista, T., Ohana, B. and Pinto, A. (2010). A randomized, placebo-controlled trial of memantine for functional disability in amyotrophic lateral sclerosis. *Amyotrophic Lateral Sclerosis*, *11*, 456-460.

[48] Di Lazzaro, V., Dileone, M., Pilato, F., Profice, P., Ranieri, F., Musumeci, G., Angelucci, F., Sabatelli, M. and Tonali, P. A. (2006). Repetitive transcranial magnetic stimulation for ALS. A preliminary controlled study. *Neuroscience Letters*, *408*, 135-140.

[49] Di Lazzaro, V., Dileone, M., Pilato, F., Profice, P., Cioni, B., Meglio, M., Papacci, F., Sabatelli, M., Musumeci, G., Ranieri, F. and Tonali, P. A. (2010). Long-term motor cortex stimulation for amyotrophic lateral sclerosis. *Brain Stimulation*, *3*, 22-27.

[50] Drory, V. E., Goltsman, E., Reznik, J. G., Mosek, A. and Korczyn, A. D. (2001). The value of muscle exercise in patients with amyotrophic lateral sclerosis. *Journal of the Neurological Sciences*, *191*, 133-137.

[51] Eisen, A. A. and Shtybel, W. (1990). Clinical experience with transcranial magnetic stimulation. *Muscle and Nerve*, *13*, 995-1011.

[52] Fattori, B., Grosso, M., Bongioanni, P., Nacci, A., Cristofani, R., AlSharif, A., Licitra, R., Matteucci, F., Rossi, B., Rubello, D., Ursino, F. and Mariani, G. (2006). Assessment of swallowing by oropharyngoesophageal scintigraphy in patients with amyotrophic lateral sclerosis. *Dysphagia*, *21*, 280-286.

[53] Ferrante, R. J., Browne, S. E., Shinobu, L. A., Bowling, A. C., Baik, M. J., MacGarvey, U., Kowall, N. W., Brown, R. H. Jr. and Beal, M. F. (1997). Evidence of increased oxidative damage in both sporadic and familial amyotrophic lateral sclerosis. *Journal of Neurochemistry*, *69*, 2064-2074.

[54] Fornai, F., Longone, P., Cafaro, L., Kastsiuchenka, O., Ferrucci, M., Manca, M. L., Lazzeri, G., Spalloni, A., Bellio, N., Lenzi, P., Modugno, N., Siciliano, G., Isidoro, C., Murri, L., Ruggieri, S. and Paparelli, A. (2008). Lithium delays progression of amyotrophic lateral sclerosis. *Proceedings of the National Academy of Sciences U.S.A.*, *105*, 2052-2057.

[55] Francis, K., Bach, J. R. and DeLisa, J. A. (1999). Evaluation and rehabilitation of patients with adult motor neuron disease. *Archives of Physical Medicine and Rehabilitation*, *80*, 951-963.

[56] Franks, M. E., Macpherson, G. R. and Figg, W. D. (2004). Thalidomide. *Lancet*, ***363***, 1802-1811.

[57] Gardiner, P., Dai, Y. and Heckman, C. J. (2006). Effects of exercise training on alpha-motoneurons. *Journal of Applied Physiology*, *101*, 1228-1236.

[58] Gibbons, C. and Beneteau, E. (2010). Functional performance using eye control and single switch scanning by people with ALS. *Perspectives on Augmentative and Alternative Communication*, *19*, 64-69.

[59] Gill, A., Kidd, J., Vieira, F., Thompson, K. and Perrin, S. (2009). No benefit from chronic lithium dosing in a sibling-matched, gender-balanced, investigator-blinded trial using a standard mouse model of familial ALS. *PLoS One*, *4*, e6489.

[60] Goodin, D. S., Rowley, H. A. and Olney, R. K. (1988). Magnetic resonance imaging in amyotrophic lateral sclerosis. *Annals of Neurology*, *23*, 418-420.

[61] Gordon, P. H., Moore, D. H., Miller, R. G., Florence, J. M., Verheijde, J. L., Doorish, C., Hilton J. F., Spitalny, G. M., MacArthur, R. B., Mitsumoto, H., Neville, H. E., Boylan, K., Mozaffar, T., Belsh, J. M., Ravits, J., Bedlack, R. S., Graves, M. C., McCluskey, L. F., Barohn, R. J. and Tandan, R. Western ALS Study Group. (2007). Efficacy of minocycline in patients with amyotrophic lateral sclerosis: a phase III randomised trial. *Lancet Neurology*, *6*, 1045-1053.

[62] Gordon, P. H. (2011). Amyotrophic lateral sclerosis: pathophysiology, diagnosis and management. *CNS Drugs*, *25*, 1-15.

[63] Great Lakes ALS Study Group. (2003). A comparison of muscle strength testing techniques in amyotrophic lateral sclerosis. *Neurology*, *61*, 1503-1506.

[64] Gros-Louis, F., Gaspar, C. and Rouleau, G. (2006). A. genetics of familial and sporadic amyotrophic lateral sclerosis. *Biochimica Biophysica Acta*, *1762*, 956-972.

[65] Guedj, E., Ber, I., Lacomblez, L., Dubois, B., Verpillat, P., Didic, M., Salachas, F., Vera, P., Hannequin, D., Lotterie, J. A., Puel, M., Decousus, M., Thomas-Antérion, C., Magne, C., Vercelletto, M., Bernard, A. M., Golfier, V., Pasquier, J., Michel, B. F., Namer, I., Sellal, F., Bochet, J., Volteau, M., Brice, A., Meininger, V., French Research Network on FTD/ FTD-MND, and Habert, M. O. (2007). Brain SPECT perfusion of frontotemporal dementia associated with motor neuron disease. *Neurology*, *69*, 488-490.

[66] Guidubaldi, A., Fasano, A., Ialongo, T., Piano, C., Pompili, M., Mascianà, R., Siciliani, L., Sabatelli, M. and Bentivoglio, A. R. (2011). Botulinum toxin A versus B in sialorrhea: a prospective, randomized, double-blind, crossover pilot study in patients with amyotrophic lateral sclerosis or Parkinson's disease. *Movement Disorders*, *26*, 313-319.

[67] Guy, N., Bourry, N., Dallel, R., Dualé, C., Verrelle, P., Lapeyre, M. and Clavelou, P. (2011). Comparison of radiotherapy types in the treatment of sialorrhea in amyotrophic lateral sclerosis. *Journal of Palliative Medicine*, *14*, 391-395.

[68] Hanson, E., Yorkston, K. and Britton, D. (2011). Dysarthria in amyotrophic lateral sclerosis: a systematic review of characteristics, speech treatment, and AAC options. *Journal of Medical Speech-Language Pathology*. In press.

[69] Hardiman O. (2011). Management of respiratory symptoms in ALS. *Journal of Neurology*, *258*, 359-365.

[70] Harris, D. and Goren, M. (2009). The ERICA eye gaze system versus manual letter board to aid communication in ALS/MND. *British Journal of Neuroscience Nursing*, *5*, 227-230.

[71] Harvey, W.T. and Martz, D. (2007). Motor neuron disease recovery associated with IV ceftriaxone and antibabesia therapy. *Acta Neurologica Scandinavica*, *115*, 129-131.

[72] Haverkamp, L. J., Appel, V. and Appel, S. H. (1995). Natural history of amyotrophic lateral sclerosis in a database population. Validation of a scoring system and a model for survival prediction. *Brain*, *118*, 707-719.

[73] Henriques, A., Pitzer, C. and Schneider, A. (2010). Neurotrophic growth factors for the treatment of amyotrophic lateral sclerosis: where do we stand? *Frontiers in Neuroscience*, 4, 32-40.

[74] Hillel, A. D., Miller, R. M., Yorkston, K., McDonald, E., Norris, F. H. and Konikow, N. (1989). Amyotrophic lateral sclerosis severity scale. *Neuroepidemiology*, *8*, 142-150.

[75] Hoagland, R., Mendoza, M., Armon, C., Barohn, R. J., Bryan, W. W., Goodpasture, J. C., Miller, R. G., Parry, G. J., Petajan, J. H. and Ross, M. A. (1997). Reliability of maximal voluntary isometric contraction testing in a multicenter study of patients with amyotrophic lateral sclerosis. Syntex/Synergen Neuroscience Joint Venture rhCNTF ALS Study Group. *Muscle and Nerve*, *20*, 691-695.

[76] Ihara, Y., Nobukuni, K., Takata, H. and Hayabara, T. (2005). Oxidative stress and metal content in blood and cerebrospinal fluid of amyotrophic lateral sclerosis patients with and without a Cu,Zn-superoxide dismutase mutation. *Neurological Research*, *27*, 105-108.

[77] Iversen, I. H., Ghanayim, N., Kübler, A., Neumann, N., Birbaumer, N. and Kaiser, J. (2008). A brain-computer interface tool to assess cognitive functions in completely paralyzed patients with amyotrophic lateral sclerosis. *Clinical Neurophysiology*, *119*, 2214-2223.

[78] Kalmar, B., Novoselov, S., Gray, A., Cheetham, M. E., Margulis, B. and Greensmith, L. (2008). Late stage treatment with arimoclomol delays disease progression and prevents protein aggregation in the SOD1 mouse model of ALS. *Journal of Neurochemistry*, *107*, 339-350.

[79] Kanai, H., Sawa, A., Chen, R. W., Leeds, P. and Chuang, D. M. (2004). Valproic acid inhibits histone deacetylase activity and suppresses excitotoxicity-induced GAPDH nuclear accumulation and apoptotic death in neurons. *Pharmacogenomics Journal*, *4*, 336-344.

[80] Kaufmann, P., Thompson, J. L., Levy, G., Buchsbaum, R., Shefner, J., Krivickas, L. S., Katz, J., Rollins, Y., Barohn, R. J., Jackson, C. E., Tiryaki, E., Lomen-Hoerth, C., Armon, C., Tandan, R., Rudnicki, S. A., Rezania, K., Sufit, R., Pestronk, A., Novella, S. P., Heiman-Patterson, T., Kasarskis, E. J., Pioro, E. P., Montes, J., Arbing, R., Vecchio, D., Barsdorf, A., Mitsumoto, H., Levin, B. and QALS Study Group (2009). Phase II trial of CoQ10 for ALS finds insufficient evidence to justify phase III. *Annals of Neurology*, *66*, 235-244.

[81] Kieran, D., Kalmar, B., Dick, J. R., Riddoch-Contreras, J., Burnstock, G. and Greensmith, L. (2004). Treatment with arimoclomol, a coinducer of heat shock proteins, delays disease progression in ALS mice. *Nature Medicine*, *10*, 402-405.

[82] Kobayashi, M., Ikeda, K., Kinoshita, M. and Iwasaki Y. (1999). Amyotrophic lateral sclerosis with supranuclear ophthalmoplegia and rigidity. *Neurological Research*, *21*, 661-664.

[83] Kriz, J., Nguyen, M. and Julien, J. (2002). Minocycline slows disease progression in a mouse model of amyotrophic lateral sclerosis. *Neurobiology of Disease*, *10*, 268-278.

[84] Lai, E. C., Felice, K. J., Festoff, B. W., Gawel, M. J., Gelinas, D. F., Kratz, R., Murphy, M. F., Natter, H. M., Norris, F. H. and Rudnicki, S. A. (1997). Effect of recombinant

human insulin-like growth factor-I on progression of ALS. A placebo-controlled study. The North America ALS/IGF-I Study Group. *Neurology*, *49*, 1621-1630.

[85] Lambert, E. H. and Mulder, D. W. (1957). Electromyographic studies in amyotrophic lateral sclerosis. *Proceedings of the staff meetings. Mayo Clinic*, *32*, 441-446.

[86] Lau D., Ogbogu, U., Taylor, B., Stafinski, T., Menon, D. and Caulfield, T. (2008). Stem cell clinics online: the direct-to-consumer portrayal of stem cell medicine. *Cell Stem Cell*, *3*, 591-594, 2008.

[87] Lefaucheur, J. P. (2008). Principles of therapeutic use of transcranial and epidural cortical stimulation. *Clinical Neurophysiology*, *119*, 2179-2184.

[88] Logemann, J. A. (2008). Treatment of oral and pharyngeal dysphagia. *Physical Medicine and Rehabilitation Clinics of North America*, *19*, 803-816.

[89] Logroscino, G., Traynor, B. J., Hardiman, O., Chiò, A., Couratier, P., Mitchell, J. D., Swingler, R. J. and Beghi, E. for EURALS. (2008). Descriptive epidemiology of amyotrophic lateral sclerosis: new evidence and unsolved issues. *Journal of Neurology, Neurosurgery and Psychiatry*, *79*, 6-11.

[90] Lombardo, F., Frijia, F., Bongioanni, P., Canapicchi, R., Minichilli, F., Bianchi, F., Hlavata, H. B., Rossi, B. and Montanaro, D. (2009). Diffusion Tensor MRI and MR Spectroscopy in long lasting upper motor neuron involvement in Amyotrophic Lateral Sclerosis. *Archives Italiennes de Biologie*, 147: 69-82.

[91] Lomen-Hoerth, C., Murphy, J., Langmore, S., Kramer, J. H., Olney, R. K. and Miller B. (2003). Are amyotrophic lateral sclerosis patients cognitively normal? *Neurology*, *60*, 1094-1097.

[92] Longstreth, W. T., Nelson, L. M., Koepsell, T. D. and van Belle, G. (1991). Hypotheses to explain the association between vigorous physical activity and amyotrophic lateral sclerosis. *Medical Hypotheses*, *34*, 144-148.

[93] Lui, A. J. and Byl, N. N. (2009). A systematic review of the effect of moderate intensity exercise on function and disease progression in amyotrophic lateral sclerosis. *Journal of Neurologic Physical Therapy*, *33*, 68-87.

[94] Lyall, R. N., Polkey, M., Leigh, P. N. and Moxham, J. (2001). Respiratory muscle strength and ventilatory failure in amyotrophic lateral sclerosis. *Brain*, *124*, 2000-2013.

[95] Matthews, R. T., Yang, L., Browne, S., Baik, M. and Beal, M. F. (1998). Coenzyme Q10 administration increases brain mitochondrial concentrations and exerts neuroprotective effects. *Proceedings of the National Academy of Sciences U.S.A.*, *95*, 8892-8897.

[96] McCrate, M. E. and Kaspar, B. K. (2008). Physical activity and neuroprotection in amyotrophic lateral sclerosis. *Neuromolecular Medicine*, *10*, 108-117.

[97] Miller, R. G., Rosenberg, J.A., Gelinas, D. F., Mitsumoto, H., Newman, D., Sufit, R., Borasio, G. D., Bradley, W. G., Bromberg, M. B., Brooks, B. R., Kasarskis, E. J., Munsat, T. L. and Oppenheimer, E. A. (1999). Practice parameter: the care of the patient with amyotrophic lateral sclerosis (an evidence-based review): report of the Quality Standards Subcommittee of the American Academy of Neurology: ALS Practice Parameters Task Force. *Neurology*, *52*, 1311-1323.

[98] Miller, R. G., Jackson, C. E., Kasarskis, E. J., England, J. D., Forshew, D., Johnston, W., Kalra, S., Katz, J. S., Mitsumoto, H., Rosenfeld, J., Shoesmith, C., Strong, M. J. and Woolley, S. C., Quality Standards Subcommittee of the American Academy of Neurology. (2009_a). Practice parameter update: The care of the patient with

amyotrophic lateral sclerosis: drug, nutritional, and respiratory therapies (an evidence-based review): report of the Quality Standards Subcommittee of the American Academy of Neurology. *Neurology*, *73*, 1218-1226.

[99] Miller, R. G., Jackson, C. E., Kasarskis, E. J., England, J. D., Forshew, D., Johnston, W., Kalra, S., Katz, J. S., Mitsumoto, H., Rosenfeld, J., Shoesmith, C., Strong, M. J. and Woolley, S. C., Quality Standards Subcommittee of the American Academy of Neurology. (2009_b). Practice parameter update: The care of the patient with amyotrophic lateral sclerosis: multidisciplinary care, symptom management, and cognitive/behavioral impairment (an evidence-based review): report of the Quality Standards Subcommittee of the American Academy of Neurology. *Neurology*, *73*, 1227-1233.

[100] Morland, C., Boldingh, K. A., Iversen, E. G. and Hassel, B. (2004). Valproate is neuroprotective against malonate toxicity in rat striatum: an association with augmentation of high-affinity glutamate uptake. *Journal of Cerebral Blood Flow and Metabolism*, *24*, 1226-1234.

[101] Mulder, D. W., Kurland, L. T., Offord, K. P. and Beard, C. M. (1986). Familial adult motor neuron disease: amyotrophic lateral sclerosis. *Neurology*, *36*, 511-517.

[102] Norris, F. H., Calanchini, P. R., Fallat, R. J., Pancharis, S. and Jewett, B. (1974). Administration of guanidine in amyotrophic lateral sclerosis. Neurology, 24, 721-728.

[103] Norris, F. H., Smith, R. A. and Denys, E. H. (1985). Motor neurone disease: towards better care. *British Medical Journal*, *291*, 259-262.

[104] Oba, H., Araki, T., Ohtomo, K., Monzawa, S., Uchiyama, G., Koizumi, K., Nogata, Y., Kachi, K., Shiozawa, Z. and Kobayashi, M. (1993). Amyotrophic lateral sclerosis: T_2 shortening in motor cortex at MR imaging. *Radiology*, *189*, 843-846.

[105] Okuda, B., Yamamoto, T., Yamasaki, M., Maya, K. and Imai, T. (1992). Motor neuron disease with slow eye movements and vertical gaze palsy. *Acta Neurologica Scandinavica*, *85*, 71-76.

[106] Osei-Lah, A. D., Turner, M. R., Andersen, P. M., Leigh, P.N. and Mills, K. R. A novel central motor conduction abnormality in D90A homozygous patients with amyotrophic lateral sclerosis. *Muscle and Nerve*, *29*, 790-794.

[107] Pasinelli, P., Belford, M. E., Lennon, N., Bacskai, B. J., Hyman, B. T., Trotti, D. and Brown, R. H. Jr. (2004). Amyotrophic lateral sclerosis-associated SOD1 mutant proteins bind and aggregate with Bcl-2 in spinal cord mitochondria. *Neuron*, *43*, 19-30.

[108] Pasquali, L., Longone, P., Isidoro, C., Ruggieri, S., Paparelli, A. and Fornai, F. (2009). Autophagy, lithium, and amyotrophic lateral sclerosis. *Muscle and Nerve*, *40*, 173-194.

[109] Patel, M. and Day, B. J. (1999). Metalloporphyrin class of therapeutic catalytic antioxidants. *Trends in Pharmacological Sciences*, *20*, 359-364.

[110] Patten, S. B., Svenson, L. W, White, C. M., Khaled, S. M. and Metz, L. M. (2007). Affective disorders in motor neuron disease: a population-based study. *Neuroepidemiology*, *28*, 1-7.

[111] Pizzasegola, C., Caron, I., Daleno, C., Ronchi, A., Minoia, C., Carrì, M. T. and Bendotti, C. (2009). Treatment with lithium carbonate does not improve disease progression in two different strains of SOD1 mutant mice. *Amyotrophic Lateral Sclerosis*, *10*, 221-228.

[112] Polkey, M. I., Lyall, R. A., Moxham, J. and Leigh, P. N. (1999). Respiratory aspects of neurological disease. *Journal of Neurology, Neurosurgery and Psychiatry*, *66*, 5-15.

[113] Pugdahl, K., Fuglsang-Frederiksen, A., de Carvalho, M., Johnsen, B., Fawcett, P. R., Labarre-Vila, A., Liguori, R., Nix, W.A. and Schofield, I. S. (2007). Generalised sensory system abnormalities in amyotrophic lateral sclerosis: an European multicentre study. *Journal of Neurology, Neurosurgery and Psychiatry*, *78*, 746-749.

[114] Qureshi, M. M., Hayden, D., Urbinelli, L., Ferrante, K., Newhall, K., Myers, D., Hilgenberg, S., Smart, R., Brown, R.H. Jr. and Cudkowicz, M. E. (2006). Analysis of factors that modify susceptibility and rate of progression in amyotrophic lateral sclerosis (ALS). *Amyotrophic Lateral Sclerosis*, *7*, 173-182.

[115] Raaphorst, J., De Visser, M., Linssen, W. H., De Haan, R. J. and Schmand, B. (2010). The cognitive profile of amyotrophic lateral sclerosis: A meta-analysis. *Amyotrophic Lateral Sclerosis*, *11*, 27-37.

[116] Ringholz, G. M., Appel, S. H., Bradshaw, M., Cooke, N. A., Mosnik, D. M. and Schulz, P. E. (2005). Prevalence and patterns of cognitive impairment in sporadic ALS. *Neurology*, *65*, 586-590.

[117] Rothstein, J.D., Martin, L. J. and Kuncl, R.W. (1992). Decreased glutamate transport by the brain and spinal cord in amyotrophic lateral sclerosis. *New England Journal of Medicine*, *326*, 1464-1468.

[118] Rothstein, J. D., Patel, S., Regan, M. R., Haenggeli, C., Huang, Y. H., Bergles, D. E., Jin, L., Dykes Hoberg, M., Vidensky, S., Chung, D. S., Toan, S. V., Bruijn, L. I., Su, Z. Z., Gupta, P. and Fisher, P. B. (2005). Beta-lactam antibiotics offer neuroprotection by increasing glutamate transporter expression. *Nature*, *433*, 73-77.

[119] Rouaux, C., Panteleeva, I., Rene, F., Gonzalez de Aguilar, J. L., Echaniz-Laguna, A., Dupuis, L., Menger, Y., Boutillier, A. L. and Loeffler, J. P. (2007). Sodium valproate exerts neuroprotective effects in vivo through CREB-binding protein dependent mechanisms but does not improve survival in an amyotrophic lateral sclerosis mouse model. *Journal of Neuroscience*, *27*, 5535-5545.

[120] Sarkar, S., Floto, R. A., Berger, Z., Imarisio, S., Cordenier, A., Pasco, M., Cook L. and J. Rubinsztein, D. C. (2005). Lithium induces autophagy by inhibiting inositol monophosphatase. *Journal of Cell Biology*, *170*, 1101-1111.

[121] Senent, C., Golmard, J. L., Salachas, F., Chiner, E., Morelot-Panzini, C., Meninger, V., Lamouroux, C., Similowski, T. and Gonzalez-Bermejo, J. (2011). A comparison of assisted cough techniques in stable patients with severe respiratory insufficiency due to amyotrophic lateral sclerosis *Amyotrophic Lateral Sclerosis*, *12*, 26-32.

[122] Siciliano, G., D'Avino, C., Del Corona, A., Barsacchi, R., Kusmic, C., Rocchi, A., Pastorini, E., Murri, L. (2002). Impaired oxidative metabolism and lipid peroxidation in exercising muscle from ALS patients. *Amyotrophic Lateral Sclerosis and Other Motor Neuron Disorders*, *3*, 57-62.

[123] Siciliano, G., Carlesi, C., Pasquali, L., Piazza, S., Pietracupa, S., Fornai, F., Ruggieri, S. and Murri, L. (2010). Clinical trials for neuroprotection in ALS. *CNS* and *Neurological Disorders - Drug Targets*, *9*, 305-313.

[124] Silani, V., Cova, L., Corbo, M., Ciammola, A. and Polli, E. (2004). Stem-cell therapy for amyotrophic lateral sclerosis. *Lancet*, *364*, 200-202.

[125] Smith, R.G., Henry, Y. K., Mattson, M. P. and Appel, S. H. (1998). Presence of 4-hydroxynonenal in cerebrospinal fluid of patients with sporadic amyotrophic lateral sclerosis. *Annals of Neurology*, *44*, 696-699.

[126] Smith, R. A., Miller, T. M., Yamanaka, K., Monia, B. P., Condon, T. P., Hung, G., Lobsiger, C. S., Ward, C. M., McAlonis-Downes, M., Wei, H., Wancewicz, E. V., Bennett, C. F. and Cleveland, D. W. (2006). Antisense oligonucleotide therapy for neurodegenerative disease. *Journal of Clinical Investigation*, *116*, 2290-2296.

[127] Sorenson, E. J., Windbank, A. J., Mandrekar, J. N., Bamlet, W. R., Appel, S. H., Armon, C., Barkhaus, P. E., Bosch, P., Boylan, K., David, W. S., Feldman, E., Glass, J., Gutmann, L., Katz, J., King, W., Luciano, C. A., McCluskey, L. F., Nash, S., Newman, D. S., Pascuzzi, R. M., Pioro, E., Sams, L. J., Scelsa, S., Simpson, E. P., Subramony, S. H., Tiryaki, E. and Thornton, C. A. (2008). Subcutaneous IGF-1 is not beneficial in 2-year ALS trial. *Neurology*, *71*, 1770-1775.

[128] Spataro, R., Ficano, L., Piccoli, F. and La Bella, V. (2011). Percutaneous endoscopic gastrostomy in amyotrophic lateral sclerosis: effect on survival. *Journal of the Neurological Sciences*, *304*, 44-48.

[129] Steele, J. C. and McGeer, P. L. (2008). The ALS/PDC syndrome of Guam and the cycad hypothesis. *Neurology*, *70*, 1984-1990.

[130] Stommel, E. W., Cohen, J. A., Fadul, C. E., Cogbill, C. H., Graber, D. J., Kingman, L., Mackenzie, T., Channon Smith, J. Y. and Harris, B. T. (2009). Efficacy of thalidomide for the treatment of amyotrophic lateral sclerosis: a phase II open label clinical trial. *Amyotrophic Lateral Sclerosis*, *10*, 393-404.

[131] Sugai, F., Yamamoto, Y., Miyaguchi, K., Zhou, Z., Sumi, H., Hamasaki, T., Goto, M. and Sakoda, S. (2004). Benefit of valproic acid in suppressing disease progression of ALS model mice. *European Journal of Neuroscience*, *20*, 3179-3183.

[132] Ticozzi, N., Tiloca, C., Morelli, C., Colombrita, C., Poletti, B., Doretti, A., Maderna, L., Messina, S., Ratti, A. and Silani, V. (2011). Genetics of familial Amyotrophic Lateral Sclerosis. *Archives Italiennes de Biologie*, *149*, 65-82.

[133] Tomik, B. and Guiloff, R. J. (2010). Dysarthria in amyotrophic lateral sclerosis: A review. *Amyotrophic Lateral Sclerosis*, *11*, 4-15.

[134] Turner, M. R., Kiernan, M. C., Leigh, P. N. and Talbot, K. (2009). Biomarkers in amyotrophic lateral sclerosis. *The Lancet Neurology*, *8*, 94-109.

[135] Uno, M., Kitazato, K. T., Suzue, A., Matsuzaki, K., Harada, M., Itabe, H. and Nagahiro, S. (2005). Inhibition of brain damage by edaravone, a free radical scavenger, can be monitored by plasma biomarkers that detect oxidative and astrocyte damage in patients with acute cerebral infarction. *Free Radical Biology and Medicine*, *39*, 1109-1116.

[136] Van Den Bosch, L., Tillkin, P., Lemmens, G. and Robberecht, W. (2002). Minocycline delays disease onset and mortality in a transgenic model of ALS. *Neuroreport*, *13*, 1067-1070.

[137] Varrato, J., Siderowf, A., Damiano, P., Gregory, S., Feinberg, D. and McCluskey, L. (2001). Postural change of forced vital capacity predicts some respiratory symptoms in ALS. *Neurology*, *57*, 357-359.

[138] Veldink, J. H., Kalmijn, S., Groeneveld, G. J., Titulaer, M. J., Wokke, J. H. and van den Berg, L. H. (2005). Physical activity and the association with sporadic ALS. *Neurology*, *64*, 241-245.

[139] Venkatachalam, K., Long, A. A., Elsaesser, R., Nikolaeva, D., Broadie, K. and Montell, C. (2008). Motor deficit in a Drosophila model of mucolipidosis type IV due to defective clearance of apoptotic cells. *Cell*, *135*, 838-851.

[140] Waragai M. (1997). MRI and clinical features in amyotrophic lateral sclerosis. *Neuroradiology*, *39*, 847-851.

[141] Worms, P. M. (2001). The epidemiology of motor neuron diseases: a review of recent studies. *Journal of the Neurological Sciences*, *191*, 3-9.

[142] Wu, D. C., Re, D. B., Nagai, M., Ischiropoulos, H. and Przedborski, S. (2006). The inflammatory NADPH oxidase enzyme modulates motor neuron degeneration in amyotrophic lateral sclerosis mice. *Proceedings of the National Academy of Sciences U. S. A.*, *103*, 12132-12137.

[143] Yang, Q. and Guan, K. L. (2007). Expanding mTOR signaling. *Cell Research*, *17*, 666-681.

[144] Yorkston K., Strand, E., Miller, R., Hillel, A. and Smith, K. (1993). Speech deterioration in amyotrophic lateral sclerosis: implications for the timing of intervention. *Journal of Medical Speech-Language Pathology*, *1*, 35-46.

[145] Yorkston, K., Beukelman, D. R., Hakel, M. and Dorsey, M. (2007). *Sentence Intelligibility Test, Speech Intelligibility Test*. Lincoln, Neb, USA: Madonna Rehabilitation Hospital.

[146] Yorkston, K., Beukelman, D. R., Strand, E. and Hakel, M. (2010). *Management of Motor Speech Disorders in Children and Adults*. Austin, Tex, USA: Pro-Ed.

[147] Yoshino, H. and Kimura, A. (2006). Investigation of the therapeutic effects of edaravone, a free radical scavenger, on amyotrophic lateral sclerosis (Phase II study). *Amyotrophic Lateral Sclerosis*, *7*, 241-245.

[148] Zoccolella, S., Beghi, E., Palagano, G., Fraddosio, A., Guerra, V., Samarelli, V., Lepore, V., Simone, I. L., Lamberti, P., Serlenga, L. and Logroscino, G. (2008). Analysis of survival and prognostic factors in amyotrophic lateral sclerosis: a population based study. *Journal of Neurology, Neurosurgery and Psychiatry*, *79*, 33-37.

In: Medical and Biological Frontiers Research Compendium ISBN: 978-1-62417-022-5
Editor: Tsisana Shartava

Chapter 10

Correlation between Serum Chromium Concentration and the Oxidative Stress Marker Malondialdehyde in Type I and Type II Diabetes

*I. H. Garba[1]**, *G. A. Ubom[2] and J. A. Chups[3]*
[1]Chemistry Programme, School of Science,
Abubakar Tafawa Balewa University, Bauchi, Nigeria
[2]Department of Biochemistry, Faculty of Medical Sciences,
University of Jos, Plateau Nigeria
[3]Department of Science Laboratory Technology, Plateau State Polytechnic,
Barkin Ladi, Plateau Nigeria

Abstract

Serum concentration of chromium and oxidative stress (malondialdehyde) were measured in Types I and II diabetic patients. The nature of the relationship between serum chromium and oxidative stress was also assessed in Types I and II diabetic patients. Results showed that both Types I and II diabetes were associated with a significantly elevated serum chromium levels. Serum chromium increased by 22.6% in Type I diabetic patients and 25.3% in their Type II counterparts, $p < 0.05$. Oxidative stress level as indicated by serum malondialdehyde (MDA) was also elevated in both Type I and Type II diabetes. Malondialdehyde concentration was 7.44 ± 0.53 μmol and 9.88 ± 0.91 μmol in Types I and II diabetic patients respectively, values that are higher than the control serum malondialdehyde concentration of 5.51 ± 0.52 μmol, $p < 0.05$.

The correlation between serum chromium and oxidative stress in both controls and Types I and II diabetic patients shows a weak relationship between these parameters. This indicates the difference in the pattern of the influence played by this metal in the phenomenon of oxidative stress induced by diabetes mellitus and the differences in the pathogenesis, etiology and severity of types I and II diabetes. The elevated levels of

* Corresponding author: hassanibrahimgarba0@gmail.com; ihgarba2002@yahoo.com.

serum chromium can potentiate further production of reactive oxygen species, and hence contribute to an increase in the oxidative stress phenomenon already found to be associated with both Types I and II diabetes.

Keywords: Diabetes, Malondialdehyde, Oxidative Stress, Chromium, Correlation, Serum

Introduction

Chromium is a naturally occurring heavy metal found in the environment, commonly in trivalent Cr (III), and hexavalent, Cr (VI) forms. Major sources of chromium for humans include foods such as vegetables, high bran breakfast cereals, broccoli, green beans and meat [1-2]. Chromium salts such as chromium polynicotinate, chromium chloride and chromium picolinate (CrP) are used widely as micronutrients and nutritional supplements and have been demonstrated to exhibit a significant number of health benefits in animals and humans [3]. In addition to its significance in maintaining the general health of humans, chromium is also an essential nutrient required by the human body to promote the action of insulin for the utilization of sugars, proteins and fats [4]. CrP in particular has been used as a nutritional supplement to control blood sugar in diabetes and help reduce cholesterol and blood pressure levels. Chromium increases insulin binding to cells, insulin receptor number and activates insulin receptor kinase leading to increased insulin sensitivity [3]. Whereas Cr (VI) is known to be cytotoxic, studies on the prolonged use of Cr (III) in dosages up to 350 times above the reference dose has shown no significant harmful effects [5]. However, with increased levels i.e. > 20 micrograms / ml, oxidative stress, reduction of cytochrome C and DNA breakages may arise [6]. This study is therefore aimed at measuring the concentration of chromium and the levels of oxidative stress (malondialdehyde) in the serum of types I and II diabetic patients and assessing the nature of the relationship between this metal and malondialdehyde in this condition.

Subjects and Methods

Subjects and Exclusion Criteria

Twenty five adult Types I and II diabetic patients (mean age, 61.8 years) were involved in this study. There were 25 age-matched healthy volunteers who served as controls. Both patients and controls were recruited from a comparable background (same geographical area and socio-sanitary status). None of the patients or control was using hormones, oral contraceptives or trace-metal containing supplements at the time of the study. All were non-smokers. Patients with concomitant diseases such as rheumatoid arthritis, Wilson's disease, cancer or liver diseases were excluded. Other exclusion criteria were as described in Dee et al., 2006 [7].

Blood Samples

Fasting blood samples (5ml) were collected from patients and controls under sterile conditions into metal-free containers by venepuncture. Serum was prepared by centrifuging the blood at 3000g for 10 minutes at room temperature. The collected sera were stored in metal-free containers at 4°C until analysis.

Determination of Malondialdehyde

Serum malondialdehyde (MDA) was assayed according to the flourometric method described in Wojciech, Neve and Peretz, [8]. Briefly, 50μL of serum of serum was introduced into 10mL test tubes containing 1 mL of distilled water. After addition of the solution of 29mmol/L thiobarbituric acid (TBA) in acetic acid (pH of the reaction mixture, 2.4 – 2.6) and mixing, the samples were placed in a water bath and heated for 1 hour at 95-100°C. After the samples were cooled, 25μL of 5mol/L HCl was added (final pH 1.6 – 1.7), and the reaction mixture was extracted by agitation for 5min with 3.5mL of *n*-butanol. The butanol phase was separated by centrifugation at 1500g for 10min, and the fluorescence of the butanol extract measured with a flourometer at wavelengths of 525nm (excitation) and 547nm (emission) using a SANCO Fluorescent Photometer – Model 930A.

Determination of Serum Chromium Concentration

All the glassware used in the determination were first dipped in 5% nitric acid for 48 hours, then washed with tap water and distilled deionized water, each three times before drying. Serum samples (0.5ml) were diluted 10-fold with 0.5% (v/v) solution of Triton-X-100 prior to analysis. [9]. The concentration of chromium was determined in duplicate using a Buck Atomic Absorption Spectrophotometer (AAS), Buck Scientific Instruments, USA.

Statistical Analysis

Data was analyzed using Stratigraphics 3.0 Software. Comparison of mean values between controls and Types I and II diabetics was done using one way Analysis of Variance (ANOVA). The method of Least Significant Difference (LSD) was used to assess the difference between means. The nature of the relationship between serum chromium and malondialdehyde was done using the Pearson's Product Moment Correlation Coefficient (r). Data were expressed as mean +/- SD. $p < 0.05$ were considered significant.

Ethics

Ethical approval for this work was obtained from the Ethics Committee of Plateau Hospital Jos, Plateau State Nigeria. In addition, the Council of International Organization of Medical Sciences / World Health Organization (CIOMS / WHO) International Guidelines for the Conduct of Research Involving Human Subjects [10] was also adhered to.

Results

The results obtained showed that both types I and II diabetes are associated with significantly elevated levels of serum chromium, table 1. Serum chromium concentration were 22.6% and 25.30% higher in Types I and II diabetics respectively when compared to the chromium level of 1.15 ± 0.19 mg/l in the controls, $p < 0.05$. No significant difference exist between the serum chromium concentration in Types I and II diabetics. Oxidative stress levels, as indicated by serum malondialdehyde concentration was found to be elevated in both types I and II diabetic patients relative to the control value of 5.51 ± 0.52 μmol.

The serum malondialdehyde concentration was highest in type II diabetics, increasing significantly by a magnitude of 79.30% above the control MDA levels, $p < 0.05$. There was a 35% increase in serum MDA in type I diabetes relative to the control, $p < 0.05$. Among the two patient groups, serum MDA was significantly higher in Type II diabetics; 9.88 ± 0.91μmol relative to the concentration of 7.44 ± 0.53 μmol in their type I counterparts, $p<0.05$.

The correlation matrix shown in table 2 indicates a shift in the pattern of relationship between serum chromium and MDA. With a shift of correlation from $r = 0.39$ in the controls to $r = -0.0012$ and $r = 0.18$ in Types I and II diabetic patients respectively, it indicates that the relationship between serum chromium and MDA is not static in these conditions.

Table 1. Serum chromium and malondialdehyde concentration in Type I and II diabetic patients and control

Subjects	Chromium (mg/l) Malondialdehyde (μmol)
Control	1.15 ± 0.19* 5.51 ± 0.52**
Type I Diabetics	1.41 ± 0.22*,[a] 7.44 ± 0.53**
Type II Diabetics	1.44 ± 0.29*,[b] 9.88 ± 0.91**

* ' ** $p < 0.05$; [a], [b] $p > 0.05$.

Table 2. Pattern of correlation between serum chromium and malondialdehyde (MDA) in Type I and II diabetic patients and control

	Chromium (mg/l)
Malondialdehyde (MDA) (μmol)	Control ($r = 0.39$, $p = 0.053$) Type I Diabetics ($r = -0.0012$, $p = 0.99$) Type II Diabetics ($r = 0.18$, $p = 0.40$)

Conclusion

Types I and II diabetes differ in their etiology. While Type I diabetes is mainly an autoimmune process, only the minority of type II diabetes is based on an autoimmune process. The major immunological process is the destruction of pancreatic insulin-producing β-cells, which is caused not only by T-cell mediated cytotoxicity, but also cytokine-induced cell death, followed by the appearance of autoantibodies [11-12]. Diabetes mellitus is characterized by chronic elevation of blood glucose (hyperglycemia) as consequence of decreased blood levels or decreased action of insulin [13], a hormone responsible for the regulation of the plasma glucose concentration and glucose utilization [14-15]. In type I diabetes, the autoimmune destruction of β-cells by the cellular and humoral immune system in the pancreatic islets of Langerhans leads to impaired insulin secretion and subsequently hyperglycemia. This type of diabetes is characterized by the appearance of antigen-specific T-cells and antibodies in peripheral blood which are directed against a variety of β-cell antigens, including glutamic acid decarboxylase, tyrosine phosphatase 1A-2 and insulin. The onset of type I diabetes frequently occurs before the age of 20 years, but disease manifestation is also common in adult patients. Exogenous administration of insulin is necessary to maintain glucose homeostasis and prevent early and late diabetic complications [12, 16]. In type II diabetes comprising approximately 90% of cases of diabetes mellitus, hyperglycemia is the consequence of relative insulin deficiency and insulin resistance of various tissues including muscle and adipose tissue. While in early type II diabetes insulin resistance and the resulting increased metabolic demand may be overcome by increased pancreatic insulin secretion, failure of β-cells to maintain adequate insulin production and decrease in β-cell mass are common in progressive disease, resulting in chronic hyperglycemia and loss of metabolic control [13, 17-18]. Hyper-insulinemia is associated with down-regulation of insulin receptors, thus further contributing to the exhaustion of insulin production in β-cells [19]. Both types I and II diabetes show a genetic predisposition although only type I diabetes is HLA dependent [12-13, 16, 20]. Complications arising from types I and II diabetes include diabetic neuropathy, retinopathy, angiopathy and nephropathy, which are mainly due to the accumulation of advanced glycosylation end products (AGES). The risk of diabetic complications increases with duration of diabetes and the grade of hyperglycemia [13, 16]. The results from this study showed significantly elevated levels of oxidative stress (malondialdehyde, MDA) in both types I and II diabetic patients. These findings are in agreement with the results of similar studies reporting an association between diabetes and increased oxidative stress [21-23]. Some workers have further postulated that oxidative stress plays a central role in the onset of diabetes mellitus as well as in the development of vascular and neurologic complications of the disease [24]. One potential source of oxidative stress in diabetes mellitus is a cascade of reactive oxygen species (ROS) leaking from the mitochondria and this process has been associated with the onset of type I diabetes via apoptosis of pancreatic β-cells, and the onset of type II diabetes via insulin resistance [25-26]. The elevated levels of oxidative stress can be accounted for by the hyperglycemia, which is a hallmark of diabetes. Hyperglycemia, defining established diabetes can induce oxidative stress by various mechanisms; excessive levels of glucose reaching the mitochondria leads to an overdrive of the electron transport chain, resulting in over-production of superoxide anions normally scavenged by mitochondrial superoxide dismutase (SOD). Failure of the latter leads to oxidative stress and it was recently proposed that this mechanism is responsible for the activation of all major pathways underlying the different components of vascular diabetic complications (glycation, PKC activation, sorbitol pathway)[27]. Another mechanism whereby high glucose can stimulate oxidative stress is the auto-oxidation of glucose in the presence of transition metals as well as generation of reactive oxygen species during the process of glycation. Indeed the development from Schiff's base to Amadori to advanced glycation end products (AGES) is accompanied by ROS-generating reactions at various steps [28]. Additional sources of increased ROS production and increased oxidative stress consequent to hyperglycemia include changes in redox potential of glutathione, although non-hyperglycemic mechanisms have also been reported e.g. increased activity of xanthine oxidase, a ROS-generating enzyme [29-30]. Furthermore decreased antioxidant defenses have also been observed in diabetes mellitus, including reduction in serum paraoxonase and in total anti-oxidant capacity of plasma. Some of these mechanisms may possibly operate simultaneously in a synergistic fashion [31]. The elevated levels of serum chromium in both types I and II diabetics indicate an altered state of chromium homeostasis in this disease. Indeed out results are in agreement with findings in several studies where subjects with diabetes were reported to have an altered chromium metabolism due to impaired chromium utilization. Diabetics absorb more chromium than non-diabetics but also have urinary losses [4, 32-33]. In addition diabetics appear to sense a need for additional chromium which is illustrated by an increased absorption of the metal, but are unable to utilize the absorbed chromium reflected by increased losses. Therefore while chromium concentration in blood and urinary losses are elevated in diabetics, tissue levels of the metal were found in some studies to be lower than those of the controls [4, 34-35]. The implications of this finding point towards caution in introducing chromium supplementation in diabetics. While chromium supplementation is has been shown to improve glucose tolerance, impaired glucose metabolism in children, adults with varying degrees of impaired glucose tolerance, elderly subjects and hyperglycemics, the relative improvement is proportional to the degrees of glucose intolerance [4]. Since diabetes is already known to be associated with high oxidative stress levels, the elevated oxidative stress can alter micronutrient requirements including chromium. Additional stresses that can further alter chromium metabolism in humans are glucose loading, high simple sugar diets, lactation, acute and chronic exercise and physical trauma [36]. Chromium once mobilized in response to stress, is not reabsorbed by the kidneys but is lost in the urine [32]. While chromium supplementation and oxidative stress appear as potential therapeutic targets in diabetes, the exploitation of these targets in diabetes should be done bearing in mind the following implications: an elevated chromium concentration in serum can convert this metal into a pro-oxidant thereby accelerating the further production of more reactive oxygen species. Targeting oxidative stress with the aim of reducing it in diabetes should also take into cognizance the fact that the phenomenon plays a role in several important cellular metabolic processes [38-40]. The variation in the nature of the correlation between oxidative stress (MDA) and serum chromium concentration in controls and types I and II diabetics indicates the relative differences in the etiology, pathogenesis and severity of types I and II diabetes.

References

[1] Hertel, R.F. (1986) Sources of exposure and biological effects of chromium. *IARC Sci. Publ. 71:* 63-77.

[2] US Environmental Protection Agency (1984) Health effects assessment for hexavalent chromium. Prepared by the office of health and Environmental Assessment. Environmental Criteria, EPA/540/1-86-019, Cincinnati, updated 1998.

[3] Shrivastava, R. Upreti, R. K. Seth, P. K. and Chaturvedi, U. C. (2002) Effects of chromium on the immune system. *FEMS Immunol Med. Microbiol. 34:*1-7.

[4] Anderson, R. A. (1997) Chromium as an essential nutrient for humans. *Reg. Toxicol Pharmacol 26:* S35-S41.

[5] Hathcock, J. N. (1996) Safety limits for nutrients. *J. Nutr. 126(Suppl):* 2386-2389.

[6] Bagchi, M. Bagchi, J. Belmori, J. et al (1997) Comparative induction of oxidative stress in cultured J77 4 A t macrophage cells by chromium picolinate and chromium nicotinate. *Res Commun Mol. Pathol. Pharmacol. 97:* 335-340.

[7] Dee, P. Chang-Hsun, H. Yi-Jen, H. et al (2006) The influence of chromium chloride-containing milk to glycemic control of patients with Type 2 diabetes mellitus: a randomized, double blind, placebo-controlled trial. *Metab Clin Exp 55:* 923-927.

[8] Wojceich, W. Neve, J. and Peretz, A. (1993) Optimized steps in flourometric determination of thiobarbituric acid-reactive substances in serum: Importance of extraction pH and influence of sample preservation and storage. *Clin. Chem. 39:* 2522-2526.

[9] Minhe, L. Huimin, J. Baiquan, X. Xi, C. and Zhengxiang, X. (1989) Relationship between viral hepatitis and trace elements in sera. *Varian AA-89:* 3p.

[10] Council of International Organization of Medical Sciences / World Health Organization (CIOMS/WHO) International Ethical Guidelines for Biomedical Research Involving Human Subjects. Geneva, Switzerland, 1993.

[11] Eizirik, D. L. and Mandrup-Poulsen, T. (2001) A choice of death-the signal transductionof immune-mediated beta-cell apoptosis. *Diabetologia 44:* 2115–2133.

[12] Daneman, D. (2006) Type 1 diabetes. *Lancet 367:* 847–858.

[13] Horton, E. S. (1995) NIDDM—the devastating disease. *Diabetes Res. Clin. Pract. 28(Suppl):* S3–S11.

[14] Halban, P. A. (1991) Structural domains and molecular lifestyles of insulin and its precursors in the pancreatic beta cell. *Diabetologia 34:* 767–778.

[15] Saltiel, A. R. and Kahn, R. C. (2001) Insulin signalling and the regulation of glucose and lipid metabolism. *Nature 414:* 799–806.

[16] Lernmark, A. (1999) Type 1 diabetes. *Clin. Chem. 45(8 Pt 2):* 1331–1338.

[17] Rhodes, C. J. (2005) Type 2 diabetes—a matter of beta-cell life and death? *Science 307:* 380–384.

[18] Mlinar, B. Marc, J. Janez, A. and Pfeifer, M. (2007) Molecular mechanisms of insulin resistance and associated diseases. *Clin. Chim. Acta 375:* 20–35.

[19] Jansen, J. Wolfram, K. and Lothar, R. (2009) Zinc and diabetes – Clinical links and molecular mechanisms. *J. Nutr. Biochem. 20:* 399-417.

[20] Lebovitz, H. E. (1999) Type 2 diabetes: an overview. *Clin. Chem. 45:*1339–1345.

[21] Stephens, J. W. Gabble, D. R. Hurel, S. J. Miller, G. J. Cooper, J. A. and Humphries, S. E. (2006) Increased plasma markers of oxidative stress are associated with coronary heart disease in males with diabetes mellitus and with 10 year risk in prospective sample of males. *Clin Chem 52:* 446-452.

[22] Mohora, M. Greabu, M. Muscurel, C. and Duta, C. (2007) The sources and the targets of oxidative stress in the etiology of diabetic complications. *Romanian J. Biophys. 17:* 63-84.

[23] Elisa, B. M. I. P. Bruno, S. P. Subrata, K. B. and Jose, B. L. F. (2009) Antioxidant SOD Mimetic Prevents NADPH Oxidase-Induced Oxidative Stress and Renal Damage in the Early Stage of Experimental Diabetes and Hypertension. *Amer. J. Nephrol. 29:* 309-318.

[24] Rosen, P. Nawoth, P. P. King, G. Moller, W. and Tritschler, H. J. (2001) The role of oxidative stress in the onset and progression of diabetes and its complications: A summary of a congress series sponsored by UNESCO-MCBN, the American Diabetes Association and the German Diabetes Society. *Diabetes Metab. Res. Rev. 17:* 189-212.

[25] Knight, J. A. (1998) Free radicals: their history and current status in aging and disease. *Ann Clin Lab Sci 28:* 331-346.

[26] Bonnefont-Rousselot, D. Bastard, J. P. Jandon, M. C. and Delattre, J. (2000) Consequences of the diabetic status on the oxidant / antioxidant balance. *Diabetes Metab 26:* 163-176.

[27] Nishikawa, T. Edelstein, D. Du, X. L. et al (2000) Normalizing mitochondrial superoxide production blocks three pathways of hyperglycemic damage. *Nature 404:* 787-790.

[28] Wiernsperger, N. F. (2003) Oxidative stress as a therapeutic target in diabetes: Revisiting the controversy. *Diabetes Metab 29:* 579-598.

[29] West, I. C. C. (2000) Radicals and oxidative stress in diabetes. *Diabetes Med. 17:* 171-180.

[30] Desco, M. C. Asensi, M. Marquez, R. et al (2002) Xanthine oxidase is involved in free radical production in type I diabetes: protection by allopurinol. *Diabetes 51:* 1118-1124.

[31] Michael, P. Renee, N. C. Taseer, C. and Joel, G. (2004) Increased breath markers of oxidative stress in diabetes mellitus. *Clin. Chim. Acta 344:* 189-194.

[32] Gurson, C. T. and Saner, G. (1971) Effect of chromium on glucose utilization in marasmic protein-calorie malnutrition. *Am. J. Clin. Nutr. 24:* 1313-1319.

[33] Morris, B. W. Griffiths, H. and Kemp, G. J. (1988) Correlations between abnormalities in chromium and glucose metabolism in group of diabetics. *Clin. Chem. 34:* 1525-1526.

[34] Harris, M. I. (1990) Non-insulin dependent diabetes mellitus in black and white Americans. *Diabetes Metab. Rev. 6:* 71-90.

[35] Riales, R. and Albrink, M. J. (1981) Effect of chromium chloride supplementation on glucose tolerance and serum lipids including high density lipoprotein of adult men. *Am. J. Clin. Nutr. 34:* 2670-2678.

[36] Anderson, R. A. (1989) Essentiality of chromium in humans. *Sci. Total Environ. 86:* 75-81.

[37] Ron, K. and Abraham, N. (2002) Oxidation of biological systems: oxidative stress phenomena, antioxidants, redox reactions and methods for their quantification. *Toxicol Pathol 30:* 620-650.

[38] Benher, M. Engelberg, D. and Levitzki, A. (2002) ROS, stress activated-kinases and stress signaling in cancer. *EMBO Rep. 3*: 420-425.

[39] Droge, W. (2002) Free radicals in the physiological control of cell function. *Physiol. Rev. 82:* 47-95.

[40] Gutteridge, J. M. Quilan, G. J. and Kovacic, P. (1989) Phagomimetic action of antimicrobial agents. *Free Rad. Res. 28:* 1-14.

In: Medical and Biological Frontiers Research Compendium ISBN: 978-1-62417-022-5
Editor: Tsisana Shartava

Chapter 11

Current Advances in Prostheses in Hernia Repair

*J. M. Suárez-Grau**
General and Abdominal Surgeon, General Hospital of Riotinto,
University Hospital Virgen del Rocío, University of Seville, Spain

The "Biomaterial Consensus Conference" in 1983, reached an agreement on the definition of biomaterial: the substance (or combination of substances), natural or synthetic, that can be used alone or in combination, and for a variable period of time, that can treat, increase or replace a function of the body. It can therefore be defined as all materials reachable as metals and alloys, ceramics, carbon derivatives, polymers and biological tissues, which have been used and are still used in surgical treatments. Only some of these are components of the prostheses used today in surgery for inguinal hernia.

Amid's classification proposed in 1997, provides three sets of synthetic prostheses in response to the diameter of the pores, but basically marking guidelines application of different prosthetic materials has now been relegated due to the emergence of next-generation prosthesis. They seek to achieve the best possible integration into the tissues, improve their performance on all interfaces and avoid complications.

The following table shows the classification of Amid:

Classification of synthetic prosthesis (Amid)		
Type I	Macroporous prosthesis: Pores>75 microns	Monofilament polypropylene mesh
Type II	Macroporous prosthesis at least one of three directions) Pores < 10 microns	e-PTFE mesh
Type III	Macroporous prosthesis with multifilament component or microporous	Polyester mesh e-PTFE perforated mesh Monofilament polypropylene mesh
Type IV	Prosthesis with submicrons pores	

* Juan Manuel graugrau@gmail.com.

Traditional Classification:

Biological materials: aponeurotic tissue, skin (dermis), muscle.
Sintetic materials: metals and alloys (titanium, iron, steel), Polymers (carbon, polyglycolic acid, polyglactin, PTFE, polivinilic acid, polyester, polypropylene).

Types of actual prostheses in surgery:

Non-absorbables prostheses: polyester, polypropylene, PTFE-e.
Absorbables prostheses: polyglactin, polyglycolic acid, Acelular collagen matrix of bovine, pig or human tissue.

Nonabsorbable Prosthesis

Polyester (Dacron)

Dacron is a polyester composed entirely biomaterial, derived from glicoethilen and terephthalic acid. It was used the first time in the United States in 1954 as a prosthesis in vascular surgery and subsequently introduced in Europe (France) in 1967 by Rives, for surgical repair of abdominal wall defects.

In general, all them are composed of tiny strands of braided polyester fibers. The mesh is displayed fine, light, soft, flexible, slightly elastic and fitted with high tensile strength.

Forgetfulness makes plastic adapted to different anatomical situations and is ideal for operations that require the placement of the mesh retromuscular or preperitoneal hernioplasty as Rives, Stoppa and Wantz. The macroporous structure encourages a lively fibroblastic reaction and rapid formation of a periprosthetic capsule. (Type III prosthesis according Amid).

Dacron is a non-resorbable biomaterial that provides excellent biological tolerance and a moderate inflammatory response, but in contact with the viscera, the intense fibroblastic reaction can lead to adhesions and it can be complicated by adhesions: sub-occlusive or obstructive syndrome, or even producing intestinal fistulaes.

The resistance to infection is less than a monofilament prosthesis because the interstices of the polyester fibers are perfect nesting niches that allow the entry of the bacteria but not of macrophages. In case of infections it is often necessary to remove the prosthesis.

Polypropylene

Usher used the first prosthesis of polypropylene in hernia surgery in 1958. Polypropylene is a synthetic derivative of polyethylene tht has undoubted advantages such as: high tensile strength, the possibility of sterilization, tolerance to infections and many chemicals products, ease of use and comfort for the patient, does not create tension and rarely shows intolerance. Since 1958 the use of polypropylene has become the principal material used for the repair of abdominal wall defects, especially for the treatment of inguinal hernia.

The polypropylene monofilament is available in various forms, which differ mainly by the kind of twisted and the dimensions of the pores.

The type of braided mesh gives its mechanical characteristics: weight, stiffness, memory plastic, two-dimensional elasticity, flexibility, surface roughness (Velcro effect ®), diameter of the pores.

All polypropylene prosthesis share some characteristics such as high tensile strength, encouraging rapid intra-and periprosthetic fibroblastic reaction and unfortunately the susceptibility to infections (prosthetic type I, according to Amid). The polypropylene creates a dense scar tissue, induced by fibroblastic reaction, which in contact with intraperitoneal structures has a high risk of adhesion formation with possibility of evolution to erosions and intestinal fistulas.

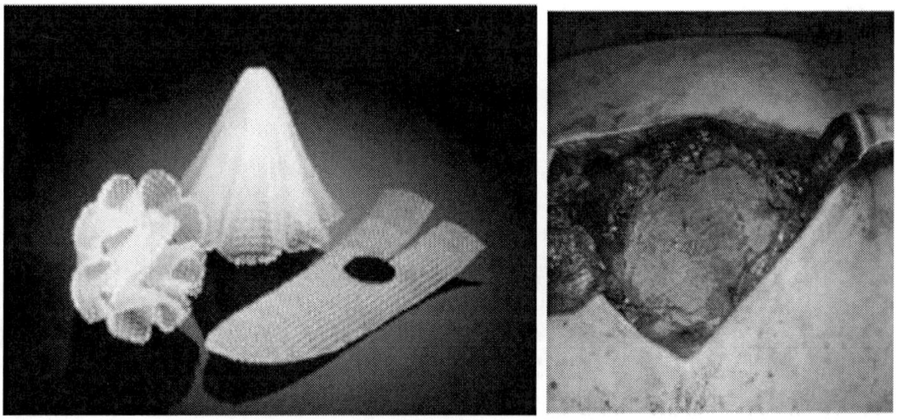

Figure 1.

Polytetrafluoroethylene (PTFE) and Expanded PTFE (PTFE-e)

The expanded polytetrafluoroethylene (PTFE-e) is a synthetic derivative of Teflon through a procedure discovered in 1963 in Japan, and subsequently redefined in 1970 by Gore in the United States. The e-PTFE has been used initially for the production of prosthetic vascular surgical use. Its use for repair of abdominal wall defects began 1983, Gore-Tex ® Soft Tissue Patch (STP).

The expanded PTFE is one of the most inert and biocompatible biomaterials among those currently available. It is not absorbed, does not cause allergies, triggers a minimal inflammatory response, is not altered by the action of tissular enzymes and it is not modificate by the presence of infections.

Its microporous structure of trabecular type, consisting of e-PTFE micronet joined together along three dimensions of microfibrils. The micropores have a diameter of 20 microns. The multi-microporous structure allows the penetration of fibroblasts and collagen formation within the mesh. The integration of PTFE by the tissues is quite slow (3-4 weeks). Other prosthesis (Gore-Tex ® Mycromesh) of microporous structure, has macropores of diameter of 0.8 microns, equidistant between them, which ensure rapid and earlier anchor integration. After 7 days of implantation, this mesh appears firmly attached to the tissue with minimal foreign body reaction and extensive vascularization.

Mechanical tests on PTFE shows extremely resistant with high tensile and suture retention, similar to that of polypropylene monofilament. If placed in contact with viscera, also after 2-4 weeks of implantation, are coated with a layer of mesothelial cells, resulting in soft and easily adhesions dissected.

Another feature of PTFE is the high biological inertness. It is a biomaterial which also allows the normal development of the tissue repair processes (there is a fibrous tissue formation rather organized which is placed horizontally along the surface of the prosthesis and perpendicularly deepens the micropores, with little foreign body reaction strange).

The behavior of PTFE-e against bacterial contamination and infection is controversial argument. Due to its hydrophobicity, the e-PTFE has the ability to slow down bacterial penetration, but there are several articles opposed to these theoretical and clinical results, which confirm the low possibility of penetration of neutrophil granulocytes, with subsequent infection and possibility of chronic infection in the mesh. (Gore-Tex ® Dual Mesh: Type II prosthesis according to Amid, Gore-Tex ® Mycromesh: Type III prosthesis according Amid).

The e-PTFE prostheses have added two antimicrobial agents (chlorhexidine diacetate and silver carbonate), (Gore-Tex ® Dual Mesh Plus), which inhibits bacterial colonization of the prosthesis until 10 days after implantation, and makes it the safest in current comparative studies with the rest of the meshes.

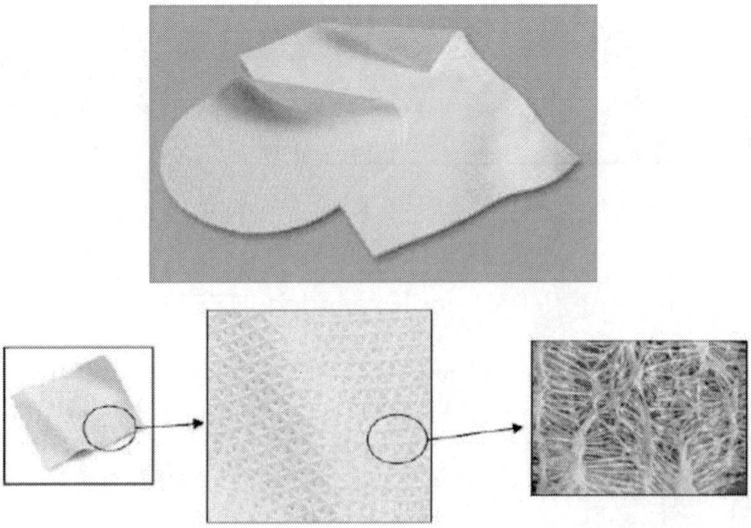

Figure 2.

Resorbable Prosthesis

The absorbable prostheses are emerging and are being widely studied subject to controversy. The principle of the use of absorbable prosthesis for hernia surgery is based on a double presupposition:

They are used as internal reinforcement (offered by the prosthesis itself) and turn cause a stimulus for fibroblast activation with subsequent production of connective tissue to enhance healing.

Resorbable synthetic prostheses are a polymer of glycolic acid esters (Dexon ®, Davis and Geck,) or a copolymer derived from the synthesis of the latter with lactic acid (polyglactin 910) (Vicryl ®, Ethicon).

Synthetic absorbable meshes are usually textured multifilament braided. Most prostheses are soft, flexible, extensible, mouldable, and biodegradable. They are gradually resorbed by hydrolysis beginning between 90 days and 6 months, with a gradual reduction in mass and resistance to stress.

Figure 3.

Other sintetic bioprostheses are made from a new material (PGA-TMC), which is conforming a mesh composed of a microporous structure of synthetic absorbable copolymer fiber (67% polyglycolide and 33% trimethylene carbonate). It is 100% absorbable prosthesis at 6 months of placement, currently marketed as a plug for inguinal hernia (Gore Bioabsorbable Hernia Plug ®). It belongs to the category of microporous mesh, with a particular character, is hydrophilic, which makes it theoretically optimal vector to absorb and release water based products on the site of fixing it.

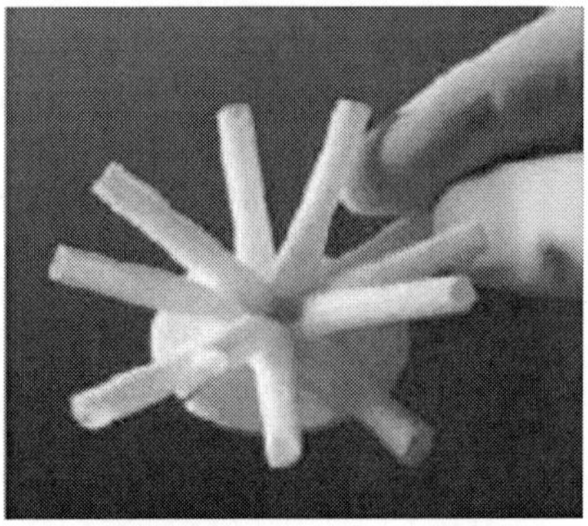

Figure 4.

Xenograft acellular collagen type I (Surgisis ®, Cook ®) from porcine submucosa, including growth factors and glycosaminoglycans. It produces very little rejection and gradually their fibers are replaced by fibroblastic cells, newly formed vessels, with the creation of extracellular matrix is gradually replacing the mesh.).

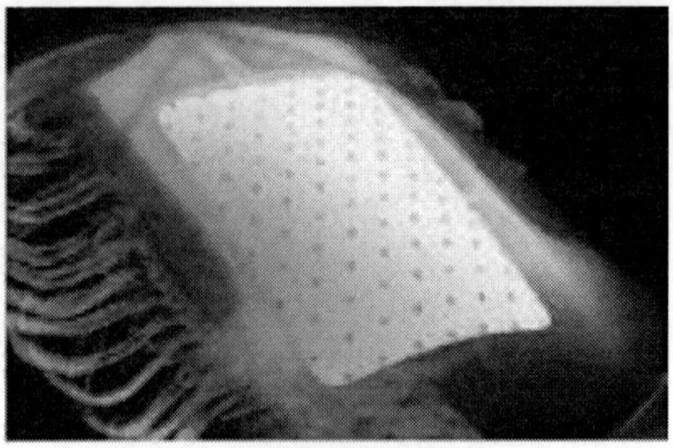

Figure 5.

Alloprostheses human acellular dermal matrix (Alloderm ®, LifeCell ®) is a mesh with excellent characteristics and without risk of intolerance or rejection.It also provides the advantages of the equivalence with the PTFE with a lower rate of adhesions if you are in contact with viscera.

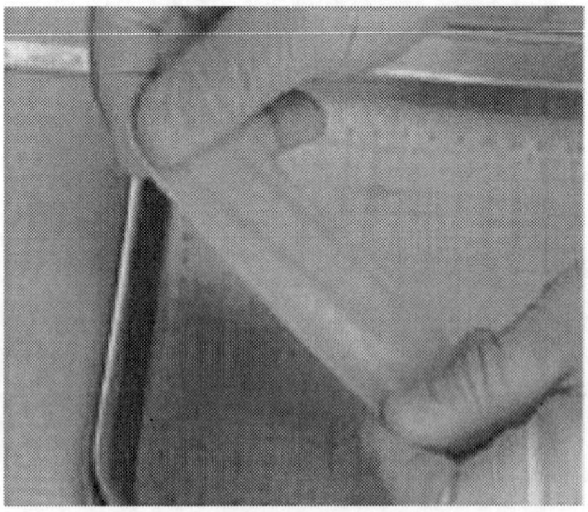

Figure 6.

Xenograft derived from bovine pericardium (Peri-Guard and Veritas ® Collagen® Matrix, Synovis Surgical Innovations), a material with excellent flexibility and resistance. It is one of the less foreign material remains in the receiver compared with others.

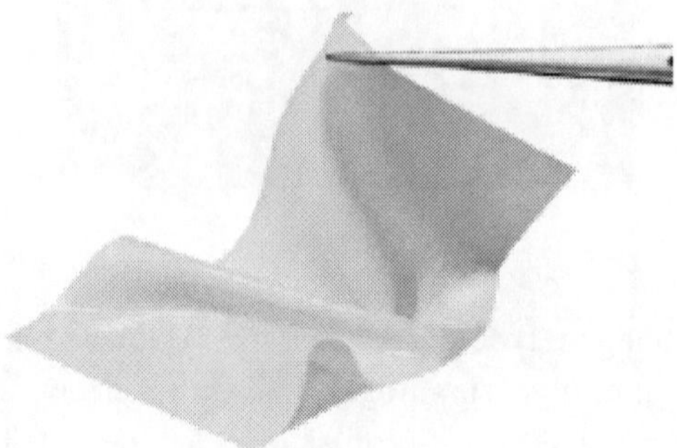

Figure 7.

Xenograft acellular collagen matrix subdermal swine (Permacol ®, TissueScience). The publications choose to use in infected areas and complicated providing an optimal solution to this problem.

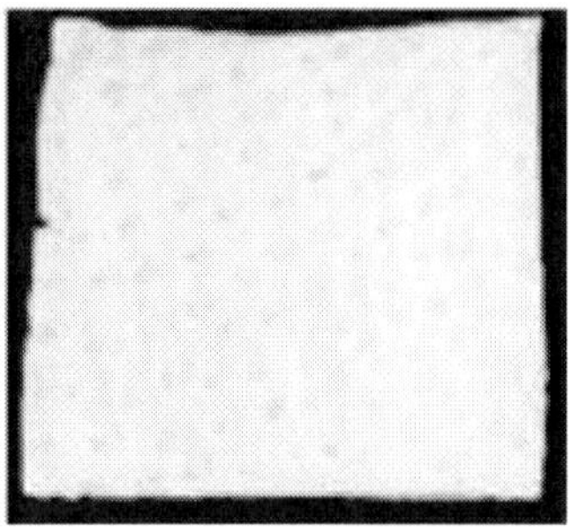

Figure 8.

The use of these biological absorbable meshes has been equated with non-absorbable meshes for hernia recurrence purposes. But the advantage offered by these meshes is when preventing or treating infection at the implant site, and is currently the main indication. The absorbable prostheses are therefore presented as a temporary alternative to polypropylene and PTFE-e in the presence of infections. The supplied mesh support reabsorbable until resolution of septic problems may in fact increase the chances of success of the permanent prosthesis.

These types of natural dentures require a very strict controls, given their origin in various animal species (cattle, pigs) for the risk of transmitting diseases, as has happened with lyophilized human dura prosthesis. The characteristics of reabsorbable prosthesis can be exploited positively for the construction of prosthetic joint, particularly useful for ventral hernia surgery.

New Trends in Prostheses Material

A new classification of the meshes in surgery attempt to: integration and peritoneum formation:

Reticular prostheses are useful for placement in a tissue interface.

The laminates are optimal prosthesis for placement in direct contact with the visceral peritoneum. The composite prosthesis can be placed on all interfaces, but its design is devised in order to be placed in a tissue and a visceral peritoneum interface.

Laminar prostheses: these meshes provoke low formation of new peritoneum, but high integration with the receptor tissues.

Non absorbable: PTFE, Silicone, Poliuretane.

Absorbable: biological material (dermis or submucosa of pig, bovine or human tissue)

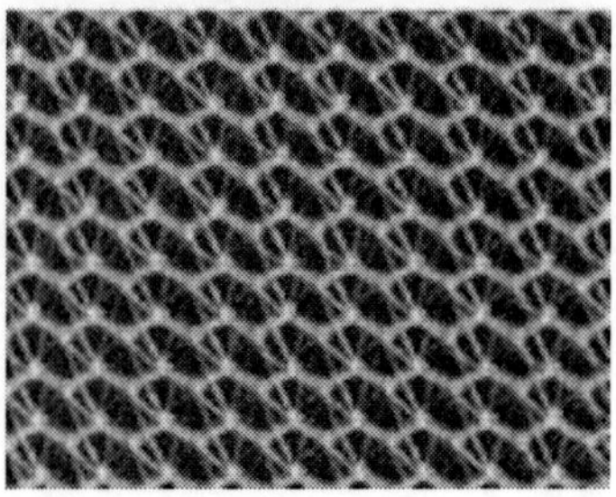

Figure 9.

Reticular prostheses: these meshes provoke a big formation of new peritoneum, and normal integration.

Non absorbable: polyester, polypropylene

Absorbable: polyglactin, polyglycolic acid

Lightweight prostheses: these meshes have a big pore and low density prostheses. This prostheses *lightweight* can be so much of material (one lonely material or mixed materials such non-absorbable and absorbable material).

These large pore and low density implants are integrated causes less strange body reaction, because have less biomaterial, with the advantage that the implant maintains the elasticity of the host tissue. Lightweight prostheses can be either non-absorbable material as absorbable material, thereby generating hybrid prostheses. These hybrid prostheses ultimately generate less fibrous reaction favoring the integration of the mesh and obtaining improved clinical outcomes compared with open surgery.

Composites prostheses: This prosthesis provokes high formation of peritoneum and high integration. Two different- materials layers: the first (superior layer) use to be prosthesis of reticular type, destined to increase the fibroblastic reaction, polypropylene or polyester usually. The second component (inferior layer) uses to be a laminar type and it can be absorbable or scarcely reactive material like the PTFE.

In ventral hernia or primary hernia surgery This prosthesis are currently hosting by a series of properties: inducing good tissue integration and prevent the formation of adhesions when placed in contact with the viscera. The composite prosthesis (composites) are generally constituted of two layers of different materials: biomaterials that form the first component (top) are usually reticular prosthesis type, destined to join the fibroblastic reaction, either polypropylene or polyester. The second component (bottom) is usually laminar and can be absorbable or poorly reactive and PTFE-e.

They are especially useful in large hernia defects repair, where is necessary a reconstruction of the abdominal wall, and does not exist resistant tissue where to fix the mesh properly. In laparoscopic surgery of abdominal hernia is useful, where the biomaterial is in contact with the visceral peritoneum.

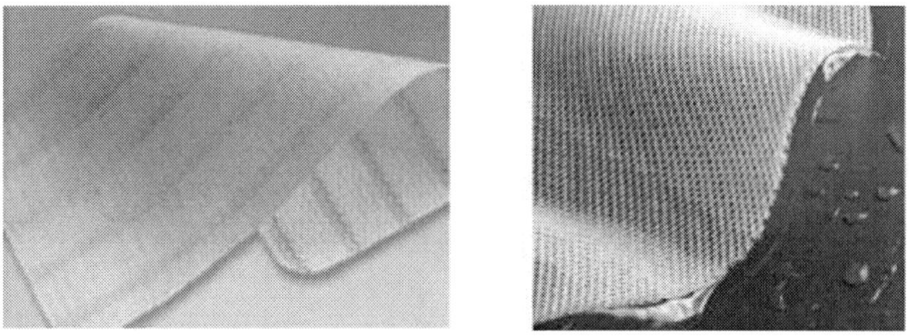

Figure 10.

Classification of prostheses used in the repair of abdominal wall hernial defects (Bellon 2005)	
Reticular prosthesis	
Non absorbables	Polypropylene (high or low density), polyester.
Partially absorbables	Polypropylene/polygalctin 910, polypoprylene/polygrecaprone
Absorbables	Polylactic, polyglactin 910
Laminar prosthesis	
Non absorbables	e-PTFE, silicone, polyurethane
Absorbables	porcine intestinal submucosa,, bovine pericardium, human acellular dermal matrix, others biological meshes.
Composite prosthesis	
Non absorbables components	Polypropylene/e-PTFE, polypropylene/polyurethane
Absorbables components	Polypropylene/polyethylene glycol , polyester/polyethylene glycol, polypropylene/hyaluronic acid, polypropylene/ polidiaxona/ cellulose

Bioprostheses: Current Studies in Surgery

The bioprostheses are used in hernia processes to cover defects. Although today is still valid herniorrhaphy in some types of hernias, it is increasingly appropriate to use these materials to prevent possible complications, mainly recurrence.

After analyzing several meta-analysis about the current herniorrhaphy (Bassini, MacVay, Shouldice Macintyre) concluded that, that the prosthetic repair is the procedure of choice for inguinal hernia.

Recurrences after repairs materials prosthetic figures have fallen to very low percentages: inguinal hernia recurrence is over 1-2%. The recurrences with no prosthetic techniques were in the 10-12% of cases.

The indication of prosthesis in hernia repair is focused on:

Big-hernia defects (hernia sac more than 10 cm).
Multi-recidive Eventrations.
Eventrations in location-special: close to lumbar bony prominences (Subcostal, in pubis or xiphoid).

Cassar reported recurrence after prosthetic repair around 0-10% in open surgery and laparoscopic surgery on a 0-9%. This accounts for half of recurrences in 4%. The recurrence without the use of prostheses is between 30 and 50%, so the placement of a bioprosthesis is the technique of choice currently.

Another indication for the use of prosthesis is temporarily closing the abdomen in cases where the closure can generate a compartment syndrome. In these cases you must use a laminar prosthesis.

Therefore the cases of recurrence after repair without prosthetic hernia defects are not acceptable and therefore the repair is imposed by biomaterials even minor defects.

Actual Analysis of Absorbable-Nonabsorbable Bioprosthetic

The apparition of new absorbable components in bioprostheses makes the debate to determine which mesh is better and in what situation to use each one. Also between absorbable and nonabsorbable mesh itself there are features that differ widely between them.

Discussed below are the main differences by analysis of current experimental studies and collection of enforcement cases with bioprostheses in vivo.

Most contentious points are:

Integration of the mesh.
Postoperative adhesions on contact with the visceral peritoneum.
Susceptibility to being infected and recover from the infection.
Biophysical characteristics that avoid hernia recurrence.

Nonabsorbable Bioprosthesis

When analyzing separately nonabsorbable meshes we focus on current articles that have been animal experiments and human studies.

Ott in the study compared resorbable mesh nonabsorbable mesh, concluded with more infection in the nonabsorbable mesh and the postoperative adhesion formation especially.

Martin Cartes and Morales in their experimental study in pigs showed ventral hernia rate of adhesions that occur with nonabsorbable, polypropylene (synthetic prosthesis as the main type lattice) and PTFE-e (as synthetic prosthesis main type lattice). Adhesions to polypropylene were mostly consistent, and the entire surface of the implant, while in PTFE-e showed a clear reduction of adhesions and in addition only the edges of the implant. By using inhibitors of adhesion formation, such as fibrin sealant (Tissucol ®) and hyaluronidase (Thiomucase ®), they found a reduction of adhesions to the prosthesis. This interface has directed many surgeons to use fibrin sealant with the abdominal wall prostheses, especially for laparoscopic surgery to minimize the possible adhesions.

In infection prosthesis, Carbonell described a study which compared the main prosthesis at that time. The prosthesis that resisted better the infection was PTFE-e, above other biomaterials, including the absorbable prostheses. It showed that levels of infection in different biomaterials were higher in synthetic nonabsorbable, except the e-PTFE, where the infection was very low, especially by its antiseptic impregnation.

The Nonabsorbable prostheses are biologically inert and have a structure that ensures unchanged in the formation of a new wall while the prosthesis remains anchored. It is evident by the many existing studies that describe how nonabsorbable meshes are widely used, but with the following problems (in a very low rate): complications in contact with abdominal viscera (adhesions, fistulas, etc.), impaired synthetic products that make the prosthesis and infection of themselves as prime examples.

These are their weaknesses, and ultimately are the source of the study and promotion of the creation of absorbable mesh, which attempt to overcome these shortcomings discussed. We can say further that in minimizing the adverse effects of a nonabsorbable bioprosthesis should be taken into account by their best results, macroporous meshes composed of monofilament that are better integrated, more histocompatibility complex, and are less infection in the mesh.

The Laminar prostheses offer great advantages in the resistance of biomaterial and to the infection, but are more likely to be intolerable and have to be removed if an infection of the mesh.

Burger analyzed 200 rats with various types of mesh: a) nonabsorbable prosthesis: polypropylene (Prolene ®) and PTFE-e (Dualmesh ®) b) Composite Prostheses: polypropylene - polyglecaprone composite (Ultrapro ®), polypropylene + titanium composite (Timesh ®) , polypropylene coated sodium carboxymethylcellulose more hyaluronidase (Sepramesh ®), polyester coated with polyethylene glycol glycerol with collagen (Parietex Composite ®), polypropylene + polydioxanone composite coated activated cellulose (Proceed ®) c) absorbable prostheses: from bovine pericardium (Tutomesh ®). This author and his research group concludes that there is no difference between them in relation to infection of the same concerns and only noteworthy is the significant decrease of adhesion in composites, as well as good integration, so Parietex® and Sepramesh Composite ® are the most appropriate of all the above for use in direct contact with viscera to have the lowest rate of adhesions combined with better integration. Dentures Dualmesh ® and Tutomesh ® also have the characteristics of having a strong retraction.

The new hybrid materials and composites, which combine with nonabsorbable material partially or fully absorbable material, in addition to forming macroporous, low density (ligthweigth) are an excellent alternative in order to minimize the adverse effects of nonabsorbable bioprosthesis.

Nowadays another advance in this type of mesh is the ability to self-adhesion of new prostheses. This is possible by three-dimensional structure or the addition of little hooks of absorbable material, which enables early stabilization of the mesh without using sutures.

Absorbable Bioprosthesis

The creation of these prostheses was born to improve the weak points of the nonabsorbable. The research level in vitro and in animal model demonstrates succeed. It has shown a decrease in the rate of adhesions when placed in contact with viscera and a lower rate of infection of the same, so much so that its current indication is primarily focused in infected or at high risk infection, despite not having antimicrobial properties.

All these advantages are demonstrated by several studies such as the Zheng experimental study: using collagen implants of pig submucosa (Pelvicol ®) in Wistar rats found along the intervals of 7, 14, 30 90 days the existence of less inflammatory response, fewer adhesions and a correct and orderly formation of collagen.

In 2007, Gaertner made an experimental study of great importance in absorbable prostheses, leaving the biomaterial at 3 and 6 months in rats. In ventral hernia repair used 4 types of reabsobable mesh 2x2 cm, in contact with viscera: two prostheses derived from bovine pericardium (Peri-Guard ® in 15 rats and Veritas ® in 13 rats) human dermal collagen matrix (allograft, Alloderm ® in 10 rats) and collagen subdermal pig (xenograft Permacol ® in 10 rats) and found that all was proper integration with minimal intraperitoneal adhesions, and no difference is in terms of tensile strength dynamometry and pneumoperitoneum applied after the sacrifice of animals. However it is notable that occurred in the prostheses infections derived from bovine pericardium (5 in Peri-Guard ® and 1 Veritas ®) and ulceration the skin also in the same prosthesis (6 in Peri-Guard ®). The prosthesis most favored in resistance, adhesion and reduced integration was Permacol ®; with similar results Peri-Guard ®, but with the disadvantages discussed before.

When searching for information on the results of absorbable prosthesis in patients highlight Franklin, who made a collection of data on infection in 23 hernioplasties potentially or actually contaminated laparoscopically, and using bovine serosa absorbable prosthesis (Surgisis ®) found no complications in the immediate postoperative patients with a normal recovering.

It follows from this study that reabsorbable mesh is a good alternative in these circumstances, although the authors acknowledge that their number is very short and studies are needed long time. However there are conflicting studies also present in humans, where it is not clear superiority of these meshes.

Ueno presented a review of 20 patients requiring hernia surgery but in the context of dirty surgery (strangulated hernia and perforated enterocutaneous fistula, infected prostheses need to remove and correct the hernia defect) using porcine submucosal collagen prosthesis (Surgisis). In this review they wanted to check whether there are harmful effects of the xenograft, and what is their behavior in dirty surgery. They conclude that there is no deterioration due to the porcine origin of the mesh, but nevertheless there is a 50% postoperative complications (8 patients presented with wound infection, including loss of mesh and fasciitis necrotizing), and a recurrence at 15 months of 30%. The bioprosthesis offers great advantages, but the problem is the infected abdominal wall and the pathologies of patients.

Van't Riet made one of the latest revisions of absorbable mesh in patients in late 2007, specifically polyglactin 910 mesh versus nonabsorbable mesh. In this study, the absorbable meshes do not perform better than non-absorbable regard to complications and mortality.

The advantage of crosslinked mesh versus non-crosslinked mesh remains a controversial area. Early investigation showed increased stiffness for two crosslinked biologic mesh products (porcine dermis and bovine pericardium) compared to the non-crosslinked bovine pericardium mesh. Greater cell infiltration was seen in the non-crosslinked mesh. Future investigation is warranted as to whether these characteristics are clinically important or if the crosslinked mesh poses an increased risk for infection by preventing collagen breakdown and macrophage migration. Chemical cross-linking of collagen is performed not only in hernia prosthetics, but also in bone, cartilage, and vascular implants, and in degrees from low to high density. The cross-linking density is bigger, so does fibroblast encapsulation and implant resistance to enzymatic degradation. However, the rate of cellular infiltration decreases. The optimum cross-linking pattern and density to balance graft strength and durability with cellular in-growth and remodeling remain unclear. A lack of quality long-term clinical experience and data makes it difficult to decide which product has the optimal balance. In conclusion: the placement of any synthetic material in the presence of intra-abdominal infection has a high risk of complications, regardless of whether the graft absorbable (polyglactin) or non-absorbable (polypropylene or polyester), so that biomaterials should be avoided if possible in the presence of infection.

Complications in Prostheses

The recurrence rates have decreased drastically thanks to prostheses, but other new problems have been presented in hernioplasty: Infection, adherences and intolerance.

We have made surgical experimentations to study these problems, and there are the most frequent solutions:

Recidive

The correct election of the prostheses is essential in the surgery.

Choose a reticular mesh (lightweight) in open surgery (without contact with viscera) is the best option. If the intraabdominal content could be in contact with thee mesh, best use a laminar or composite mesh is justified.

A laminar or composite mesh in laparoscopic surgery is the most extended and correct option.

The good election of the mesh, according with the hernia characteristics, reduces the recurrence.

Infection

The antisepsis methods and a correct technique could be completed with antibiotic prophylaxis. In the infection of prostheses several actions could be attempts: remove the laminar mesh, cures in reticular meshes, and finally use the absorbable (biological essentially) meshes to repair the defect in infected tissue or after remove the infected mesh. The use of antimicrobial drugs in the infection place is a new concept that can be useful in this complication.

In the case of reticular mesh:

If the infection is not in all the mesh, it is possible remove only the infected area of the mesh and washing it several times to decrease the grown rate of the bacteria.
If the mesh shows a complete infection the best choice is to remove all the mesh and use another surgical procedure (placing a new biological mesh, using a VAC therapy or performing an anatomical reconstruction such a herniorrhaphy or separation of components).

In the case of laminar mesh:

Although the infection was only a small portion of the mesh, the most often treatment is removes all the mesh and uses the anterior surgical procedures.
A new generation of mesh has an antibiotic impregnation (Vancomicin), and they can be used in the infection in hernia repair.

Adhesions

The laminar and composites meshes have low rates of adhesion to the intraperitoneal organs. Substances such fibrin glue or hialuronidasa cream decreases the adhesion.

The adhesion with intraperitoneal organs when using a reticular mesh must be repaired with a redo to remove the mesh and looking for any perforation or erosion of bowels and the others intraabdominal organs.
The adhesion using a laminar mesh is not frequent. The best option is a composite mesh to avoid the adhesion when the mesh is or could be in contact with viscera.

Intolerance

This problem was frequent in the past, nowadays the prostheses are very good tolerates without this problem.

If the intolerance appears it could be a chronic infection of the mesh. The existence of infection must be investigating (blood test, cultures, imaging test…).
If despite of all this, the intolerance is confirmed, the best option is replace it for other kind of mesh (depending of the place of the anterior mesh and the contact with viscera).

The new advances in prostheses go to use one material (or mixed material) with medium or big pore and low molecular weight, which increases a proper integration in the receptor and minimize de foreign inflammatory response. This material must to be elastic and strong enough to use it in laparoscopic approach in the hernia surgery.

References

[1] Bellon JM, Garcia-Honduvilla N, Carnicer E, Serrano N, Rodriguez M, Bujan J. Temporary closure of the abdomen using a new composite prosthesis (PLPU99). *Am. J. Surg*. 2004 Sep;188(3):314-20.

[2] Bellón JM, Rodríguez M, García-Honduvilla N, Pascual G, Buján J. Partially absorbable meshes for hernia repair offer advantages over nonabsorbable meshes. *Am. J. Surg*. 2007 Jul;194(1):68-74.

[3] Bellon JM, Serrano N, Rodriguez M, Garcia-Honduvilla N, Pascual G, Bujan J. Composite prostheses used to repair abdominal wall defects: physical or chemical adhesion barriers? *J. Biomed. Mater. Res. B Appl. Biomater*. 2005 Aug;74(2):718-24.

[4] Bellon-Caneiro JM, Carnicer-Escusol E, Rodriguez-Mancheno M, Garcia- Honduvilla N, Serrano-Amarilla N, Bujan-Varela J. Use of a composite prosthesis (PL-PU99) versus a biological prosthesis (Surgisis) in na experimental model of temporary abdominal closure. *Cir. Esp*. 2005 Aug;78(2):103-8.

[5] Burger JW, Halm JA, Wijsmuller AR, ten Raa S, Jeekel J. Evaluation of new prosthetic meshes for ventral hernia repair. *Surg. Endosc*. 2006 Aug;20(8):1320- 5.

[6] Carbonell AM, Kercher KW, Sing RF, Heniford BT. Susceptibility of prosthetic biomaterials to infection. *Surg. Endosc*. 2005 Dec;19(12):1670.

[7] Carbonell AM, Matthews BD, Dreau D, et al. The susceptibility of prosthetic biomaterials to infection. *Surgical Endoscopy* 2005;19:430-435.

[8] Chastan P. Tension-free open hernia repair using an innovative self-gripping semi-resorbable mesh. *Hernia*. 2009 Apr;13(2):137-42. Epub 2008 Nov 13.

[9] Diaz JJ Jr, Guy J, Berkes MB, Guillamondegui O, Miller RS. Acellular Dermal Allograft for Ventral Hernia Repair in the Compromised Surgical Field. *Am. Surg*. 2006 Dec;72(12):1181-1188.

[10] Franklin ME Jr, Gonzalez JJ Jr, Glass JL. Use of porcine small intestinal submucosa as a prosthetic device for laparoscopic repair of hernias in contaminated fields: 2-year follow-up. *Hernia*. 2004 Aug;8(3):186-9.

[11] Gaertner WB, Bonsack ME, Delaney JP. Experimental evaluation of four biologic prostheses for ventral hernia repair. *J. Gastrointest Surg*. 2007 Oct;11(10):1275-85.

[12] Gilbert AI. The importance of fixing onlay patches. *Hernia*. 2003 Dec;7(4):171.

[13] Holtom PD, Shinar Z, Benna J, Patzakis MJ. Porcine small intestine submucosa does not show antimicrobial properties. *Clin. Orthop. Relat Res*. 2004 Oct;(427):18-21

[14] Kim H, Bruen K, Vargo D. Acellular dermal matrix in the management of highrisk abdominal wall defects. *Am. J. Surg*. 2006 Dec; 192(6): 705-9.

[15] Liang HC, Chang Y, Hsu CK, Lee MH, Sung HW. Effects of crosslinking degree of an acellular biological tissue on its tissue regeneration pattern. *Biomaterials*. 2004; 25:3541–3552.

[16] Losanoff JE, Millis JM. Susceptibility of prosthetic biomaterials to infection. *Surg. Endosc.* 2006 Jan;20(1):174-5. Epub 2005 Oct 24.

[17] Martin-Cartes J, Morales-Conde S, Suarez-Grau J, Lopez-Bernal F, Bustos- Jimenez M, Cadet-Dussort H, Socas-Macias M, Alamo-Martinez J, Tutosaus- Gomez JD, Morales-Mendez S. Use of hyaluronidase cream to prevent peritoneal adhesions in laparoscopic ventral hernia repair by means of intraperitoneal mesh fixation using spiral tacks. *Surg. Endosc*. 2007 Jun 26.

[18] Martin-Cartes JA, Morales-Conde S, Suarez-Grau JM, Bustos-Jimenez M, Cadet-Dussort H, Socas-Macias M, Lopez-Bernal F, Alamo-Martinez JM, Tutosaus-Gomez JD, Morales-Mendez S. Prevention of peritoneal adhesions to intraperitoneal prostheses. An experimental study in pigs. *Cir. Esp*. 2006 Oct;80(4):214-9.

[19] Melman L et al. Proceedings of World Hernia Congress. Berlin, Germany. 2009.

[20] Melman L et al. Histologic Evaluation of Crosslinked and Non-crosslinked Biologic Mesh Materials in a Porcine Model of Mature Ventral Incisional Hernia Repair. Proceedings of American Hernia Society: *Hernia Repair* 2010. Orlando, FL. 2010.

[21] Ott R, Hartwig T, Tannapfel A, Blatz R, Rodloff AC, Madaj-Sterba P, Möbius Ch, Köckerling F. Biocompatibility of bacterial contaminated prosthetic meshes and porcine dermal collagen used to repair abdominal wall defects. *Langenbecks Arch. Surg*. 2007 Jul;392(4):473-8.

[22] Patton JH Jr, Berry S, Kralovich KA. Use of human acellular dermal matrix in complex and contaminated abdominal wall reconstructions. *Am. J. Surg.* 2007 Mar;193(3):360-3; discussion 363.

[23] Schumpelick V, Klinge U. Prosthetic implants for hernia repair. *Br. J. Surg*. 2003 Dec; 90(12):1457-8.

[24] Ueno T, Pickett LC, de la Fuente SG, Lawson DC, Pappas TN. Clinical application of porcine small intestinal submucosa in the management of infected or potentially contaminated abdominal defects. *J. Gastrointest Surg*. 2004 Jan;8(1):109-12.

[25] Van't Riet M, van Steenwijk PJ, Bonjer HJ, Steyerberg EW, Jeekel J. Mesh repair for postoperative wound dehiscence in the presence of infection: is absorbable mesh safer than non-absorbable mesh? *Hernia.* 2007 Oct;11(5):409- 13.

[26] Zheng F, Lin Y, Verbeken E, Claerhout F, Fastrez M, De Ridder D, Deprest J. Host response after reconstruction of abdominal wall defects with porcine dermal collagen in a rat model. *Am. J. Obstet. Gynecol.* 2004 Dec;191(6):1961-70.

In: Medical and Biological Frontiers Research Compendium ISBN: 978-1-62417-022-5
Editor: Tsisana Shartava

Chapter 12

Melanogenesis and Natural Hypopigmentation Agents

H. M. Chiang, H. W. Chen, Y. H. Huang, S. Y. Chan, C. C. Chen, W. C. Wu and K. C. Wen*
Department of Cosmeceutics, China Medical University,
Taichung, Taiwan

Abstract

Human melanin is synthesized in melanosomes located in melanocytes of the skin, hair, eyes, ears, and leptomeninges. Melanin not only determines skin color, but also protects the skin from UV damage by absorbing UV light. Congenital pigmentary disorders that result in skin and hair depigmentation, such as Hermenksky Pudluk Syndrome, Chediak Higashi Syndrome, and Griscelli Syndrome are due to various gene mutations that cause defects in melanin synthesis. Excessive production of melanin, which occurs in response to UV-induced DNA damage, inflammation, or other skin injuries, however, can result in skin hyperpigmentation including freckles, melasma, solar lentigo, age spots, and post-inflammatory hyperpigmentation. In this article we review the synthesis of melanin, the signaling pathways related to the regulation of melanogenesis, the factors influencing melanogenesis and various pigmentation disorders, as well as the effectiveness of various natural products at reducing hyperpigmentation.

Abbreviations

ACTH, adrenocorticotropin melanocyte stimulating hormone;
AHA, α-hydroxy acids;

* Correspondence to: Professor Kuo-Ching Wen. Department of Cosmeceutics. China Medical University. Taichung, Taiwan 404. E-mail: kcwen0520@mail.cmu.edu.tw. Telephone: 886-4-22053366 ext. 5302. Fax: 886-4-22078083.

ASP, agouti signaling protein;
ATP, adenosine 5'-triphosphate;
BBI, Bowman Birk inhibitor;
bFGF, basic fibroblast growth factor;
BHAs, β-hydroxy acids;
cAMP, cyclic AMP;
CRE, cAMP response element;
CREB, cAMP-response element binding protein;
CRH, corticotropin-releasing hormone;
DCT, TRP2,DOPAchrome tautomerase;
DHI, 5,6-dihydroxyindole;
DHICA, 5,6-dihydroxyindole-2-carboxylic acid;
DKK 1, dickkopf-related protein 1;
DPPH, 1,1-diphenyl-2-picryl-hydrazyl;
ECE, ET converting enzyme;
ERK2, extracellular signal-regulated kinase 2;
ET-1, endothelin-1;
ETBR, endothelin B receptor;
FOXD3, forkhead-box transcription factor D3;
GM-CSF, granulocyte-macrophage colony-stimulating factor;
GSK3β, glycogen synthase kinase-3β;
HGF, hepatocyte growth factor;
HPS, Hermansky-Pudlak syndrome;
HQ, hydroquinone;
IL, interleukin;
ITF2, immunoglobulin transcription factor-2;
L-DOPA, 3,4-dihydroxyphenylalanine;
LEF-1, lymphoid-enhancing factor-1;
LIF, leukemia inhibitory factor;
LT, leukotrienes;
MAP kinase, mitogen-activated protein kinase;
MC1R, melanocortin 1 receptor;
MITF, microphthalmia-associated transcription factor;
MOPB, methylophiopogonanone B;
NGF, nerve growth factor;
NHKC, normal human keratinocytes;
NHMC, normal human melanocytes;
NO, nitric oxide;
NRG, neuregulin;
PAR-2, protease activated receptor 2;
PAX3, paired box 3;
PGs, Prostaglandins;
PIAS3, protein inhibitor of activated STAT3;
PKA, protein kinase A;
PKC, protein kinase C;
PLA2, phospholipase A2;

POMC, pro-opiomelanocortin;
ROS, reactive oxygen species;
RSK, ribosomal S6 kinase;
SA, salicylic acid;
SCCE, stratum corneum chemotrypic enzyme;
SCF, Stem cell factor;
SEM, skin equivalent model;
SOX, Sry-related HMG box;
STAT3, signal transducer and activator of transcription 3;
STI, soybean trypsin inhibitor;
TGF-β1, transforming growth factor-β1;
TNF-α, tumor necrosis factor α;
TPA, 12-*O*-tetradecanoylphorbol-13-acetate;
TRP1, tyrosinase-related protein 1;
UV, ultraviolet;
α-MSH, α-melanocyte-stimulating hormone;

Introduction

Variations in human skin, hair, and eye color are due to the type, amount, stage, and distribution of melanin[1]. Melanin, one of the most widely distributed pigments, is a heterogeneous polyphenol-like biopolymer with a complex structure and color varying from yellow to black[2]. More than 150 genes regulate and contribute to skin pigmentation[3, 4]. In addition to contributing to the color of skin and hair, melanin also protects skin from physical (such as ultraviolet (UV) irradiation damage), chemical (such as environmental pollutants, heavy metals, and oxidative stress), and biochemical (such as bacteria) challenges[5, 6]. Overexposure to solar UV irradiation can result in photoaging, mutagenesis, and photocarcinogenesis in human skin[7, 8].

The incidence of skin cancer is increasing at a rate of 3% to 4% per year, and the mortality rate associated with skin cancer (melanoma) is increasing more rapidly than the mortality rate associated with any other cancer[9]. Melanocytes transfer melanosomes through their dendrites to surrounding kerotinocytes where they form melanin caps. This accumulation of melanin plays a protective role against UV irradiation by absorbing and transforming UV energy into harmless heat. Melanin can also scavenge toxic xenobiotics and reactive oxygen species (ROS) as well as bind to drugs, thereby protecting human skin against chemical and biochemical challenges[5, 6, 10-12]. However, excessive production of melanin and its accumulation in the skin can cause pigmentation disorders, including melasma, solar lentigo, and post-inflammatory hyperpigmentation[13]. Overproduction of melanin is not only a dermatological issue but also poses esthetic problems, especially among patients in Asian cultures.

In this article we review the synthesis of melanin, the signaling pathways related to the regulation of melanogenesis, the factors influencing melanogenesis and various pigmentation disorders, as well as the effectiveness of various natural products at reducing hyperpigmentation.

Melanosynthesis

Variations in dermal pigmentation depend on the number, size, composition, and distribution of melanocytes as well as the activity of melanogenic enzymes.

Melanin synthesis by melanocytes within membrane-bound organelles (melanosomes) and their transfer to keratinocytes within the epidermal melanin unit determines cutaneous pigmentation.

Melanin synthesis is characterized by an increased number of melanocytes in the basal layer of the epidermis, the size, maturation, and number of melanosomes, the production of melanin, the dendricity of melanocytes, the transfer of melanosomes from melanocytes to keratinocytes, the proliferation of keratinocytes, and the thickening of the epidermis and stratum corneum.

Melanocytes and Melanosomes

Melanin is synthesized in melanocytes, which are localized at the basal layer of the epidermis.

Each melanocyte is functionally related to underlying fibroblasts in the dermis and to keratinocytes in the epidermis. Each melanocyte transfers pigment-containing melanosomes via dendritic melanocytes to approximately 36 basal and suprabasal keratinocytes – the so-called epidermal melanin unit[3, 14, 15] (Figure 1).

This inter-cell cross-talk regulates the function and phenotype of human skin[16]. Protease-activated receptor 2 (PAR-2) plays an important role in melanosomal transfer[17, 18]. PAR-2, a G protein-coupled receptor, mediates the phagocytosis of melanosomes in a Rho-dependent manner[19]. The amount and type of melanin produced and transferred to the keratinocytes with subsequent incorporation, aggregation, and degradation influences skin complexion coloration[20]. Melanoblasts, melanocyte precursor cells, are derived from the neural crest and migrate to target sites such as dermis and eyes[21]. Melanoblasts differentiate into melanocytes when they reach their destination and start to produce melanosomes, the organized elliptic membrane-bound organelles where melanin is synthesized. Melanin synthesis starts with the exportation of structural proteins from the endoplasmic reticulum to the cytosol, where they fuse with melanosome-specific regulatory glycoproteins that have been released in coated vesicles from the Golgi apparatus. Melanin synthesis ensues subsequent to the sorting and trafficking of these proteins to melanosomes[22, 23]. Melanosomes are divided into four maturation stages according to their structure and to the type and amount of melanin produced[24, 25]. 'Early' melanosomes (stages I and II) present with little or no pigment, while 'late' melanosomes (stages III and IV) present with some to complete pigment. Stage I melanosomes are spherical vacuoles lacking tyrosinase activity and internal structural components. Stage II melanosomes are elongated, fibrillar organelles containing tyrosinase and little melanin[26, 27]. After stage II, melanin synthesis starts. Stage III melanosomes have uniformly deposited pigment on the internal fibrils. Mature melanosomes (stage IV) are either elliptical or ellipsoidal in shape, are electron-opaque due to complete melanization, and have minimal tyrosinase activity. Highly pigmented melanocytes are rich in Stage IV melanosomes which are transferred by melanocyte dentrites to keratinocytes [16].

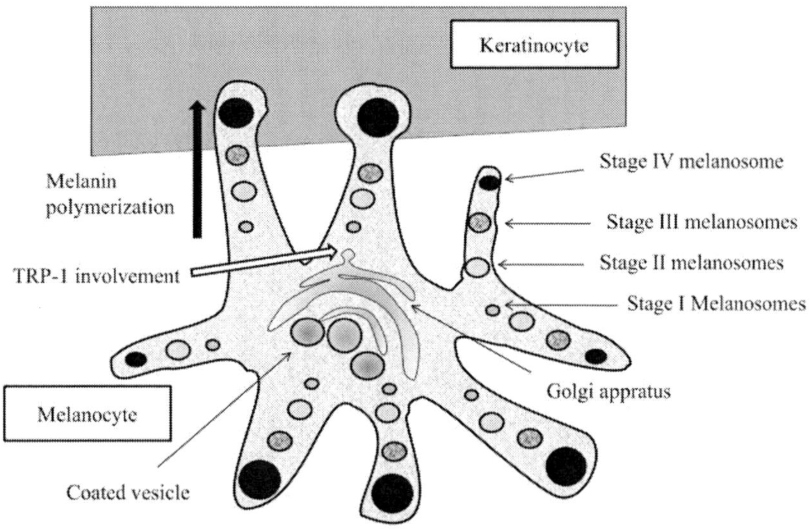

Figure 1. Melanosome transfer.

The trafficking of sorting vesicles to their target organelles is controlled by two classes of microtubule-associated motor proteins – kinesins and cytoplasmic dyneins[28]. Kinesins power plus-end-directed microtubule-based motility, while cytoplasmic dyneins drive minus-end-directed motility [29, 30]. Dyneins and kinesins also play roles in retrograde and in anterograde transport of melanosomes [31-34], whereas dyneins and spectrin dominate the movement of early melanosomes [35].

The methods of melanosome transfer from melanocytes to keratinocytes include cytophagocytosis of melanocyte dendrite tips[36, 37] and exocytosis of melanosomes into the extracellular space and their subsequent uptake by phagocytosis into keratinocytes[38, 39], either by filopodia-mediated melanosome transfer[40-42] or the filopodial-phagocytosis model[43]. Rab, melanophilin, and myosin Va have been shown to be involved in the movement of melanosomes[37, 44].

Melanin biosynthesis

Melanins are polymorphous, multifunctional biopolymers. The major types of melanins include eumelanin, pheomelanin, a combination of eumelanin and pheomelanin (mixed melanin), and neuromelanin (Figure 2). Eumelanin is a blackish-brown heterogeneors polymer consisting of 5,6-dihydroxyindole (DHI) and 5,6-dihydroxyindole-2-carboxylic acid (DHICA). Pheomelanin is yellowish-red in color and consists of sulfur-containing benzothiazine derivatives[2, 45].

Neuromelanin is produced in dopaminergic neurons of the human substantia nigra, the dorsal motor nucleus of the vagus nerve, and the median raphe nucleus of the pons. Neuromelanin has the capacity to chelate redox-active metals such as Cu, Mn, and Cr as well as toxic metals such as Cd, Hg, and Pb to avoid neuron degeneration[46]. If the level of neuromelanin decreases, dopamine synthesis may be diminished, resulting in diseases associated with neuronal degradation. Massive loss of dopamine-producing pigmented neurons in the substantia nigra has been found in patients with Parkinson's disease[47].

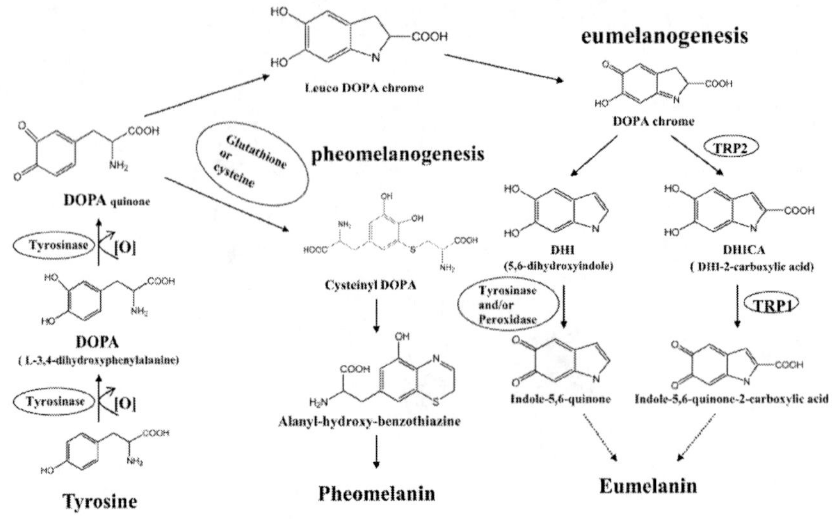

Figure 2. Pathway of melanin biosynthesis.

The biosynthetic pathway governing melanin formation is well established[48-52] (Figure 2). Synthesis of melanin starts with the conversion of the amino acid L-tyrosine to dopaquinone by tyrosinase, a copper-containing glycosylated type I membrane-bound glycoprotein that catalyzes the rate-limiting step of melanin biosynthesis[53, 54]. Tyrosinase is synthesized by melanosomal ribosomes on the rough endoplasmic reticulum[55]. The enzyme is glycosylated en route to and within the Golgi apparatus, and subsequently delivered to melanosomes via coated vesicles[55, 56]. Tyrosinase is the most common target for therapeutic agents intended to alleviate hyperpigmentation[57-59]. Tyrosinase catalyzes two distinct oxidation reactions. First, tyrosinase catalyzes the oxidation of monophenol (L-tyrosine) to o-diphenol (3,4-dihydroxyphenylalanine, L-DOPA (monophenolase activity)). Second, L-DOPA is oxidized to o-quinone (dopaquinone) (diphenolase activity). Tyrosinase gene transcription has been shown to correlate with the differentiation of lysosomes and/or peroxisomes into melanosomes[60, 61]. Tyrosinase-related protein 1 (TPR-1) and DOPAchrome tautomerase (DCT, also known as TRP-2) subsequently metabolize dopaquinone into eumelanin through a process referred to as eumelanogenesis. Dopaquinone is transferred to DHI via multiple processes including decarbxylation, oxidation, and polymerization and DOPAchrome is converted to DHICA. Pheomelanogenesis refers to the process through which dopaquinones conjugate with thiol-containing cysteines or glutathiones to form pheomelanin. As mentioned above, dopaquinone plays pivotal roles both in eumelanogenesis and pheomelanogenesis[16]. Eumelanogenesis involves the activation of tyrosinase, TRP-1, and TRP-2 whereas the synthesis of pheomelanin only requires the activation of tyrosinase[16, 62]. Following the synthesis of those pigments, melanin-containing melanosomes are transferred to neighboring keratinocytes. However, without successful transfer of melanosomes to keratinocytes, the skin can appear essentially unpigmented[63].

Factors Regulating Melanin Biosynthesis

UV radiation from the sun stimulates melanin synthesis in skin. After UV exposure, melanocytes increase their expression of pro-opiomelanocortin (POMC, the precursor of α-MSH) and its receptor melanocortin 1 receptor (MC1R), tyrosinase, TRP-1, protein kinase C (PKC), and other signaling factors[64-66] (Figure 3). Upon exposure to UV irradiation, fibroblasts release the above-mentioned cytokines, growth factors, and inflammatory factors, which then stimulate melanin production and/or stimulate melanin transfer. UV also stimulates the production of endothelin-1 (ET-1) and POMC in keratinocytes, factors that then act in a paracrine manner to stimulate melanocyte function[67, 68]. Other keratinocyte-derived factors that regulate the proliferation and/or differentiation of melanocytes include α-MSH, adrenocorticotropin melanocyte stimulating hormone (ACTH), basic fibroblast growth factor (bFGF), nerve growth factor (NGF), endothelins, granulocyte-macrophage colony-stimulating factor (GM-CSF), steel factor, leukemia inhibitory factor (LIF), and hepatocyte growth factor (HGF)[69]. Melanocytes have been shown to increase the production of intracellular nitric oxide (NO), which in turn triggers signal transduction cascades to initiate melanogenesis[70, 71] through the enzyme tyrosinase. In addition, human melanocyte proliferation requires cross-talk between several signaling pathways including the cAMP/PKA, PKC, and tyrosine kinase pathways; therefore, the mechanisms by which various factors increase skin pigmentation are closely inter-related[52, 72-75].

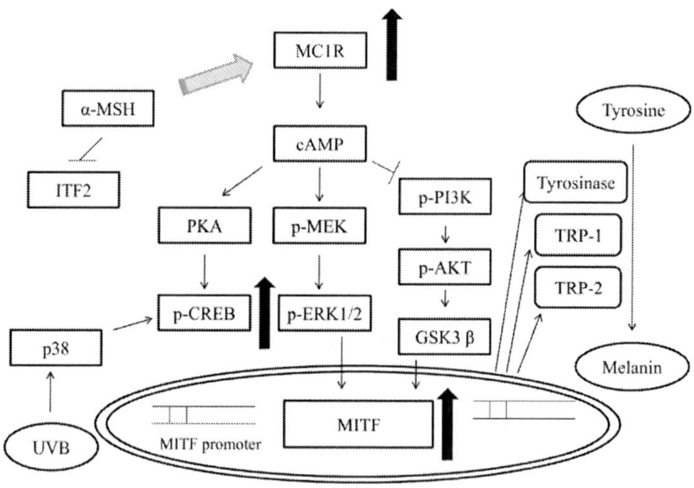

Figure 3. Factors regulating melanin biosynthesis.

UV radiation has been shown to influence melanogenesis through a paracrine regulation process involving keratinocytes[52, 76](Figure 3). Both autocrine and paracrine cytokine networks are involved in UV-induced upregulation of melanogenesis[77]. α-MSH is a major mediator of the response of melanocytes to UV[78]. The POMC gene is activated in the pituitary gland but POMC-derived peptides are also generated in keratinocytes and melanocytes[79, 80]. The POMC gene encodes a large precursor protein, which is then enzymatically cleaved to form several different peptides including α-MSH, ACTH, melanocortin, and β-endorphin[80]. The binding of α-MSH and ACTH to MC1R on the melanocyte membrane[81] activates intracellular adenylate cyclase through G proteins, which then catalyze the conversion of adenosine triphosphate to cyclic AMP (cAMP)[82]. cAMP exerts its function through protein kinase A (PKA)[83]. The intracellular elevation of cAMP increases the protein expression of microphthalmia-associated transcription factor (MITF), tyrosinase, and TRP-2, but not tyrosinase or TRP-2 mRNAs[84]. PKA promotes the activation of the cAMP-response element binding protein (CREB) that binds to the cAMP response element (CRE) that is present in the M promoter of the MITF gene[85, 86]. MITF is a transcription factor with a basic helix-loop-helix-leucine zipper motif. MITF regulates melanocyte cellular differentiation and the transcription of melanogenic enzymes such as tyrosinase, TRP-1, and TRP-2 and the transcription of melanosome structural proteins including MART-1 and Pmel17[87-90]. Pmel17 is a structural matrix protein and an amyloid protein required for the generation of the internal fibril[91]. The promoter sequences of tyrosinase, TRP-1, and TRP-2 share a highly conserved motif known as the M-box, which contributes to their melanocyte-specific expression[92, 93](Figure 4). TRP-1 promoter activity is up regulated by paired box 3 (PAX3)[94]. The M-box (AGTCATGTGCT) is an extended E-box (ACATGTGA) and is necessary for promoter up-regulation by MITF[16, 95]. The E-box is more important than the M-box in promoting the transcription factor MITF[96](Figure 4). MITF is exclusively expressed in melanocytes. It binds to the M-box promoter elements of tyrosinase and modulates TRP-1 and TRP-2, resulting in hyperpigmentation[97-99]. In addition to the process of melanization, MITF also regulates melanocyte proliferation, differentiation, development, apoptosis, and survival[100-102].

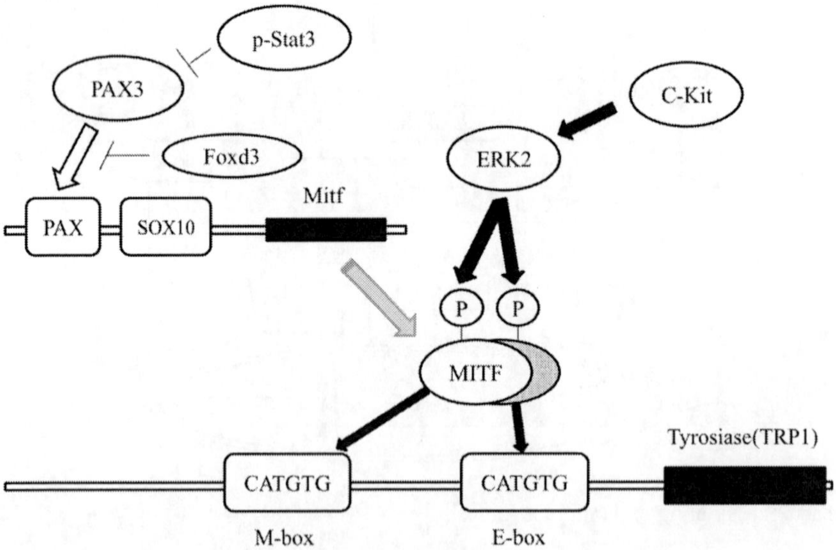

Figure 4. Tyrosinase gene expression.

A transient increase in MITF leads to the up-regulation of tyrosinase, TRP-1, and TRP-2[103] as well as to increased dendricity[88]. Many transcription factors including Sry-related HMG box (SOX) 9 and 10, PAX3, signal transducer and activator of transcription 3 (STAT3), protein inhibitor of activated STAT3 (PIAS3), lymphoid-enhancing factor-1 (LEF-1), immunoglobulin transcription factor-2 (ITF2), and forkhead-box transcription factor D3 (FOXD3) are able to modulate the expression and/or transcriptional activity of MITF in vivo[104] (Figure 4). The transcription factor SOX9 may play an important role in UVB-induced melanocyte differentiation and pigmentation through MITF regulation[105]. SOX10 regulates the expression of MITF and TRP-2. SOX10 has been demonstrated to activate the TRP-2 promoter-reporter construct and to work in synergy with MITF[106, 107]. PAX3 binds to the MITF gene promoter to regulate MITF expression[108]. In addition, PAX3 has been shown to act in synergy with SOX10 to up regulate the expression of MITF[109]. The transcriptional activity of MITF is regulated through the interaction between STAT3 and PIAS3. LEF-1, a transcription factor involved in the Wnt signal transduction pathway, initiates and facilitates MITF expression, while ITF2 and FOXD3 down regulate MITF expression[104, 110-112].

The transcriptional activity of MITF is regulated by phosphorylation of tyrosinase residues on extracellular signal-regulated kinase 2 (ERK2) following signals from c-kit (tyrosinase-type receptor) and then by phosphorylation of the 73rd serine residue in the N terminal domain of MITF[113] (Figure 4). The tyrosinase gene and TRP-1 promoter zones share a CATGTG motif. When MITF is activated, binding to the formed dimmers serves to regulate the expression of the tyrosinase gene TRP-1. MITF is also regulated at the transcriptional level by interleukin-6 (IL-6) and the Wnt signaling pathway and it is post-transcriptionally regulated by phosphorylation via ribosomal S6 kinase (RSK), glycogen synthase kinase-3β (GSK3β), p38 stress signaling, and the mitogen-activated protein kinase (MAP kinase) pathways[89, 90, 98, 114-116](Figure3). α-MSH also stimulates p38 MAP kinase, which in turn phosphorylates upstream transcription factors that bind to the tyrosine promoter[52].

Human placental lipid upregulates p38 activation and subsequent tyrosinase expression, thereby promoting melanogenesis[117]. Down-regulation of p38 expression leads to an increase in expression of biomarkers associated with differentiation such as tyrosinase and tyrosinase-related proteins.

The mechanism involved in the p38-mediated regulation of melanogenesis is the ubiquitin–proteasome pathway, through which melanogenic enzymes are degraded[118]. In addition, inhibition of ERK and AKT signaling via MITF up-regulation plays a key role in inducing hyperpigmentation[119]. ERK activation results in phosphorylation of MITF and its subsequent ubiquitination and degradation[120]. Sphingosine-1-phosphate, C2-ceramide, and sphingosylphosphorylcholine activate ERK and may play important roles in the inhibition of melanogenesis[120-122].

Transforming growth factor-β1 (TGF-β1) inhibits melanogenesis by mediating the down-regulation of MITF promoter activity as well as by reducing the production of tyrosinase, TRP-1, TRP-2, and MITF protein levels. In addition, TGF-β1 inhibits the expression of PAX 3, which in turn inhibits melanogenesis[123]. It has been reported that TGF-β1 influences the ERK pathway and down regulates MITF and the production of melanogenic enzymes[115, 124, 125].

The agouti signaling protein (ASP) can down regulate MITF gene expression and compete with α-MSH in binding to MC1R, causing inhibition of α-MSH signaling on the MC1R receptor. ASP modulates the frequency, rate, and extent of eumelanin and pheomelanin generation[4].

Studies have demonstrated that high levels of ASP are associated with yellow-pigmented bands in mouse hair because ASP inhibits α-MSH binding to MC1R [16]. Thus, MC1R and its ligands, α-MSH and ASIP, regulate the switch between eumelanin and pheomelanin synthesis in melanocytes[79, 126].

UVB exposure activates the transcription factor p53, which in turn induces the expression of POMC. Expression of that α-MSH precursor leads to the secretion of α-MSH and the up-regulation of melanogenesis via MC1R in keratinocytes[127, 128]. In addition, p53 directly stimulates the expression of the genes encoding tyrosinase and TRP1 in melanocytes[129]. UVB also induces the expression of corticotropin-releasing hormone (CRH) in melanocytes, which is mediated by the CREB–PKA signaling pathway with consequent stimulation of POMC expression through the CRH-R1 receptor. The POMC gene has been shown to be p53-responsive following UV irradiation[130].

Kichina et al. demonstrated that stable transfection of wild-type p53 into pigmented melanoma cells leads to overexpression of wild-type p53 and a decrease in tyrosinase mRNA levels and tyrosinase activity[131].

Khlgatian et al. have shown that UV irradiation results in increased p53-dependent tyrosinase mRNA levels in melanoma cells and that p53 is required for the thymidine dinucleotide-induced increase in tyrosinase function in mouse epidermis[132]. They also reported that tanning is part of a p53-mediated adaptive response of mammalian skin to UV-induced DNA damage[132].

Other hormones, such as steroids and sex hormones, can influence pigmentation[79, 127, 133], and it has been reported that cholesterol is capable of increasing the expression of MITF and its target genes in melanocytes through the up-regulation of the CREB protein[134]. Two fibroblast-derived paracrine factors, namely dickkopf-related protein 1 (DKK1) and neuregulin-1 (NRG1), regulate melanogenesis. DKK1 is a factor secreted by fibroblasts. DKK1 has been shown to suppress growth of melanocytes, strongly inhibit melanin production, and inhibit binding of Wnt proteins to their receptors, which results in down-regulation of melanogenesis[102, 135].

In addition, DKK1 suppresses melanocyte growth and function by inhibiting the Wnt/b-catenin signaling pathway[136, 137]. DKK1 has also been shown to regulate the expression of PAR-2[137].

Pigmentary Disorders

Hyperpigmentation disorders are characterized by the overproduction of melanin and include melasma, postinflammatory hyperpigmentation, freckles, moles, chloasma, age spots, and lentigines[138-140]. Hypopigmentation disorders are characterized by the underproduction of melanin and include disorders such as oculocutaneous albinism, Hermansky–Pudlak syndrome, Griscelli syndrome, Chediak-Higashi syndrome, and Waardenburg syndrome.

Oculocutaneous albinism is an inherited autosomal recessive disorder characterized by deficiency or complete absence of melanin[61]. At least 10 types of oculocutaneous albinism exist. Patients with the disorder present with hypopigmention of the skin, hair, and eyes as well as reduced visual acuity with nystagmus and photophobia. Furthermore, in these patients there is often complete lack of tyrosinase activity[141, 142].

Oculocutaneous albinism type 2, which is characterized by a congenital reduction or absence of melanin pigment in the skin, hair, and eyes, is the most common type and the incidence is highest in black Africans[16].

Hermansky-Pudlak syndrome (HPS) is a genetically heterogeneous group of related autosomal recessive conditions. It is divided into eight types according to the HPS genes that carry mutations[143].

Defects in proteins encoded by these genes can affect the biogenesis or function of intracellular organelles such as melanocytes and retinal pigment epithelial cells. HPS is also associated with lung disease, inflammatory bowel disease, renal disease, and bleeding problems due to platelet dysfunction[16].

Griscelli syndrome is an autosomal recessive disorder characterized by pigmentary dilution of the skin and the accumulation of large and abnormal end-stage melanosomes in the center of melanocytes[144].

It may be caused by defects in the formation of the Rab27a–Mlph–MyoVa protein complex in melanocytes, an important protein that connects melanosomes to the actin network[144]. Chediak-Higashi syndrome is an autosomal recessive disorder similar to oculocutaneous albinism[145].

Patients with this syndrome are susceptible to infection because they lack natural killer cell function and are at risk for developing lymphofollicular malignancy and peripheral neuropathies[146, 147].

Mutations in the human homolog of the MITF gene are associated with auditory and pigmentary abnormalities in patients with Waardenburg syndrome type IIA[109, 148, 149]. Mutations in the PAX3 gene are associated with Waardenburg syndrome type I, while SOX 10 mutations are characteristic of Waardenburg syndrome type IV[4, 51].

Mechanisms of Depigmentation

Studies on the processes of cellular melanogenesis and the response of pigment-producing cells to UV radiation have been instrumental in promoting the development of depigmenting agents[57, 58, 114, 150, 151].

The mechanisms of action by which biological and chemical agents cause hypopigmentation include (i) tyrosinase inhibition, maturation, and enhancement of its degradation; (ii) inhibition of tyrosinase mRNA transcription; (iii) inhibition of MAP kinases, TRP-1, TRP-2, and MITF; (iv) downregulation of MC1R activity; (v) interference with melanosome maturation and transfer; and (vi) melanocyte loss and desquamation[57, 114, 150-153].

Tyrosinase inhibition is the most common approach to achieve skin hypopigmentation as this enzyme catalyses the rate-limiting step of pigmentation[114, 152]. Tyrosinase inhibitors can be classified as competitive, uncompetitive, mixed type, and non-competitive inhibitors[57, 154].

Tyrosinase can be inhibited at the transcriptional and post-transcriptional levels by inhibiting tyrosinase mRNA transcription and disrupting tyrosinase glycosylation by using competitive or non-competitive inhibitors to attenuate the catalytic activity of tyrosinase, by accelerating tyrosinase degradation, and by modulating tyrosinase stability[155, 156].

Natural Hypopigmentation Agents

Hydroquinone, ascorbic acid, and retinoic acid have been shown to be effective skin-whitening agents; however, they are associated with harmful side effects, thereby limiting their clinical use[155]. Compounds derived from natural products, on the other hand, have been shown to be as effective as chemical-based products at reducing hyperpigmentation. Some natural skin-depigmenting products have been reported to directly effect melanogenesis; enhance tyrosinase degradation; interfere with melanosome maturation and its transfer; inhibit inflammation-induced melanogenesis; and accelerate skin desquamation[51, 154, 157-159].

Effect on Melanogenesis

As shown in Table 1, whitening agents derived from natural products can be divided into three groups: phenols, polyphenols, and others [58]. Table 1 also presents the plants from which the compounds are derived, the mode of action including tyrosinase inhibition, other enzyme inhibition (OEI (TRP1 and TRP2), melanin inhibition (MI), and other mechanisms of action, as well as the IC_{50} values of said compounds. The mechanisms of tyrosinase inhibition can be evaluated by measuring enzyme inhibition kinetics using Lineweaver-Burk plots with varying concentrations of L-DOPA as the substrate. Moraceae, Anacardiaceae, Chloranthaceae, Ericaceae, Lamiaceae, Sapindaceae, and Fabaceae are rich in phenols and polyphenols that have anti-melanogenesis activity. Most studies used B16 melanoma cells as a model to investigate the mechanism of action governing melanin inhibition. Some of the studies used mouse melan-a or mel-ab melanocyte cultures or normal human melanocytes (NHMC) as experimental models. Data from studies that involved the use of NHMC cells are probably more reliable because those cells mimic the response to stimuli seen *in vivo*. Human melanocyte proliferation and enhancement of melanin synthesis require cross-talk between several cytokines and hormones that are released from keratinocytes. Co-cultures of melanocytes and keratinocytes from mouse[160, 161] or human skin[162] also more closely mimic the response seen *in vivo*.

The brownish guinea pig (GP) model is commonly used to study the effects of skin-whitening agents on reducing hyperpigmentation induced by UV or exposure to exogenous α-MSH (Table 1). In human studies, the activities of skin-whitening agents are normally investigated by evaluating skin color changes using a Chromameter or a Mexameter or by histochemical investigations of DOPA positive cells [163, 164]. Beginning in September 2009, the Commission of the European Communities established a prohibition to test finished cosmetic products and cosmetic ingredients on animals (European Commission - Consumer Affairs). Commercially available skin equivalent models (SEMs), a keratinocyte and melanocyte co-culture system [165], and MatTek's MelanoDerm™ (MatTek Corporation), a human three dimensional skin-like tissue structure, are useful *in vitro* models for evaluating the ability of cosmetic and pharmaceutical agents to modulate skin pigmentation. A common vertebrate model organism that is used for whitening studies is the zebrafish, which has been [165, 166] proved to be a useful model for demonstrating the *in vivo* toxicity of whitening agents.

Table 1. Whitening ingredients from natural sources effect on melanogenesis

Compounds (phenol, polyphenols, others)	Source	Mode of action				Refs.
		TI	OEI (TRP-1, TRP-2)	other	MI	
Phenols						
Anacardic acid, 6-[8(Z),11(Z),14-pentadecatrienyl]-salicylic acid, 5-[8(Z),11(Z),14-pentadecatrienyl] resorcinol	*Anacardium occidentale* cashew fruit (Anacardiaceae)	Yes (c)				**[249]**
10'(Z)-heptadecenylhydroquinone [HQ17(1)]	*Rhus succedanea* (Anacardiaceae)	Yes IC_{50}= 37 μM			Yes IC_{50}= 40 μM	**[250]**
2-hydroxy-4-methoxybenzaldehyde	*Rhus vulgaris* Meikle *Sclerocarya caffra* Sond (Anacardiaceae) *Mondia whitei* (Hook) Skeels (Asclepiadaceae)	Yes (m) IC_{50}=0.03 mM				[251]
3,4-Dihydroxyacetophenone	Ilex pubescens (Aquifoliaceae)	Yes IC_{50}= 10 μM		Reduction of TYR and MITF protein level	Yes	**[252]**
p-Coumaric acid	*Panax ginseng* (Araliaceae)	Yes (m) IC_{50}= 3.65 mM				**[253]**
p-Coumaric acid	*Sasa quelpaertensis* (Gramineae)	Yes (c)		Reduction of TYR protein level	Yes	[254]
2',4',6'-trihydroxydihydrochalcone	*Greyia flanaganii* (Greyiaceae)	Yes IC_{50}= 69.15 μM				[255]
protocatechuic aldehyde	*Salvia miltiorrhiza* (Lamiaceae)	Yes (c) IC_{50}=19.92 μM				[256]

Table 1. (Continued)

Compounds (phenol, polyphenols, others)	Source	Mode of action				Refs.
		TI	OEI (TRP-1, TRP-2)	other	MI	
protocatechualdehyde	*Phellinus linteus* (Hymenochaetaceae)	Yes (c)				[257]
protocatechuic acid methyl ester	Black Rice Bran	Yes IC_{50}= 0.28 μM				[258]
phloroglucinol (1), eckstolonol (2), eckol (3), hlorofucofuroeckol A (4), ieckol (5)	*Ecklonia stolonifera*. brown alga extracts (Laminariaceae)	Yes [(1) and (2), -- (c)] (1) IC_{50}= 92.8 μg/mL (2) IC_{50}= 126 μg/mL Yes [(3) , (4) and (5) -- (n)] (3) IC_{50}=33.2 μg/mL (4) IC_{50}=177 μg/mL (5) IC_{50}=2.16 μg/mL			Yes	[259]
Phloroglucinol, dieckol, eckol,	*Ecklonia cava* (Lessoniaceae)	Yes Dieckol (88.9% of TYR at 50 μM)		Reduction of UV-B induced cell damages	Yes	[260]
7-phloroeckol	*Ecklonia cava* (Lessoniaceae)	Yes (nc) IC_{50} =0.85 μM			Yes	[261]
cinnamaldehyde(1), 2-methoxy cinnamaldehyde (2) cinnamic acid (3) O-coumaric acid (4) , icariside DC (5), dihydromelilotoside (6), dihydromelilotoside (7)	*Cinnamomum cassia* (Lauraceae)	Yes (1) IC_{50}=0.52 ±0.03 mM, (2) IC_{50}=0.42 ±0.02 mM, (3) IC_{50}=0.41 ±0.01 mM, (4) IC_{50}=0.67 ±0.03 mM,				

Compounds (phenol, polyphenols, others)	Source	Mode of action				Refs.
		TI	OEI (TRP-1, TRP-2)	other	MI	
		(5) IC_{50}=0.71 ±0.03 mM, (6) IC_{50}=0.57 ±0.01 mM, (7) IC_{50}=0.63 ±0.02 mM				[262]
Mulberroside F (moracin M-6, 39-di-O-β-D-glucopyranoside)	*Morus alba* leaves (Moraceae)	Yes TYR (mushroom) IC_{50}=0.29 µg/mL ; TYR (mammalian) IC_{50}=68.3 µg/mL		Superoxide Scavenging Activity	Yes (30.6% of MI at 1 mg/mL)	[263]
4-Substituted resorcinols	*Artocarpus incises* (Moraceae)	Yes (c)				[264]
Macelignan	*Myristica fragrans* (Myristicaceae)	Yes IC_{50}=30 µM	TRP-1 TRP-2	Reduction of TYR, TRP-1 and TRP-2 protein level	Yes IC_{50}=13 µM	[265]
Americanin A (1), 3,3'-bisdemethylpinoresinol (2)	*Morinda citrifolia* seeds (Rubiaceae)	Yes (1) IC_{50} =2.7 mM (2) IC_{50} =0.3 mM		SOD-like activity		[266]
3-caffeoylquinic acid 4-caffeolyquinic acid 5-caffeoylquinic acid 5-feruloylquinic acid 3,4-dicaffeoylquinic acid 3,5-dicaffeoylquinic acid 4,5-dicaffoylquinic acid	green coffee beans (Rubiaceae)	Yes				[267]
3,4-dihydroxycinnamic acid (1), 4-Hydroxy-3-methoxycinnamic acid (2)	*Pulsatilla cernua* (Ranunculaceae)	Yes (nc) (1) IC_{50}=0.97 mM (2) IC_{50}=0.33 mM				[268]

Table 1. (Continued)

Compounds (phenol, polyphenols, others)	Source	Mode of action				Refs.
		TI	OEI (TRP-1, TRP-2)	other	MI	
4-acetonyl-3,5-dimethoxy-*p*-quinol (1), cis-*p*-coumaric acid (2), trans-*p*-coumaric acid (3), *p*-hydroxybenzoic acid (4), Vanillic acid (5)	*Synsepalum dulcificum* (Sapotaceae)	Yes (1) IC_{50}=208.1 μM, (2) IC_{50}=197.9 μM, (3) IC_{50}=168.7 μM, (4) IC_{50}=358.6 μM, (5) IC_{50}=174.4 μM				[269]
Cardamonin	*Alpinia katsumadai Hayata* (Zingiberaceae)	Yes		MITF	Yes	[270]
Isopanduratin A (1) , 4-hydroxypanduratin A (2)	*Kaempferia pandurata.* (Zingiberaceae)	Yes (1) IC_{50}=10.5 μM (2) IC_{50}>30 μM		Reduction of TYR protein level	Yes (1) IC_{50}= 10.64 μM (2) IC_{50}= 23.25 μM	[271]
Curcumin, yakuchinone A, yakuchinone B, eugenol ferulic acid	Chouji Syzygium aromaticum (Myrtaceae) and Yakuchi Alpinia oxyphylla (Zingiberaceae)	Yes (c) (Curcumin and yakuchinone B)				[272]
polyphenols						
1,2,3,4,6-penta-O-galloyl-â-D-glucose	*Galla rhois* (Anacardiaceae)	Yes (nc)				[273]
2,3,4,6-tetra-O-galloyl-D-glucopyranose (1), 1,2,3,6-tetra-O-galloyl-beta-D-glucopyranose (2), 1,2,3,4,6-penta-O-galloyl-beta-D-glucopyranose (3)	*Rhus chinensis* (Anacardiaceae)	Yes (nc) (1) IC_{50} = 54 μM, (2) IC_{50} = 30 μM, (3) IC_{50} = 15 μM			Yes	[274]
Tannic acid	*Rhus javanica* leaves (Anacardiaceae)	Yes (c) IC_{50}= 22 μM				[275]

Compounds (phenol, polyphenols, others)	Source	Mode of action				Refs.
		TI	OEI (TRP-1, TRP-2)	other	MI	
Icariside I (1), Icariside II (2), Icaritin (3)	*Epimedium grandiflorum* (Berberidaceae)				Yes (1) IC_{50}= 49.04 µM, (2) IC_{50}= 10.53 µM, (3) IC_{50}= 11.13 µM	[276]
Xanthohumol	*Humulus lupulus* L. (Cannabaceae)	Yes	Reduction of TRP-1 and TRP-2 mRNA level	Reduction of cAMP, MITF protein and its mRNA expression and TYR protein expression	Yes	[277]
GB-2 (biflavanones)	*Garcinia kola* Seed (Clusiaceae)	Yes IC_{50} = 582 µM				[278]
GS contained 2 biflavonoids; 2R,3S-5,7,4',5",7",3"',4"'-heptahydroxy-flavanone[3-8"] flavone (1), 5,7,4',5",7",3"',4"'-heptahydroxy[3-8"] biflavanone (2)	*Garcinia subelliptica* (Clusiaceae)	Yes (1) IC_{50} = 2.5 µM (2) IC_{50} = 26 µM				[279]

Table 1. (Continued)

Compounds (phenol, polyphenols, others)	Source	Mode of action				Refs.
		TI	OEI (TRP-1, TRP-2)	other	MI	
3 flavonols: Quercetin (1), Kaempferol (2), Morin (3), 2 flavones: Luteolin (4), Luteolin 7-*O*-glucoside (5)	*Heterotheca inuloides* (Asteraceae)	3 favonols-(c) (1) $ID_{50} = 0.07$ mM (2) $ID_{50} = 0.23$ mM (3) $ID_{50} = 2.32$ mM 2 flavones-(n) (1) $ID_{50} = 0.19$ mM (2) $ID_{50} = 0.50$ mM				[280]
Luteolin		Yes		Inhibition of adenyl cyclase activity	Yes	[281]
N-feruloylserotonin (1), N-(*p*-coumaroyl)serotonin (2), acacetin (3)	*Carthamus tinctorius* L. (Asteraceae)	Yes (1) $IC_{50} = 0.023$ mM (2) $IC_{50} = 0.074$ mM (3) $IC_{50} = 0.779$ mM			Yes (1) $IC_{50} = 0.191$ mM (2) $IC_{50} = 0.245$ mM (3) $IC_{50} > 20$ mM	[282]
Inulavosin	*Inula nervosa* (Asteraceae)			Mistargeting of tyrosinase to lysosomes	Yes	[283]

Anastatin A (1), Isosilybin A (2), Isosilybin B (3), Luteolin (4), Quercetin (5), (+)-Dehydrodiconiferyl alcohol (6), (+)-Balanophonin (7), 3,4-Dihydroxybenzaldehyde (8)	*Anastatica hierochuntica* (Cruciferae)			Isosilybin A (2) and Isosilybin B (3) inhibit the mRNA expression of TRP-2.	Yes (1) IC_{50} = 16 μM, (2) IC_{50} = 10 μM, (3) IC_{50} = 6.1 μM, (4) IC_{50} = 14 μM, (5) IC_{50} = 15 μM, (6) IC_{50} = 16 μM (7) IC_{50} = 15 μM (8) IC_{50} = 17 μM	[284]
Silymarin	*Silybum marianum* (milk thistle) (Asteraceae)	Yes		Reduction of TYR protein levels	Yes IC_{50}= 28.2 μg/mL	[285]
5,2',4'-trihydroxy-2'',2''-dimethylchromene-(6,7:5'',6'')-flavanone	*Dalea elegans* (Fabaceae)	Yes [(m) L-tyrosine IC_{50}= 0.26 μM] [(nc) L-DOPA IC_{50}= 18.61 μM]				[286]
Kuraridin (1), Kurarinone (2), Norkurarinol (3)	*Sophora flavescens* (Fabaceae)	Yes (1) IC_{50}= 1.1 μM (2) IC_{50}= 1.3 μM (3) IC_{50}= 2.1 μM				[287]
Sophoraflavanone G (1), Kurarinone (2) Kurarinol (3)	*Sophora flavescens* (Fabaceae)	Yes (1) nc- IC_{50} = 4.7 μM, (2) nc- IC_{50} = 2.2 μM (3) c- IC_{50} = 0.1 μM				[288]
Sophoraflavanone G (1), Kuraridin (2), Kurarinone (3)	*Sophora flavescens* (Fabaceae)	Yes (1) IC_{50} = 6.6 μM (2) IC_{50} = 0.6 μM (3) IC_{50} = 6.2 μM				[289]

Table 1. (Continued)

Compounds (phenol, polyphenols, others)	Source	Mode of action				Refs.
		TI	OEI (TRP-1, TRP-2)	other	MI	
Kurarinone (1) Kushnol F (2)	*Sophora flavescens* (Fabaceae)	Yes (1)-nc (1) IC_{50} = 4.6 μg/mL (2) IC_{50} = 9.0 μg/mL				[290]
Kurarinol (1), Kuraridinol (2)	*Sophora flavescens* (Fabaceae)	Yes (1,2)-nc (1) IC_{50} =8.60±0.51 μM (2) IC_{50} =0.88±0.06 μM			Yes (1) IC_{50}=29 μM, (2) IC_{50}=17 μM	[291]
5,2',4'-trihydroxy-2'',2''-dimethylchromene-(6,7:5'',6'')-flavanone	*Dalea elegans* (Fabaceae)	Yes [(m) L-tyrosine IC_{50}= 0.26 μM] [(nc) L-DOPA IC_{50}= 18.61 μM]				[286]
Kuraridin (1), Kurarinone (2), Norkurarinol (3)	*Sophora flavescens* (Fabaceae)	Yes (1) IC_{50}= 1.1 μM (2) IC_{50}= 1.3 μM (3) IC_{50}= 2.1 μM				[287]
N-Feruloyl-N′-cis-feruloyl-putrescine	*Sophora japonica* (Fabaceae)	Yes (m) IC_{50} = 85.0 μM				[292]
Dalbergioidin	*Lespedeza cyrtobotrya* (Fabaceae)	Yes (nc) IC_{50} =20 μM			Yes IC_{50} =27 μM	[293]
Haginin A	*Lespedeza cyrtobotrya* (Fabaceae)	Yes (nc) IC_{50} =5.0 μM	TRP-1 protein level	Reduction of TYR, and MITF protein level, Induction of ERK and Akt/PKB protein level	Yes Melan-a cells IC_{50} = 3.3 μM ; HEMn cells IC_{50} = 2.7 μM	[294]

Compounds (phenol, polyphenols, others)	Source	Mode of action				Refs.
		TI	OEI (TRP-1, TRP-2)	other	MI	
Glycyrrhisoflavone (1), Glyasperin C (2)	*Glycyrrhiza uralensis* (Fabaceae)	Yes (2) IC_{50} = 0.13 μg/mL			Yes (1) 63.73 ± 6.8 % inhibition at 5 μg/mL (2) 17.65 ± 8.8 % at 5 μg/mL	[295]
Licuraside (1), Isoliquiritin(2), Licochalcone A (3)	*Glycyrrhiza uralensis* (1-2) *Glycyrrhiza inflate* (3) (Fabaceae)	Yes 1, 2 and 3 (c) (1) IC_{50} =0.072 mM (2) IC_{50} =0.038 mM (3) IC_{50} =0.0258 mM				[296]
Calycosin	*Astragalus membranaceus* (Fabaceae)	Yes IC_{50} = 38.4 μM			Yes IC_{50} = 40 μM	[297]
Butin	*Spatholobus suberectus* (Fabaceae)	Yes IC_{50} = 35.9 μM	Reduction of TRP-1 and TRP-2 protein and mRNA level	Reduction of TYR protein and mRNA level	Yes 29.26% at 100 μM	[298]
Gallocatechin (1), Epi-gallocatechin gallate(2), Quercitrin (3)	*Distylium racemosum* (Hamamelidaceae)	Yes (1) IC_{50} = 4.8 μg/ mL, (2) IC_{50} = 30.2 μg/ mL, (3) IC_{50} = 37.7 μg/ mL				[299]
Quercetin(1) Tiliroside (2)	*Marrubium velutinum* and *Marrubium cylleneum* (Lamiaceae)	Yes Yes 100% inhibition (1) 49.67 ± 1.16 mM (2) 30.19 ± 9.60 mM				[300]
Kaempferol	*Crocus sativus* L. (Iridaceae)	Yes (c) ID_{50} =0.23 mM				[301]

Table 1. (Continued)

Compounds (phenol, polyphenols, others)	Source	Mode of action				Refs.
		TI	OEI (TRP-1, TRP-2)	other	MI	
Aloesin		Yes		in vitro pigmented skin equivalent model	Yes	[305]
Bibenzyl xyloside-1 (1), Bibenzyl xyloside-2 (2), Bibenzyl xyloside-3 (3)	*Chlorophytum arundinaceum* (Liliaceae)	Yes (1) IC_{50}=1.6 μM (2) IC_{50}=0.43 μM (1) IC_{50}=0.73 μM				[302]
Resveratrol (1), Oxyresveratrol (2)	*Veratrum patulum* (Liliaceae)	Yes (1) IC_{50} = 43.5 μM (2) IC_{50} = 1.2 μM				[303]
2"- O-Feruloylaloesin, aloesin	Aloe extracts Aole vera (Liliaceae)	Yes (n)				[304]
Artocarpfuranol(1), dihydromorin (2), steppogenin (3), norartocarpetin (4), artocarpanone (5), artocarpesin (6), isoartocarpesin (7)	*Artocarpus heterophyllus* (Moraceae)	Yes (1) IC_{50} = 47.93 μM (2) IC_{50} = 10.34 μM (3) IC_{50} = 0.57 μM (4) IC_{50} = 0.46 μM (5) IC_{50} = 1.54 μM (6) IC_{50} = 0.52 μM (7) IC_{50} = 0.66 μM				[306]
Norartocarpetin (1), Resveratrol (2)	*Artocarpus gomezianus* (Moraceae)	Yes				[307)
3-prenyl luteolin	*Artocarpus heterophyllus* (Moraceae)	Yes IC_{50} = 76.3 μM			Yes IC_{50} = 57.6 μM	[308]

Compounds (phenol, polyphenols, others)	Source	Mode of action				Refs.
		TI	OEI (TRP-1, TRP-2)	other	MI	
1,3-diphenylpropanes: kazinol C (1), kazinol F (2), broussonin C (3), kazinol S (4)	*Broussonetia kazinoki.* (Moraceae)	Yes (c) (1) $IC_{50} = 15.5$ µM (2) $IC_{50} = 0.96$ µM (3) $IC_{50} = 0.43$ µM (4) $IC_{50} = 17.9$ µM				[309]
chlorophorin	*Chlorophora excelsa* (Moraceae)	Yes (c) $IC_{50} = 1.3$ µM				[310]
4-[(2''*E*)-7''-hydroxy-3'',7''-dimethyloct-2''-enyl]-2',3,4',5-tetrahydroxy-*trans*-stilbene	*Chlorophora excelsa* (Moraceae)	Yes (c) $IC_{50} = 96$ µM				[310]
(±)2,3-cis-dihydromorin (1), 2,3-trans-dihydromorin (2), Oxyresveratrol (3)	*Cudrania cochinchinensis* (Moraceae)	Yes (1) $IC_{50} = 31.1$ µM (2) $IC_{50} = 21.1$ µM (3) $IC_{50} = 2.33$ µM				[311]
2,4,2',4'-Tetrahydroxy-3-(3-methyl-2-butenyl)-chalcone	*Morus nigra* (Moraceae)	Yes (c) $IC_{50} = 0.95$ µM			Yes	[312]
Oxyresveratrol	*Morus alba* L. (Moraceae)	Yes (nc) $IC_{50} = 1$ µM				[313]
Polyphenols: Compound 1,5,9	*Morus lhou* (Moraceae)	Yes (c) (1) $IC_{50} = 1.3$ µM (5) $IC_{50} = 1.2$ µM (9) $IC_{50} = 7.4$ µM				[314]
Betulinic acid	*Morus alba* L. *and Morus rotundiloba* K. (Moraceae)	Yes				[315]
Crude extract (C-AP) Anthocyanins: cyanidin-3-alpha-O-rhamnoside (1), pelargonidin-3-alpha-O-rhamnoside (2)	*Malpighia emarginata.* acerola fruit (Malpighiaceae)	Yes (C-AP) IC_{50}=15 µg/mL, (1) (2) – (nc) (1) IC_{50}=40 µM, (2) IC_{50}=19.1 µM			Yes (data no shown)	[316]

Table 1. (Continued)

Compounds (phenol, polyphenols, others)	Source	Mode of action				Refs.
		TI	OEI (TRP-1, TRP-2)	other	MI	
2R,3S-5,7,4',5",7",3"',4"'-heptahydroxy- flavanone[3-8"] flavone, and 5,7,4',5",7",3"',4"'-heptahydroxy[3-8"] biflavanone	*Hibiscus tiliaceus* (Malvaceae)	Yes				[279]
Globulusin A (1), Eucaglobulin (2)	*Eucalyptus globules* (Myrtaceae)				Yes	[194]
Kaempferol (1), quercetin (2), mudanpioside B (3), benzoyl-oxypaeoniflorin (4), mudanpioside H (5), pentagalloyl-β-D-glucose (6)	*Paeonia suffruticosa* (Paeoniaceae)	Yes (1) to (5) --(c) (1) IC_{50} = 0.12 μM (2) IC_{50} = 0.11 μM (3) IC_{50} = 0.37 μM (4) IC_{50} = 0.45 μM (5) IC_{50} = 0.32 μM (6) -- (nc) (6) IC_{50} = 0.06 μM				[317]
2,3-dihydro-4',4'''-di-O-methylamentoflavone	*Podocarpus macrophyllus var. macrophyllus* (Podocarpaceae)	Yes IC_{50}=0.10 mM	Reduction of TRP-2 mRNA		Yes	[318]
Anthraquinones	*Polygonum cuspidatum* (Polygonaceae)	Yes				[319]
(2R,3R)-(+)-taxifolin	*Polygonum hydropiper* L. (Benitade) (Polygonaceae)	Yes IC_{50}=0.24 mM				[320]
3,4-Dihydroxycinnamic acid (1), 4-hydroxy-3-methoxycinnamic acid (2)	*Pulsatilla cernua* (Ranunculaceae)	Yes (nc) (1) IC_{50} = 0.97 mM (2) IC_{50} = 0.33 mM				[268]

Compounds (phenol, polyphenols, others)	Source	Mode of action				Refs.
		TI	OEI (TRP-1, TRP-2)	other	MI	
Quercetin	*Rosa canina* L. (Rosaceae)	Yes			Yes Reducing melanin content to 64% at 10 μM, 34.5% at 20 μM, 17.5% at 17.7% at 40 μM	[321]
3,3'-Bisdemethylpinoresinol (1), Quercetin (2)	*Morinda citrifolia* (Rubiaceae)	Yes (1) IC_{50} = 0.3 mM, (2) IC_{50} = 0.1 mM				[266]
Nobiletin	Peel of *Citrus* fruit (Rutaceae)	Yes IC_{50}=46.2 μM				[322]
Betulin, Lupeol, Soyacerebroside I	*Guioa villosa* (Sapindaceae)	Yes				[323]
(+)-*epi*-Syringaresinol (1), *N*-cis-Feruloyltyramine (2)	*Synsepalum dulcificum* (Sapotaceae)	Yes (1) IC_{50}=200 μM, (2) IC_{50}=215.5 μM				[269]
Acetone extract, epigallocatechin gallate (1), Procyanidin B_1(2)	*Sideroxylon inerme* (Sapotaceae)	Yes Acetone extract IC_{50}=63 μg/mL, (1)IC_{50}=30 μg/mL (2)IC_{50}>200 μg/mL			yes	[324]
isopanduratin A (1), 4-hydroxypanduratin A (2)	*Kaempferia pandurata* (Zingiberaceae)	Yes (1) IC_{50}=10.5 μM (2) IC_{50} > 30 μM			Yes (1) IC_{50} = 10.64 μM, (2)IC_{50} = 23.25 μM	[271]

Table 1. (Continued)

Compounds (phenol, polyphenols, others)	Source	Mode of action				Refs.
		TI	OEI (TRP-1, TRP-2)	other	MI	
Negundin A (1), Negundin B (2), 6-hydroxy-4-(4-hydroxy-3-methoxy)-3-hydroxymethyl-7-methoxy-3,4-dihydro-2-naphthaledehyde (3), Vitrofolal E (4), (+)-lyoniresinol (5), (+)-lyoniresinol-3α-O-β-D-glucoside (6), (+)-(−)-pinoresinol (7), (+)-diasyringaresinol (8)	*Vitex negundo Linn.* (Verbenaceae)	Yes (1) IC_{50} = 10.06 μM (2) IC_{50} = 6.72 μM (3) IC_{50} = 7.81 μM (4) IC_{50} = 9.76 μM (5) IC_{50} = 3.21 μM (6) IC_{50} = NA (7) IC_{50} = 15.13 μM (8) IC_{50} = 5.61 μM				[325]
Gentol	*Gnetum* genus (Zingiberaceae)	Yes IC_{50}=4.5 μM			Yes	[326]
(-)-epigallocatechin gallate (EGCG) (1) (-)-gallocatechin 3-0-gallate (GCG) (2) (-)-epicatechin gallate (ECG) (3)	Green tea	Yes (c) (1) IC_{50} = 34.10 μM (2) IC_{50} = 17.34 μM (3) IC_{50} = 34.58 μM				[327]
1,2,3,6-Tetra-Ogalloyl-b-D-glucose (1), 1,2,3,4,6-Penta-O-galloyl-b-D-glucose, (2) 2,3,4,6-Tetra-O-galloyl-D-glucose (3)	10 Chinese Galls	Yes (nc) (1) IC_{50}=30 μM (2) IC_{50}=15 μM (3) IC_{50}=54 μM			Yes	[274]

Compounds (phenol, polyphenols, others)	Source	Mode of action				Refs.
		TI	OEI (TRP-1, TRP-2)	other	MI	
N,N′-dicoumaroyl-putrescine (DCP), N,N′-diferuloyl-putrescine (DFP)	Corn bran	yes (DCP) IC_{50}=181.73 μM (DFP) IC_{50}=291.3 μM			Yes (DCP) IC_{50}=3169.5 μM (DFP) IC_{50}=733.64 μM	[328]
7,8,4'-Trihydroxyisoflavone (1), 7,3',4'-Trihydroxyisoflavone (2), Genistein (3)	Korean fermented soybean paste (Doenjang)	Yes (1) IC_{50} = 11.21 ± 0.8 μM (2) IC_{50} = 5.23 ±0.6 μM			Yes (1) IC_{50} = 12.23±0.7 μM (2) IC_{50} = 7.83 ±0.7 μM (3) IC_{50}= 57.83 ±0.5 μM	[329]
5,7-dihydroxyflavone (chrysin)	propolis			Blocking adenylyl cyclase activity	Yes (51.6% at10 μM, 40.90% at 100μM)	[330]
Others						
Extract	*Salicornia herbacea* (Amaranthaceae)	Yes			Yes	[331]
70% Acetone extract	*Rhus chinensis* (Anacardiaceae)	Yes IC_{50}= 22 μg/mL			Yes	[274]
Isoimperatorin Imperatorin	*Angelica dahurica* (Apiaceae)	Yes		Reduction of TYR mRNA levels	Yes	[332]
Anisic acid	*Pimpinella anisum* (Apiaceae)	Yes (u) IC_{50}=0.68 mM				[268]
Anisaldehyde	*Pimpinella anisum* (Apiaceae)	Yes (nc) IC_{50}=0.38 mM				[268]

Table 1. (Continued)

Compounds (phenol, polyphenols, others)	Source	Mode of action				Refs.
		TI	OEI (TRP-1, TRP-2)	other	MI	
Cumic acid (1), Cuminaldehyde (2)	*Cuminum cyminum* (Apiaceae)	Yes (nc) (1) $IC_{50} = 0.26$ mM (2) $IC_{50} = 0.05$ mM				[333]
ethanolic extract	*Areca catechu* (Arecaceae)	Yes $IC_{50} = 0.48$ mg/mL			Yes	[334]
	Lichen species: *Graphina glaucorufa,* *Graphina multistriata,* *Graphina salacinilabiata,* *Graphis assamensis,* *Graphis nakanishiana,* *Phaeographopsis indica*	Yes				[335]
(2Z,8Z)-Matricaria acid methyl ester	*Erigeron breviscapus* (Asteraceae)	Yes			Yes IC_{50}=25.4 μM	[336]
selina-4(14),7(1)-dien-8-one	*Atractylodis Rhizoma Alba.* (Asteraceae)	Yes	TRP-1, TRP-2		yes	[337]
Extract	*Lepidium apetalum* (Brassicaceae)	Yes		Reduction of TYR mRNA and MITF protein level	yes	[338]
2 germacrane-type sesquiterpenes	*Chloranthus henryi* (Chloranthaceae)	Yes IC_{50}=325 μM and 269 μM				[339]
Tianmushanol (1), 8-O-methyltianmushanol (2)	*Chloranthus tianmushanensis* (Chloranthaceae)	Yes (1) IC_{50}=358 ±3 μM (2) IC_{50}=312 ±3 μM				[340]

Compounds (phenol, polyphenols, others)	Source	Mode of action				Refs.
		TI	OEI (TRP-1, TRP-2)	other	MI	
3β,21,22,23-tetrahydroxycycloart-24(31),25(26)-diene	*Amberboa ramosa* (Asteraceae)	Yes IC_{50}=1.32 μM				[341]
1β-Hydroxy arbusculin A (1), costunolide (2), reynosin (3)	*Saussurea lappa* Clarke (Asteraceae)				Yes (1) IC_{50} = 11 μg/mL, (2) IC_{50} = 3.0 μg/mL (3) IC_{50} = 2.5 μg/mL	[342]
methanolic extract fraction	*Arbutus andrachne* L. (Ericaceae)	Yes IC_{50}=1000 mg/mL				[343]
Esculetin	*Euphorbia lathyris* L. (Euphorbiaceae)	Yes(c) IC_{50} = 43 μM				[344]
three steroids: stigmast-5-ene-3 beta,26-diol (1), stigmast-5-ene-3-ol (2), campesterol (3)	*Trifolium balansae* (Fabaceae)	Yes (1) stronger than (2) and (3) (1) IC_{50} =2.39 μM				[345]
	Stryphnodendron barbatimao, *Entada africana* *Prosopis africana* (Fabaceae) *Cariniana brasiliensis*, (Lecythidaceae) *Portulaca pilosa*, (Portulacaceae)	Yes				[346]
Trifolirhizin	*Sophora flavescens* *(Fabaceae)*	Yes IC50 =506.77±4.49 μM			Yes (3) IC50 = 36 μM	[291]
methyl gallate	*Distylium racemosum branches* *(Hamamelidaceae)*	Yes IC50 = 40.5 μg/ mL				[299]

Table 1. (Continued)

Compounds (phenol, polyphenols, others)	Source	Mode of action				Refs.
		TI	OEI (TRP-1, TRP-2)	other	MI	
5-hydroxymethyl-2-furaldehyde	*Phellinus linteus* (Hymenochaetaceae)	Yes (nc) $IC_{50} = 90.8$ μg/mL				[257]
crocusatin-K	*Crocus sativus* (Iridaceae)	Yes $IC_{50}= 260$ μM				[347]
Trans-cinnamaldehyde	*Cinnamomum cassia* (Lauraceae)	Yes (c)				[348]
linderanolide B and subamolide A	*Cinnamomum subavenium* (Lauraceae)	Yes			Yes	[349]
Extract	*Portulaca pilosa* (Lecythidaceae)	Yes				[346]
(-)-N-formylanonaine	*Michelia alba* D.C. (Magnolianceae)	Yes $IC_{50}= 74.3$ μM		DPPH, reducing power, and chelating metal ions.	yes	[350]
1',3'-dilinolenoyl-2'-linoleoylglycerol	*Flammulina velutipes* (Marasmiaceae)	Yes $IC_{50} =16.1 \pm 0.5$μg/mL				[351]
ethanolic extract of mulberry twigs (EEMT), ethanolic extract of mulberry root bark (EEMR)	*Morus alba* (Moraceae)	Yes				[352]
A series of α,β-unsaturated aldehydes	*Olea europaea L. (Oleaceae)*	Yes(n)		their ability to form a Schiff base with a primary amino group in the enzyme		[353]
(2E)-alkenal (C 7)	*Oliva olea L. (Oleaceae)*	Yes (nc)				[353]
acetonic extract	*Osmanthus fragrans (Oleaceae)*	Yes (u) IC50= 2.314 mg/mL			Yes	[354]

Compounds (phenol, polyphenols, others)	Source	Mode of action				Refs.
		TI	OEI (TRP-1, TRP-2)	other	MI	
methanol extract	Lichen species: *Usnea ghattensis* (Parmeliaceae)	Yes IC_{50}= 8.5 μg/mL				[355]
methanol extract	Lichen species: *Arthothelium awasthii* (Parmeliaceae)	Yes IC_{50}= 17.8 μg/mL				[355]
Sesamol (3,4-methylenedioxyphenol)	*Sesamum indicum* L. (Pedaliaceae)	Yes(c) IC_{50} = 1.9 μM			Yes 63% decreased in 100 mg/mL	[356]
5-(Hydroxymethyl)-2-furfural	*Dictyophora indusiata* (Phallaceae)	Yes (nc) ID_{50}=0.98 mM				[357]
piperlonguminine	*Piper longum* (Piperaceae)	Yes		Reduction of TYR mRNA, and MITF protein level, phosphorylates CREB	Yes	[358]
geranic acid	*Cymbopogon citrates* (Poaceae)	Yes IC_{50}=0.14 mM (trans) IC_{50}=2.3 mM (cis)				[359]
Extract	*Coccoloba uvifera* (Polygonaceae)	Yes IC_{50}= 68.84 μg/ml				[360]
Ethanol extract and distilled water extract	*Ganoderma lucidum (Polyporaceace)*	Yes IC50 =0.32 mg/mL				[361]
Dichloromethane fraction	*Cimicifuga heracleifolia (Ranunculaceae)*	Yes	TRP1	Phosphorylates MEK, ERK1/2 and Akt, MITF	Yes	[362]
50% ethanolic extract	*Citrus hassaku (Rutaceae)*	Yes IC50=4.7 mg/mL			Yes	[363]
Extract	*Dimocarpus longan (Sapindaceae)*	Yes IC50= 2.9–3.2 mg/mL				[364]

Table 1. (Continued)

Compounds (phenol, polyphenols, others)	Source	Mode of action				Refs.
		TI	OEI (TRP-1, TRP-2)	other	MI	
1-O-methyl-fructofuranose	*Schisandra chinensis* (Turcz.) Baill (Schisandraceae)	Yes		via activation of MEK/ERK and PI3K/Akt signaling pathway and subsequent MITF downregulation	Yes	[365]
ethanol extract, water extract, adenosine (1), Ethyl-α-D-glucopyranoside (2)	*Stichopus japonicas* (Stichopodidae)	Yes (m) ethanol extract 0.49–0.61 mg/mL, water extract 1.80–1.99 mg/mL, (1) IC_{50}= 0.13 mg /mL, (2) IC_{50}=0.19 mg /mL				[366]
hirsein A, hirsein B	*Thymelaea hirsuta* (Thymelaeaceae)	Yes	TRP1, TRP2	Decrease PKC activity, MITF, TRP1, TRP2,	Yes	[367]
Metallothionein (protein)	*Aspergillus niger (Trichocomaceae)*	Yes (m)				[368]
9-Hydroxy-4-methoxypsoraln	*Angelica dahurica (Umbelliferae)*	Yes (nc) IC50=2.0 μg/mL				[369]
Alpinia galanga extract	*Alpinia galanga Rhizome (Zingiberaceae)*	Yes IC30=18.5 μg/mL			Yes	[370]
Extract	*Curcuma aromatica Rhizome (Zingiberaceae)*	Yes IC30=8.9 μg/mL			Yes	[370]

Compounds (phenol, polyphenols, others)	Source	Mode of action				Refs.
		TI	OEI (TRP-1, TRP-2)	other	MI	
partial purification	*Curcuma longa* (Zingiberaceae)	Yes	TRP	Phosphorylates MEK, ERK1/2 and Akt, MITF, and TRP-2 protein level	Yes	[371]
triacylglycerols; triolein (1), trilinolein (2)	Sake lees	Yes (nc) TI 2 > 1 (1) IC_{50}=30 μM (2) IC_{50}=8.4 μM				[372]
aqueous extracts	green asparagus	Yes (m) IC_{50}= 1.21 mg/mL		radical scavenging, chelating activities and protected liposome against oxidative damage.		[373]
rsolic acid		Yes		Tyrosinase mRNA and protein	Yes	[374]
San-bai-tang	San-bai-tang	Yes IC_{50}= 215.6 ± 10.3 μg/mL	TRP1, TRP2	MITF	Yes IC_{50}= 254.8 ± 14.5 μg/mL	[375]

TI: tyrosinase inhibiton, (c) competitive (u) uncompetitive (nc) noncompetitive and (m) mixed mode, OEI: other enzyme inhibition, MI: melanin inhibition, TRP-1: tyrosinase related protein-1, TRP-2: tyrosinase related protein-2, PKC: protein kinase C, MITF: microphthalmia-associated transcription factor.

Enhancing Tyrosinase Degradation

Fatty acids are ubiquitous components of cell membranes and serve as a biological energy source. They also play important roles in intracellular signaling and as precursors for ligands that bind to nuclear receptors[152, 167-169]. Fatty acids act as intrinsic factors that modulate the proteasomal degradation of membrane glycoproteins such as tyrosinase. In addition, they regulate the selective degradation of melanogenic enzymes through the ubiquitin-proteasome pathway[170]. Ando et al. found that fatty acids regulate the ubiquitination of tyrosinase and are responsible for modulating the proteasomal degradation of the enzyme[170] and that they had remarkable regulatory effects on melanogenesis in cultured B16F10 murine melanoma cells by modulating proteolytic degradation of tyrosinase[171]. Physiological doses of oleic acid and linoleic acid have been shown to increase the proteolytic activity of 20S proteasomes in rat skeletal muscle [172].

Interference with Melanosome Maturation and Transfer

Table 2 presents the natural products that have been shown to interfere with melanosome maturation and transfer.

Table 2. Whitening agents from natural sources interference with melanosome maturation and transfer

Source	Compounds	Mode of action			Refs.
		maturation	transfer	others	
Soybean extract	Bowman Birk inhibitor (BBI), soybean trypsin inhibitor (STI)		yes		[175]
Achillea millefolium, Yarrow	Centaureidin	Yes	Yes	Inhibition of melanogenesis and reduction the amount of tyrosinase.	[177, 179]
Ophiopogon japonicus	Methylophiopogonanone B	Yes	Yes		[179]
Root of vegetable and yeast	Niacinamide		Yes		[162, 180-182]
	Lectins and Neoglycoproteins		Yes		[162, 376, 377]

Soybean Extract

Protease-activated receptors (PARs) are a subfamily of related G protein-coupled transmembrane receptors that are proteolytically activated by serine proteases (including trypsin or mast cell tryptase). PAR-2 is expressed in keratinocytes but not in melanocytes.

Stimulation of this receptor enhances the rate of phagocytosis of keratinocytes, which in turn leads to increased melanin transfer[173]. Soybean contains small serine proteases, such as Bowman Birk inhibitor (BBI) and soybean trypsin inhibitor (STI, Kunitz-type trypsin inhibitor), that have been shown to inhibit the PAR-2 pathway in keratinocytes.

Interference with the PAR-2 pathway was shown to induce depigmentation by reducing the phagocytosis of melanosomes by keratinocytes, thereby diminishing melanin transfer [17, 174-176]. Interestingly, only unpasteurised soybean milk exhibits this activity.

Centaureidin

Centaureidin (5,7,3'-trihydroxy-3,6,4'-trimethoxyflavone), a flavone from yarrow, has been shown to reduce melanosome transfer and melanocyte dentrite outgrowth[177]. Centaureidin either directly or indirectly activates Rho, a small GTP-binding protein that acts as a master regulator of dendrite formation. Ito et al. reported that activation of Rho in cells exposed to centaureidin resulted in dendrite retraction and reduced melanocyte trafficking of melanin to keratinocytes[178]. In addition, Saeki et al. found that centaureidin inhibited melanogenesis and reduced the total amount of tyrosinase, but not TRP-1[177].

Methylophiopogonanone B (5,7-Dihydroxy-6,8-Dimethyl-3-(4-Methoxybenzyl)Chroman-4-One, MOPB)

Studies have shown that MOPB-induced activation of Rho causes reversible dendrite retraction, microtubule disorganization, and tubule depolymerization, which in turn leads to reduced melanosome transfer. The effect MOPB has on melanogenesis, however, is not the same as the effect centaureidin has on melanin synthesis. Ito et al. showed that MOPB did not influence melanin synthesis or the expression of melanogenic enzymes[179].

Niacinamide

Niacinamide (nicotinamide; 3-pyridinecarboxamide), the amide form of vitamin B_3, is a biologically active form of niacin found in many root vegetables as well as in yeast. Studies have shown that niacinamide down regulates melanogenesis via inhibiting the transfer of melanosomes from melanocytes to keratinocytes[162, 180]. Other studies have reported that niacinamide is a tyrosinase inhibitor[181, 182].

Lectins and Neoglycoproteins

Cellular recognition between melanocytes and keratinocytes is an important process in melanosome transfer. Lectins and neoglycoproteins are glycosylated residues on melanocyte and keratinocyte membranes that play inhibitory roles in the process of receptor-mediated endocytosis, a process that facilitates melanosome transfer[63]. Specifically, plasma membrane lectins and their glycoconjugates are thought to interrupt melanocyte and keratinocyte contact and interaction by binding to their specific plasma membrane receptors, resulting in inhibition of melanosome transfer[183]. This inhibition is reversible and has been shown to be enhanced in the presence of niacinamide[162].

Inhibition of Inflammation-Induced Melanogenesis

Some mediators produced by keratinocytes after exposure to primary inflammatory stimuli or UV exposure, such as interleukin-1α (IL-1α), tumor necrosis factor α (TNF-α), ET-1, and Stem cell factor (SCF) are able to promote melanogenesis. ET-1 shows a unique behavior in exerting stimulatory effects both on DNA synthesis and melanization in human melanocytes[65, 184-186]. Activation of epidermal ETs is determined by the enzymatic cleavage of inactive prepolypeptides by an endopeptidase termed ET converting enzyme (ECE), which is regulated by the primary inflammatory cytokine IL-1α[187]. The SCF expressed in keratinocytes is involved in melanocyte growth and the synthesis, migration, and maintenance of melanin. UV exposure stimulates the overexpression of SCF, which binds to its receptor, c-kit, resulting in enhanced melanogenesis[188]. Arachidonate-derived chemical mediators, namely the cysteinyl leukotrienes (LTC) LTC4 and LTD4, and thromboxanes, such as TXB2, are released from membrane phospholipids by phospholipase A2 (PLA2). Leukotrienes not only significantly up-regulate tyrosinase, but also enhance the transfer of melanosomes to keratinocytes. These results suggest that PLA2 itself triggers melanin synthesis following UV irradiation or inflammation, thereby resulting in hyperpigmentation[52, 189]. Prostaglandins (PGs) synthesized from arachidonic acid by cyclooxygenase are responsible for regulating cellular growth, differentiation, and apoptosis. In the skin, PGs (especially PGE2, PGF2α) are produced and rapidly released by keratinocytes after exposure to UV irradiation, resulting in hyperpigmentation[190]. Therefore, anti-inflammatory compounds could be useful for the prevention or treatment of post-inflammatory hyperpigmentation. Table 3 lists some natural products that have been shown to be effective treatments for inflammation-induced hyperpigmentation. Topical application of *Matricaria chamomilla* extract has been shown to inhibit UVB-induced pigmentation by suppressing ET-1-induced DNA synthesis. The extract, however, did not affect IL-α-induced ET-1 production or tyrosinase activation[184]. Hachiya et al. reported that a 50% ethanol extract of *Sanguisorba officinalis* root inhibited UVB-induced pigmentation of brownish guinea pig skin. The results of their study suggest that the mechanism governing the inhibition of ET-1 production in human keratinocytes is via the suppression of endothelin-converting enzyme-1α[191]. Kobayashi et al. reported that a 45% 1,3-butylene glycol extract of *Althaea officinalis* roots inhibited both the secretion of ET-1 from normal human keratinocytes (NHKC) and the action of ET-1 on NHMC, mainly by suppressing ET-1-induced calcium mobilization. They found that binding of ET-1 to the endothelin B receptor (ETBR) on the cell surface of NHMC induced the mobilization of intracellular calcium [192]. Fucoxanthin, a carotenoid derived from edible sea algae, exhibited anti-pigmentary activity when applied either topically or orally in an animal model of UVB-induced melanogenesis. This effect of fucoxanthin may be due to suppression of

PGE2 synthesis and melanogenic stimulant receptors (neurotrophin, PGE2 and MC1R) [193, 194].

Table 3. Whitening agents from natural sources inhibiting on inflammation-induced melanogenesis

Source	Compounds	Mode of action	Refs.
Matricaria chamomilla	*Matricaria chamomilla* extract	Antagonist for ET-receptor (*in vitro* and *in vivo*)	[184]
Sanguisorba officinalis L.		Suppression of endothelin-converting enzyme-1α (*in vitro* and *in vivo*)	[191]
Althaea officinalis L.	roots extract	Inhibits both the secretion and action of ET-1 (*in vitro*)	[192]
sea algae	fucoxanthin	Suppression of prostaglandin (PGE2) synthesis and melanogenic stimulant receptors (neurotrophin, PGE2 and α-MSH). (*p.o.*)	[193]
Fenugreek seed (*Trigonella foenum-graecum* L.)	steroidal saponins	Inhibition of TNF-α and melanogenesis (*in vitro*)	[195]
Eucalyptus globulus	Globulusin A and eucaglobulin	Anti-inflammatory and anti-melanogenesis activity (*in vitro*)	[194]
Azadirachta indica seed	nimolicinol	Inhibition of melanogenesis (*in vitro*) and TPA-induced inflammation (*in vivo*)	[378]
Guava (Psidium guajava L.*)*	leaves extract	Suppression of skin inflammation and melanogenesis (*p.o.*)	[196]
ANTI-melanogenesis may due to antioxidant activity			
glabridin	superoxide anion productions and cyclooxygenase activities	Inhibition of UVB-induced pigmentation and erythema (*in vivo*), inhibition of superoxide anion productions and cyclooxygenase activities (*in vitro*)	[379]
	luteolin	Inhibiting adenyl cyclase induced by MSH, anti-oxidant activity in DPPH, NBT/XO and intracellular ROS and xanthine oxidase (*in vitro*)	[281]
pine bark	Pycnogenol (catechin, epicatechin and epicatechin-4-(2-hydroxyethyl)thio ether)	Inhibition of tyrosinase and melanin biosynthesis, suppressing ·O2, NO·, ONOO−, and ·OH in (*in vitro*)	[380]
Ecklonia cava (brown alga)	Phlorotannins (dieckol)	Inhibition of tyrosinase activity and reduction of intracellular ROS induced by UV-B radiation (*in vitro*)	[381]
Ishige okamurae (marine algae)	diphlorethohydroxycarmalol	Inhibition of tyrosinase activity and reduction of intracellular ROS induced by UV-B radiation (*in vitro*)	[382]
ginger	[6]-Gingerol	Decreasing ROS level and suppressing TYR activity (*in vitro*)	[383]

Globulusin A and eucaglobulin, monoterpene glycosides isolated from *Eucalyptus globules,* not only have DPPH free radical scavenging activity, thereby inhibiting phorbol myristate acetate-induced expression of tumor-necrosis factor-α and interleukin-1β, but also inhibit melanogenesis *in vitro*.[194] In addition, a methanolic extract and its steroidal saponins, 26-*O*-*β*-*D*-glucopyranosyl-(25*R*)-furost-5(6)-en-3*β*,22*β*,26-triol-3-*O*-*α*-*L*-rhamno-pyranosyl-(1″→ 2′)-*O*-[*β*-*D*-glucopyranosyl-(1‴ → 6′)-*O*]-*β*-*D*-glucopyranoside, minutoside B, and pseudoprotodioscin isolated from Fenugreek seed (*Trigonella foenum-graecum* L. Fabaceae) inhibited the production of phorbol-12-myristate-13-acetate-induced inflammatory cytokines, namely TNF-*α* and melanogenesis *in vitro*[195]. Guava leaf extracts have been shown to suppress UVB-induced skin inflammation. Takashi et al. found that the skin color of guinea pigs that had been exposed to UVB irradiation followed by treatment with guava extract (p.o.) became lighter as a result of the tyrosinase inhibitory activity of guava leaf extract[196]. Nimolicinol, a limonoid isolated from *Azadirachta indica* seeds, shows inhibitory effects both on melanogenesis in B16 melanoma cells and on 12-*O*-tetradecanoylphorbol-13-acetate (TPA)-induced inflammation in mice.

Many studies have found that compounds with potent free radical scavenging activities inhibit tyrosinase expression. Some of the most potent compounds with free radical scavenging ability and tyrosinase inhibiting activity include glabridin, diarylheptanoids and phenolic compounds from *Acer nikoense*; luteolin and pycnogenol from pine bark; phlorotannins from *Ecklonia cava*; diphlorethohydroxycarmalol from *Ishige okamurae*; and [6]-gingerol from ginger (Table 3).

Accelerating Skin Desquamation

Desmosomes, which are classified as a molecular complex of cell adhesion proteins consisting of desmoglein and desmocollin, are mainly responsible for the adhesion between epidermal cells. As the cells move upward from the basal layers to the stratum corneum, the desmosome attachments become weaker. This weakening action is accelerated by enzymes, namely the stratum corneum chemotrypic enzyme (SCCE) and Cathepsin D, by breaking the bonds of the desmosomes, resulting in the sloughing off of cells. Keratinization refers to the turnover of the stratum corneum and begins at the basal layer and gradually moves upward to the stratum corneum corneocytes. This desquamation process normally takes about four weeks and is normally more efficient in younger skin. The process stimulates the growth of newer cells at a deeper level; however, in skin of advanced age, the intercellular desmosomes become glue-like in their ability to cement cells together. As a result, cell sloughing becomes more difficult, which leads to a thicker skin with a dull appearance. The stratum corneum has a pH of 7 at the bottom layer and a pH ranging from 4.5-5.4 at the surface[(197)]. The optimal pH for SCCE and Cathepsin D activity in the final desquamation stage *ranges from 4 to 6*, which explains why those enzymes are most active at the surface of the stratum corneum[198-200].

The capability of a compound to accelerate the turnover of epidermal layers and/or disperse melanin pigment can result in skin lightening. Depigmenting agents lighten the skin by stimulating the removal of pigmented keratinocytes[155, 201]. Pigmented spots, such as freckles or actinic lentigines, melasma spots, and post-inflammatory hypermelanosis macules may be removed by the peeling of corneocytes and epidermal keratinocytes.

Chemical Exfoliants And Their Mode Of Action

(1) α-Hydroxyacids

α-Hydroxyacids (AHA, i.e. lactic acid, glycolic acid, and malic acid) are weak organic acids found in fruits, plants, and milk[202]. Studies on cell cohesion and skin pH changes indicate that keratin bonds may became weaker at low pH values. AHA solution is activated under low pH conditions and may dissolve the desmosome protein linkages causing a burst in skin exfoliation. AHAs have also been used to successfully treat pigmentary lesions such as solar lentigenes, lesions caused by melasma, and post-inflammatory hyperpigmentation macules. AHAs promote exfoliation by decreasing corneocyte cohesion and by stimulating dermal cell growth in the basal layer at low concentrations, while at higher concentrations AHAs promote epidermolysis and dispersal of basal layer melanin. The accelerated desquamation of the stratum corneum by AHAs is complemented by a direct inhibition of tyrosinase, without influencing mRNA or protein expression[201-203]. Lactic acid can be isolated from sour milk[201]. Glycolic acid can be isolated from natural sources, such as sugarcane, sugar beets, pineapple, cantaloupe, and unripe grapes. Both glycolic acid and lactic acid affect the skin layers in the same manner as described above. Furthermore, additional beneficial effects unique to lactic acid include an increase in dermal glycosaminoglycans (GAGs-natural moisturizers) and ceramides (epidermal barrier lipids), and improved water barrier properties. Glycolic acid stimulates collagen synthesis in a manner similar to that of lactic acid[204]. Yamamoto et al. studied the histological differences between patients who received a six-week treatment of topical AHA, glycolic acid, lactic acid, or citric acid as treatment for photo-aged skin and found that patients who had received AHA showed increased epidermal thickness, decreased melanin deposition, and up-regulated collegen levels relative to patients who received topical glycolic acid, lactic acid, or citric acid[205]. In addition, the authors found that AHA treatment not only decreased melanin deposition, but also resulted in the remodeling of the epidermis and the acceleration of desquamation[205]. The Cosmetic Ingredient Review, a panel endorsed by the Esthetics Manufacturers and Distributors Alliance of the American Beauty Association suggests that consumers should not use glycolic acid or lactic acid products with concentrations exceeding 10% or at a pH of 3.5; for professional use, the limits are extended to 30% and the lowest advisable pH value is 3.0.

(2) β-hydroxyacids (BHAs)

Salicylic acid (SA) is a β-hydroxyacid (BHA) found in willow bark and sweet birch. It is also a phytohormone that acts similar to hormones that regulate cell growth and differentiation. SA functions as a desquamating agent by penetrating and dissolving the intercellular matrix of the stratum corneum[114, 202]. Unlike lactic acid, salicylic acid does not hydrate the skin and does not help to normalize epidermal anatomy or physiology. Salicylic acid, which is primarily a keratolytic agent, dissolves the stratum corneum layer by layer from the outside in, resulting in a thinning of the stratum corneum. The effect of salicylic acid on hyperpigmentation inhibition has been demonstrated in a number of studies, but only at very high concentrations (50%). SA is more lipophilic than AHAs, enabling it to penetrate sebaceous substances in the hair follicles and exfoliate the pores. The water solubility of AHAs is lower than that of SA. Since SA has a much stronger comedolytic effect than AHAs, it can be used in acne therapy.

(3) Retinol

Retinol (Vitamin A) is a potent skin exfoliant and antiaging agent. Retinol has been shown to improve the visible signs of photoaging as well as normal chronological aging when used on a daily basis. Studies have shown that retinol slows down collagen degradation in skin that has been chronically exposed to sunlight. In addition, retinol has been demonstrated to inhibit enzymes that are responsible for the degradation of collagen, such as collagenase[206].

(4) Liquiritin

Liquiritin, a flavonoid glycoside derived from liquorice, significantly reduces hyperpigmentation in patients with bilateral and symmetrical idiopathic epidermal melasma[207]. Zhu et al. found that a 20% liquiritin cream was effective at inducing skin lightening by dispersing melanin in a clinical trial involving patients with melasma [208]. The proposed mechanisms involve melanin dispersion by means of the pyran ring of its flavonoidal nucleus and acceleration of epidermal renewal.

Whitening Agents Verified by Clinical Trials

Whitening agents derived from natural products that have been tested in clinical trials are listed in Table 4 and described below:

Arbutin and its Derivatives

The compound 4-hydroxyanisole has been shown to act as an alternative substrate for tyrosinase both *in vivo* and *in vitro*[209]. However, 4-hydroxyanisole and other phenolic compounds have the potential to generate toxic quinone products and have, therefore, been used in various studies to evaluate the toxic effects mediated by tyrosinase in melanoma cells[210, 211].

Hydroquinone (HQ) was widely used as an effective skin-whitening agent before it was banned by the US Food and Drug Administration in 2006 because animal studies in South Africa, the United Kingdom, and the USA revealed that HQ was a potential carcinogen and was associated with an increased incidence of ochronosis. HQ is defined as a drug since its cancer-causing properties have not yet been proved in humans. Other phenolic compounds that have been used to evaluate the toxic effects mediated by tyrosinase include arbutin, kojic acid and ascorbic acid derivatives (Table 4).

Table 4. The effect of whitening agents have been verified by clinical trials

Compounds	Indication of clinical trials	Refs.
3% Arbutin	Treating hyperpigmentary disorders, such as melasma	[212]
3% Deoxyarbutin	Acceleration of the fading of UV-induced tan	[384]
1% Kojic acid	Treating hyperpigmentary disorders, such as melasma, post-inflammatory hyperpigmentation, age spots, and freckles	[216]
10% Magnesium L-ascorbic acid 2-phosphate	Effective for reducing melasma and age spots	[220]
SLM (skin lightening moisturizer containing 3% magnesium ascorbyl phosphate	Reduction of hyperpigmented spots on the face	[385]
0.3% Rucinol	Treating hyperpigmentary disorders, such as melasma	[222]
0.5% Ellagic acid	Effective for treating UVB-induced hyperpigmentation of the skin	[224]
Ellagic Acid (200 mg, 100 mg/oral administration)	Inhibitory effect on a slight pigmentation in the human skin caused by UV irradiation	[386]
Ellagic acid	Melasma	[387]
0.5% Chamomilla extract	Effective for treating UVB-induced hyperpigmentation of the skin	[225, 226]
0.5% 5,5'-Dipropyl-biphenyl-2,2'-diol	Effective for treating UVB-induced hyperpigmentation of the skin	[228]
0.5% 5,5'-Dipropyl-biphenyl-2,2'-diol	Effective in treating hyperpigmentary disorders, such as melasma and senile lentigo	[229]
2 % Rhododendrol	Effective for treating UVB-induced hyperpigmentation of the skin	[153]
20% Azelaic acid	Melasma	[115]
Tranexamic acid	Treating melasma	[388]
3% adenosine Monophosphate Disodium Salt	Effective for treating hyperpigmentary disorders, such as melasma	[239]
4% N-acetyl-4-S-cysteaminylphenol (4-S-CAP)	Melasma	[240]
0.1% Linoleic acid	Effective for treating melasma and to lighten UVB-induced hyperpigmentation of the skin	[241-243]
5 % Glycolic acid	Whitening	[244]
10% Glycolic acid	Melasma	[245]
Lactic acid, full strength (92%; pH 3.5),	Peeling agent in the treatment of melasma	[246]
8% Glycolic acid and 8% lactic acid	Hypopigmentation	[247]
30% Salicylic acid peels	Skin whitening	[248]

Arbutin is a glycosylated form of HQ that is present in bearberry extracts but it can also be synthesized from HQ by glucosidation. Its principal modes of action are competitive inhibition of tyrosinase and TRP-1 activity, inhibition of UV-induced formation and elongation of melanocyte dendritic processes and inhibition of production of $^{\cdot}O_2^-$ and ·OH. It has been shown that a 3% arbutin-containing formulation is effective for treating hyperpigmentary disorders, such as melasma[212]. A combination therapy comprising a YAG laser and 7% α-arbutin solution has been shown to be an effective and well-tolerated treatment for refractory melasma [213]. Deoxyarbutin inhibits tyrosine hydroxylase and DOPA oxidase activities of tyrosinase. In vitro studies have demonstrated that the inhibition constant (Ki) of mushroom-derived tyrosinase is 350-fold lower than the Ki of arbutin. In a human clinical trial, topical treatment with Deoxyarbutin for 12 weeks resulted in a significant reduction in overall skin lightness in a population of light-skinned individuals and a slight reduction in overall skin lightness and improvement in solar lentigines in a population of darkskinned individuals[214, 215].

Kojic Acid

Kojic acid is a γ-pyrone compound produced during the fermentation of aspergillus species, penicillium species and filiform bacteria. Kojic acid exerts a slow-binding inhibition of tyrosinase activity, mainly by chelating copper, and inhibits the polymerization of DHI and DHICA. In a clinical trial, Mishima et al. showed that a 1% kojic acid-containing formulation was effective at treating melasma, post-inflammatory hyperpigmentation, age spots and freckles[216]. In 2003, however, the Japanese Ministry of Health, Labor and Welfare notified suppliers of kojic acid to delay manufacture or import of the product because of concerns about possible carcinogenic effects in animals [217]. However, in 2005, kojic acid was deemed to be a safe cosmetic ingredient and continues to be used as a skin-lightening quasi-drug [218].

Ascorbic Acid and its Derivatives

Ascorbic acid is highly unstable when exposed to heat or highly acidic conditions; derivatives of ascorbic acid, however, are much more stable. Some of the more commonly administered ascorbic acid derivatives include magnesium ascorbyl phosphate, ascorbyl glucoside, sodium ascorbyl phosphate and 3-O-ethyl ascorbic acid. Ascorbic acid is a potent reducer of DOPA quinone and melanin.

It has been reported that ascorbyl glucoside releases ascorbic acid gradually through hydrolysis due to the action of α-glucosidase in living organisms[219].

In a clinical trial, Kameyama et al. found that a 10% magnesium ascorbyl phosphate-containing formulation was shown to be effective at reducing the number of melasma patches and age spots[220]. In another clinical trial, Miyai et al. found that a 2% ascorbyl glucoside-containing cream was effective at accelerating the disappearance of UVB-induced hyperpigmentation[221].

Rucinol

Rucinol (4-n-butylresorcinol) has been reported to be an inhibitor of tyrosinase and TRP1 activity. Katagiri et al. found that a 0.3% Rucinol®-containing lotion was effective at alleviating UV-induced pigmentation and melasma patches[222].

Potassium Methoxysalicylate

Hideya et al. found that potassium methoxysalicylate inhibits melanin synthesis via a mechanism involving competitive inhibition of tyrosinase activity.

This mechanism is similar to the mechanisms governing the modes of action of arbutin and Rucinol[153].

Ellagic Acid

Ellagic acid, a polyphenolic compound, is found in strawberries, apples and a variety of plants.

Shimogaki et al. demonstrated that ellagic acid is a potent antioxidant and that it inhibits tyrosinase activity through copper chelation[223]. Kamide et al. showed that application of 0.5% ellagic acid-containing cream was effective for treating UVB-induced hyperpigmentation and melasma patches[224].

Chamomilla Extract

Chamomilla extract is a crude plant extract.

It inhibits melanin synthesis by binding to endothelin receptors and by inducing the synthesis of inositol triphosphate. Ichihashi et al. demonstrated that a 0.5% chamomilla extract-containing cream was effective at treating UVB-induced hyperpigmentation in humans[225, 226].

5,5′-Dipropyl-Biphenyl-2,2′-Diol (Magnolignan®)

5,5'-Dipropyl-biphenyl-2,2'-diol is a biphenyl compound isolated from *Magnolia heptapeta.*

It has been shown to inhibit melanin synthesis by interfering with the process of tyrosinase maturation[227]. Takeda et al. found that a 0.5% Magnolignan®-containing formulation was effective at treating melasma, senile lentigo and UVB-induced hyperpigmentation in humans[228, 229].

Rhododendrol (4-(4-Hydroxyphenyl)-2-Butanol)

Rhododendrol is a phenolic compound derived from White Birch and Nikko Maple. Rhododendrol inhibits melanin synthesis through competitive inhibition of tyrosinase activity.

In 2010, Kanebo Cosmetics Inc. obtained approval from the Japanese Ministry of Health, Labor and Welfare to use Rhododendrol as a whitening agent[153].

Azelaic Acid

Azelaic acid is a naturally occurring saturated nine-carbon dicarboxylic acid. Its use originated from the finding that Pityrosporum species can oxidize unsaturated fatty acids to dicarboxylic acids, which competitively inhibit tyrosinase. Azelaic acid was initially developed as a topical drug for the treatment of acne. However, because of its effect on tyrosinase, it has also been used to treat melasma, lentigo maligna and other hyperpigmention disorders[230, 231]. In addition, azelaic acid has been shown to be effective at treating postinflammatory hyperpigmentation due to acne by inhibiting the production of free radicals[232, 233]. In the USA, 20% azelaic acid is only indicated for treatment of acne, although it has off-label use for hyperpigmentation. However, studies have found that 20% azelaic acid is equivalent to or better than 2% hydroquinone for the treatment of melasma[233, 234].

Tranexamic Acid and Tranexamic Acid Cetyl Ester Hydrochloride

Plasmin, a protease found in blood serum, not only enhances the intracellular release of arachidonic acid, a precursor of prostaglandins[235], but also elevates the levels of α-MSH[236]. Tranexamic acid has been shown to inhibit UV-induced plasmin activity in keratinocytes by preventing the binding of plasminogen to keratinocytes, which ultimately results in less free arachidonic acid and a diminished ability to produce PGs, thereby decreasing the activity of tyrosinase in melanocytes[189, 237]. Both arachidonic acid and α-MSH can activate melanin synthesis in melanocytes. Therefore, the anti-plasmin activity of tranexamic acid is thought to play a role in its topical effectiveness at treating melasma. The effect of tranexamic acid cetyl ester hydrochloride in treating hyperpigmentary disorders is due to its ability to inhibit UVB-induced inflammation, leading to the quiescence of active melanocytes. This mechanism is similar to the mechanisms of action of chamomilla extract and tranexamic acid.

Adenosine Monophosphate Disodium Salt

Adenosine is the building block of adenosine 5'-triphosphate (ATP), the main intracellular source of energy. Since energy is essential for cell proliferation and maturation, supporting ATP levels with topical adenosine safely accelerates epidermal turnover[238]. Adenosine monophosphate has the potency to increase the amount of intracellular glucose uptake, which is necessary for the biosynthesis of adenosine triphosphate. Therefore, adenosine monophosphate disodium salt accelerates epidermal turnover by elevating intracellular energy metabolism, which leads to the excretion of melanin from the skin. A clinical trial found that topical administration of a 3% adenosine monophosphate disodium salt-containing formulation was effective at treating hyperpigmentary disorders, such as melasma[239].

N-Acetyl-4-S-Cysteaminylphenol

N-acetyl-4-S-cysteaminylphenol is a tyrosinase substrate, and, on exposure to tyrosinase, it forms a melanin-like pigment. The depigmentation effect of *N*-acetyl-4-S-cysteaminylphenol is associated with a decrease in the number of functioning melanocytes and in the number of melanosomes transferred to keratinocytes. A 4% N-acetyl-4-S-cysteaminylphenol emulsion (O/W) was shown to be effective for treating melasma[240].

Linoleic Acid

Linoleic acid accelerates tyrosinase degradation, resulting in the down-regulation of melanin synthesis. In clinical trials, topical application of a 0.1% linoleic acid-containing liposomal formulation alleviated melasma symptoms[241] and UVB-induced hyperpigmentation of the skin[242, 243].

AHAs and BHAs

Many clinical studies on the effectiveness of AHAs such as glycolic acid and lactic acid as peeling agents for accelerating skin desquamation have been conducted in patients with pigmentation disorders. For example, a 5% glycolic acid topical cream was shown to improve skin texture and photoaging-induced discoloration[244]. In addition, a 10% glycolic acid lotion has been reported to be effective at improving symptoms of melasma [245]. Furthermore, a 92% lactic acid (pH 3.5) formulation has been shown to be effective at treating melasma[246]. A combination of 8% glycolic acid and 8% lactic acid creams has been shown to be modestly useful in ameliorating mottled hyperpigmentation, sallowness, and roughness due to chronic cutaneous photodamage[247].A clinical trial showed that 30% salicylic acid in absolute ethanol was effective at treating acne and postinflammatory hyperpigmentation[248].

Conclusion

In this article we have reviewed the synthesis of melanin, the signaling pathways related to the regulation of melanogenesis, the factors influencing melanogenesis and various pigmentation disorders, as well as the effectiveness of various natural products at reducing hyperpigmentation. An important issue regarding crude extracts or fractions from natural products used in cosmetics is the standardization of cultivation, harvesting, collecting, storage and extraction processes of the plants. Isolation of the active components from natural products for skin-whitening formulations will clarify the effect and mechanism on hypopigmentation. In addition, multi-functional formulations may increase the efficacy of skin-whitening products.

References

[1] Spritz, R. A. & Hearing, V. J. Jr. (1994). Genetic disorders of pigmentation. *Advances in human genetics, 22,* 1-45.

[2] Prota, G. (1992). *Melanins and Melanogenesis*. New York, Academic.

[3] Bennett, D. C. & Lamoreux, M. L. (2003). The color loci of mice--a genetic century. *Pigment Cell Melanoma Res., 16,* 333-344.

[4] Yamaguchi, Y. & Hearing, V, J. (2009). Physiological factors that regulate skin pigmentation. *Biofactors, 35,* 193-199.

[5] Frenk, E. (1995) Treatment of melasma with depigmenting agents. *In: Melasma: New Approaches to Treatment (London, Martin Dunitz)*, 9-15.

[6] Hamilton, A. J. & Gomez, B. L. (2002). Melanins in fungal pathogens. *J. Med. Microbiol., 53,* 189-191.

[7] Honigsmann, H. (2002). Erythema and pigmentation. *Photodermatol. Photoimmunol. Photomed., 18*, 75-81.

[8] Garcia-Borron, J. C. (2008). SOX9 and the tanning response: something new under the sun. *Pigment Cell Melanoma Res., 21,* 3-4.

[9] Howe, H. L., Chen, V. W., Hotes, J. L., Wu, X. C., Correa, N. C. & Fulton, J. P. (2001). Cancer in North America, 1994-1998. *North American Association of Central Cancer Registries, 1: Incidence.*

[10] Perluigi, M., De Marco, F., Foppoli, C., Coccia, R., Blarzino, C., Marcante, M. L. & Cini, C. (2003). Tyrosinase protects human melanocytes from ROS-generating compounds. *Biochem. Biophys. Res. Commun., 305,* 250-256.

[11] Herrling, T., Jung, K & Fuchs, J. (2008). The role of melanin as protector against free radicals in skin and its role as free radical indicator in hair. *Spectroc. Acta Pt. A-Molec. Biomolec. Spectr., 69,* 1429-1435.

[12] Ortonne, J. P. (2002). Photoprotective properties of skin melanin. *Br. J. Dermatol., 61,* 7-10.

[13] Hearing, V. J. Jr. (1987). Mammalian monophenol monooxygenase (tyrosinase): purification, properties, and reactions catalyzed. *Methods Enzymol, 142*, 154-165.

[14] Raposo, G. & Marks, M. S. (2007). Melanosomes--dark organelles enlighten endosomal membrane transport. *Nat. Rev. Mol. Cell Biol., 8,* 786-797.

[15] Jiménez-Cervantes, C., Solano, F., Kobayashi, T., Urabe, K., Hearing, V. J., Lozano, J. A. & García-Borrón, J. C. (1994). A new enzymatic function in the melanogenic pathway. The 5,6-dihydroxyindole-2-carboxylic acid oxidase activity of tyrosinase-related protein-1 (TRP1). *J. Biol. Chem., 269,* 17993-18000.

[16] Kondo, T., Hearing, V. J. (2011). Update on the regulation of mammalian melanocyte function and skin pigmentation. *Expert. Rev. Dermat., 6,* 97-108.

[17] Seiberg, M., Paine, C., Sharlow, E., Andrade-Gordon, P., Costanzo, M., Eisinger, M. & Shapiro, S. S. (2000). Inhibition of melanosome transfer results in skin lightening. *J. Dermatol., 115,* 162-167.

[18] Seiberg, M. (2001). Keratinocyte-melanocyte interactions during melanosome transfer. *Pigment Cell Melanoma Res.,14,* 236-242.

[19] Scott, G., Leopardi, S., Parker, L., Babiarz, L., Seiberg, M. & Han, R. (2003). The proteinase-activated receptor-2 mediates phagocytosis in a Rho-dependent manner in human keratinocytes. *J. Invest. Dermatol., 121,* 529-541.

[20] Boissy, R. E. (2003). Melanosome transfer to and translocation in the keratinocyte. *Exp. Dermatol., 12,* 5-12.

[21] Nordlund, J. J., Boissy, R. E., Hearing, V. J., King, R. A., Oetting, W. S. & Ortonne, J. P. (2006). Chemistry of Melanins. *The Pigmentary System. Physiology and Pathophysiology (2nd Edition).* 282-310.

[22] Turner, W. A., Taylor, J. D. & Tchen, T. T. (1975). Melanosome formation in the goldfish: the role of multivesicular bodies. *J. Ultrastruct Res., 51,* 16-31.

[23] Boissy, R. H., Gahl, W., Nordlund, J. J., Boissy, R. E., Hearing, V. J., King, R. A., Oetting, W. S., Ortonne, J. P. (2006). Biogenesis of melanosomes., *In The Pigmentary System: Physiology and Pathophysiology, 2nd ed.* 155-170.

[24] Ozeki, H., Ito, S., Wakamatsu, K. & Hirobe, T. (1995). Chemical characterization of hair melanins in various coat-color mutants of mice. *J. Invest. Dermatol., 105*, 361-366.

[25] Lamoreux, M. L., Wakamatsu, K. & Ito, S. (2001). Interaction of major coat color gene functions in mice as studied by chemical analysis of eumelanin and pheomelanin. *Pigment Cell Melanoma Res., 14,* 23-31.

[26] Berson, J. F., Harper, D. C., Tenza, D., Raposo, G. & Marks, M. S. (2001). Pmel17 initiates premelanosome morphogenesis within multivesicular bodies. *Mol. Biol. Cell., 12,* 3451-3464.

[27] Kushimoto, T., Basrur, V., Valencia, J., Matsunaga, J., Vieira, W. D., Ferrans, V. J., Muller, J., Appella, E. & Hearing, V. J. (2001). A model for melanosome biogenesis based on the purification and analysis of early melanosomes. *Proc. Natl. Acad. Sci. U. S. A, 98,* 10698-10703.

[28] Watabe, H., Valencia, J. C., Pape, E. L., Yamaguchi, Y., Nakamura, M., Rouzaud, F., Hoashi, T., Kawa, Y., Mizoguchi, M. & Hearing, V. J. (2008). Involvement of dynein and spectrin with early melanosome transport and melanosomal protein trafficking. *J. Invest. Dermatol., 128,* 162-174.

[29] Vallee, R. B., Wall, J. S., Paschal, B. M. & Shpetner, H. S. . (1988). Microtubule-associated protein 1C from brain is a two-headed cytosolic dynein. *Nature, 32*, 561-563.

[30] Schnapp, B. J. & Reese, T. S. (1989). Dynein is the motor for retrograde axonal transport of organelles. *Proc. Natl. Acad. Sci. USA, 86,* 1548-1552.

[31] Byers, H. R., Yaar, M. Y., Eller, M. S., Jalbert, N. L. & Gilchrest, B. A., (2000). Role of cytoplasmic dynein in melanosome transport in human melanocytes. *J. Invest. Dermatol., 114,* 990-997.

[32] Hara, M., Yaar, M., Byers, H. R., Goukassian, D., Fine, R. E., Gonsalves, J. & Gilchrest, B. A. (2000). Kinesin participates in melanosomal movement along melanocyte dendrites. *J. Invest. Dermatol., 114,* 438-443.

[33] Vancoillie, G., Lambert, J., Haeghen, Y. V., Westbroek, W., Mulder, A., Koerten, H. K., Mommaas, A. M., Van, Oostveldt. P. & Naeyaert, J. M. (2000). Colocalization of dynactin subunits P150Glued and P50 with melanosomes in normal human melanocytes. *Pigment Cell Res., 13*, 449-457.

[34] Wu, M., Hemesath, T. J., Takemoto, C. M., Horstmann, M. A., Wells, A. G., Price, E. R., Fisher, D. Z. & Fisher, D. E. (2000). c-Kit triggers dual phosphorylations, which couple activation and degradation of the essential melanocyte factor Mi. *Genes. Dev., 14,* 301-312.

[35] Watabe, H., Valencia, J. C., Le Pape, E., Yamaguchi, Y., Nakamura, M., Rouzaud, F., Hoashi, T., Kawa, Y., Mizoguchi, M. & Hearing, V. J. (2007). Involvement of dynein and spectrin with early melanosome transport and melanosomal protein trafficking. *J. Invest. Dermatol., 128,* 162-174.

[36] Seiberg, M., Paine, C., Sharlow, E., Andrade-Gordon, P., Costanzo, M., Eisinger, M. & Shapiro, S. S. (2000). Inhibition of melanosome transfer results in skin lightening. *J. Invest. Dermatol., 115,* 162-167.

[37] Van Den Bossche, K., Naeyaert, J. M. & Lambert, J. (2006). The quest for the mechanism of melanin transfer. *Traffic, 7,* 769-778.

[38] Marks, M. S. & Seabra, M. C. (2001). The melanosome: membrane dynamics in black and white. *Nat. Rev. Mol. Cell. Biol., 2,* 738-748.

[39] Virador, V. M., Muller, J., Wu, X., Abdel-Malek, Z. A., Yu, Z. X., Ferrans, V. J., Kobayashi, N., Wakamatsu, K., Ito, S., Hammer, J. A. & Hearing, V. J. (2002). Influence of alpha-melanocyte stimulating hormone and ultraviolet radiation on the transfer of melanosomes to keratinocytes. *FASEB. J., 16,* 105-107.

[40] Singh, S. K., Nizard, C., Kurfurst, R., Bonte, F., Schnebert, S. & Tobin, D. J. (2008). The silver locus product (Silv/gp100/Pmel17) as a new tool for the analysis of melanosome transfer in human melanocyte-keratinocyte co-culture. *Exp. Dermatol., 17*, 418-426.

[41] Scott, G., Leopardi, S., Printup, S. & Madden, B. C. (2002). Filopodia are conduits for melanosome transfer to keratinocytes. *J. Cell Sci., 115*, 1441-1451.

[42] Zhang, R. Z., Zhu, W. Y., Xia, M. Y. & Feng, Y. (2004). Morphology of cultured human epidermal melanocytes observed by atomic force microscopy. *Pigment Cell Res., 17,* 62-65.

[43] Singh, S. K., Kurfurst, R., Nizard, C., Schnebert, S., Perrier, E & Tobin, D. J. (2010). Melanin transfer in human skin cells is mediated by filopodia--a model for homotypic and heterotypic lysosome-related organelle transfer. *FASEB. J., 24*, 3756-3769.

[44] Kuroda, T. S. & Fukuda, M. (2004). Rab27A-binding protein Slp2-a is required for peripheral melanosome distribution and elongated cell shape in melanocytes. *Nat. Cell Biol., 6*, 1195-1203.

[45] Ito, S., Wakamatsu, K., & Ozeki, H. (2000). Chemical analysis of melanins and its application to the study of the regulation of melanogenesis. *Pigment Cell Res., 13 Suppl. 8*, 103-109.

[46] Zecca, L., Shima, T., Stroppolo, A., Goj, C., Battiston, G. A., Gerbasi, R., Sarna, T. & Swartz, H. M. (1996). Interaction of neuromelanin and iron in substantia nigra and other areas of human brain. *Neuroscience, 73,* 407-415.

[47] Grossman, M. (1999). Sentence processing in Parkinson's disease. *Brain Cogn., 40,* 387-413.

[48] Raper, H. S. (1928). The anaerobic oxidases. *Physiol. Rev., 8,* 245-282.

[49] Mason, H. S. (1948). The chemistry of melanin. III. Mechanism of the oxidation of trihydroxyphenylalanine by tyrosinase. *J. Biol. Chem., 172,* 83-99.

[50] Lerner, A. B., Fitzpatrick, T. B., Calkins, E. & Summerson, W. H. (1949). Mammalian tyrosinase-preparation and properties. *J. Biol. Chem., 178,* 185-190.

[51] Lin, J. Y., Fisher, D. E. (2007). Melanocyte biology and skin pigmentation. *Nature, 445,* 843-850.

[52] Costin, G. E., Hearing, V. J. (2007). Human skin pigmentation: melanocytes modulate skin color in response to stress. *FASEB. J., 21*, 976-994.

[53] Hearing, V. J. & Tsukamoto, K. (1991). Enzymatic control of pigmentation in mammals. *FASEB. J., 5,* 2902-2909.

[54] Cooksey, C. J., Garratt, P. J., Land, E. J., Pavel, S., Ramsden, C. A., Riley, P. A. & Smit, N. P. (1997). Evidence of the indirect formation of the catecholic intermediate substrate responsible for the autoactivation kinetics of tyrosinase. *J. Biol. Chem., 272,* 26226-26235.

[55] Halaban, R., Patton, R. S., Cheng, E., Svedine, S., Trombetta, E. S., Wahl, M. L., Ariyan, S. & Hebert, D. N. (2002). Abnormal acidification of melanoma cells induces tyrosinase retention in the early secretory pathway. *J. Biol. Chem., 277,* 14821-14828.

[56] Halaban, R., Cheng, E., Svedine, S., Aron, R. & Hebert, D. N. (2001). Proper folding and endoplasmic reticulum to golgi transport of tyrosinase are induced by its substrates, DOPA and tyrosinase. *Biol. Chem., 276,* 11933-11938.

[57] Chang, T. S. (2009). An updated review of tyrosinase inhibitors. *Int. J. Mol. Sci., 10,* 2440-2475.

[58] Lin, J. W., Chiang, H. M., Lin, Y. C. & Wen, K. C. (2008). Natural Products with Skin-Whitening Effects. *J. Food Drug Anal., 16,* 1-10.

[59] Chiang, H. M., Ko. Y. L., Shih, I. C. & Wen, K. C. (2011). Development of wine cake as a skin-whitening agent and humectant. *J. Food Drug Anal., 19,* 223-229.

[60] Ando, H., Itoh, A., Mishima, Y. & Ichihashi, M. (1995). Correlation between the number of melanosomes, tyrosinase mRNA levels, and tyrosinase activity in cultured murine melanoma cells in response to various melanogenesis regulatory agents. *J. Cell Physiol., 163,* 608-614.

[61] Oetting, W. S. (2000). The tyrosinase gene and oculocutaneous albinism type 1 (OCA1): a model for understanding the molecular biology of melanin formation. *Pigment Cell Res., 13*, 320-325.

[62] Costin, G. E., Valencia, J. C., Wakamatsu, K., Ito, S., Solano, F., Milac, A. L., Vieira, W. D., Yamaguchi, Y., Rouzaud, F., Petrescu, A. J., Lamoreux, M. L. & Hearing, V. J. (2005). Mutations in dopachrome tautomerase (Dct) affect eumelanin/pheomelanin synthesis, but do not affect intracellular trafficking of the mutant protein. *Biochem. J., 391,* 249-259.

[63] Minwalla, L., Zhao, Y., Cornelius, J., Babcock, G. F., Wickett, R. R., Le Poole, I. C. & Boissy, R. E. (2001). Inhibition of melanosome transfer from melanocytes to

keratinocytes by lectins and neoglycoproteins in an in vitro model system. *Pigment. Cell Res., 14,* 185-194.

[64] Chakraborty, A. K., Funasaka, Y., Slominski, A., Ermak, G., Hwang, J., Pawelek, J. M. & Ichihashi, M. (1996). Production and release of proopiomelanocortin (POMC) derived peptides by human melanocytes and keratinocytes in culture: regulation by ultraviolet B., *Biochim. Biophys. Acta, 1313,* 130-138.

[65] Funasaka, Y., Chakraborty, A. K., Hayashi, Y., Komoto, M., Ohashi, A., Nagahama, M., Inoue, Y., Pawelek, J. & Ichihashi, M. (1998). Modulation of melanocyte-stimulating hormone receptor expression on normal human melanocytes: evidence for a regulatory role of ultraviolet B, interleukin-1 alpha, interleukin-1 beta, endothelin-1 and tumor necrosis factor-alpha. *Br. J. Dermatol., 139*, 216-224.

[66] Wakamatsu, K., Graham, A., Cook, D. & Thody, A. J. (1997). Characterisation of ACTH peptides in human skin and their activation of the melanocortin-1 receptor. *Pigment Cell Melanoma Res., 10*, 288-297.

[67] Tada, A., Suzuki, I., Im, S., Davis, M. B., Cornelius, J., Babcock, G., Nordlund, J. J. & Abdel-Malek, Z. A. (1998). Endothelin-1 is a paracrine growth factor that modulates melanogenesis on human melanocytes and participates in their responses to ultraviolet radiation. *Cell Growth Differ., 9*, 575-584.

[68] Abdel-Malek, Z., Scott, M. C., Suzuki, I., Tada, A., Im, S., Lamoreux, L., Ito, S., Barsh, G. & Hearing, V. J. (2000). The melanocortin-1 receptor is a key regulator of human cutaneous pigmentation. *Pigment Cell Melanoma Res., 13 Suppl. 8*, 156-162.

[69] Hirobe, T. (2005). Role of keratinocyte-derived factors involved in regulating the proliferation and differentiation of mammalian epidermal melanocytes. *Pigment Cell Melanoma Res., 18*, 2-12.

[70] Romero-Graillet, C., Aberdam, E., Biagoli, N., Massabni, W., Ortonne, J. P. & Ballotti, R. (1996). Ultraviolet B radiation acts through the nitric oxide and cGMP signal transduction pathway to stimulate melanogenesis in human melanocytes. *J. Biol. Chem., 271*, 28052-28056.

[71] Weller, R. (2003). Nitric oxide: a key mediator in cutaneous physiology. *Clin. Exp. Dermatol., 28*, 511-514.

[72] Abdel-Malek, Z. A., Swope, V. B., Amornsiripanitch, N. & Nordlund, J. J. (1987). *In vitro* modulation of proliferation and melanization of S91 melanoma cells by prostaglandins. *Cancer Res., 47*, 3141-3146.

[73] Hunt, G., Todd, C., Cresswell, J. E. & Thody, A. J. (1994). α-MSH and its analog Nle4Dphe7 α-MSH affect morphology, tyrosinase activity and melanogenesis in cultured human melanocytes. *J. Cell Sci., 107*, 205-211.

[74] Hara, M., Yaar, M. & Gilchrest, B. A. (1995). Endothelin-1 of keratinocyte origin is a mediator of melanocyte dendricity. *J. Invest. Dermatol., 105*, 744-748.

[75] Ancans, J., Flanagan, N., Hoogduijn, M. J. & Thody, A. J. (2003). P-locus is a target for the melanogenic effects of MC-1R signaling: a possible control point for facultative pigmentation. *Ann.N. Y. Acad. Sci., 994*, 373-377.

[76] Hirobe, T. (2004). Role of keratinocyte-derived factors involved in regulating the proliferation and differentiation of mammalian epidermal melanocytes. *Pigment Cell Melanoma Res., 18*, 2-12.

[77] Masaki, H. (2003). The measuring method of tyrosinase activity and the evaluation method of whitening effect up-to-date. *Fragrance J., special issue 18*, 35-41.

[78] Kadekaro, A. L., Kavanagh, R., Kanto, H., Terzieva, S., Hauser, J., Kobayashi, N., Schwemberger, S., Cornelius, J., Babcock, G., Shertzer, H. G., Scott, G. & Abdel-Malek, Z. A. (2005). Alpha-melanocortin and endothelin-1 activate antiapoptotic pathways and reduce DNA damage in human melanocytes. *Cancer Res., 65*, 4292-4299.

[79] Slominski, A., Tobin, D, J., Shibahara, S. & Wortsman, J. (2004). Melanin pigmentation in mammalian skin and its hormonal regulation. *Physiol. Rev., 84*, 1155-1228

[80] Rousseau, K., Kauser, S., Pritchard, L. E., Warhurst, A., Oliver, R. L., Slominski, A., Wei, E. T., Thody, A. J., Tobin, D. J. & White, A. (2007). Proopiomelanocortin (POMC), the ACTH/melanocortin precursor, is secreted by human epidermal keratinocytes and melanocytes and stimulates melanogenesis. *Faseb. J., 21,* 1844-1856.

[81] Cone, R. D., Lu, D., Koppula, S., Vage, D. I., Klungland, H., Boston, B., Chen, W., Orth, D. N., Pouton, C. & Kesterson, R. A. (1996). The melanocortin receptors: agonist, antagonist, and the hormonal control of pigmentation. *Recent. Prog. Horm. Res., 51*, 287-317.

[82] Im, S., Moro, O., Peng, F., Medrano, E. E., Cornelius, J., Babcock, G., Nordlund, J. J. & Abdel-Malek, Z. A. (1998). Activation of cyclic AMP pathway by α-melanotropin mediates the response of human melanocytes to ultraviolet B radiation. *Cancer Res., 58*, 47-54.

[83] Insel, P. A., Bourne, H. R., Coffino, P. & Tomkins, G. M. (1975). Cyclic AMP-dependent protein kinase: pivotal role in regulation of enzyme induction and growth. *Science, 190*, 896-898.

[84] Newton, R. A., Cook, A. L., Roberts, D. W., Leonard, J. H. & Sturm, R. A. (2007). Post-transcriptional regulation of melanin biosynthetic enzymes by cAMP and resveratrol in human melanocytes. *J. Invest. Dermatol., 127*, 2216-2227.

[85] Busca, R. & Ballotti, R. (2000). Cyclic AMP a key messenger in the regulation of skin pigmentation. *Pigment Cell Melanoma Res., 13*, 60-69.

[86] Tachibana, M. (2000). MITF: a stream flowing for pigment cells. *Pigment Cell Melanoma Res., 13*, 230-240.

[87] Shibahara, S., Takeda, K., Yasumoto, K., Udono, T., Watanabe, K., Saito, H. & Takahashi, K. (2001). Microphthalmia-associated transcription factor (MITF): Multiplicity in structure, function, and regulation. *J. Investig. Dermatol. Symp. Proc., 6*, 99-104.

[88] Tachibana, M., Takeda, K., Nobukuni, Y., Urabe, K., Long, J. E., Meyers, K., Aaronson, S. A., & Miki, T. (1996). Ectopic expression of MITF, a gene for Waardenburg syndrome type 2, converts fibroblasts to cells with melanocyte characteristics. *Nature Genet., 14*, 50-54.

[89] Levy, C., Khaled, M. & Fisher, D. E. (2006). MITF: Master regulator of melanocyte development and melanoma oncogene. *Trends Mol. Med., 12*, 406-414.

[90] Ebanks, J. P., Wickett, R. R. & Boissy, R. E. (2009). Mechanisms Regulating Skin Pigmentation: The Rise and Fall of Complexion Coloration., *Int. J. Mol. Sci., 10*, 4066-4087.

[91] Theos, A. C., Truschel, S. T., Raposo, G. & Marks, M. S., (2005). The *Silver* locus product Pmel17/gp100/Silv/ME20: controversial in name and in function. *Pigment Cell Melanoma Res., 18*, 322-336.

[92] Yasumoto, K., Yokoyama, K.,Takahashi, K.,Tomita. Y. & Shibahara, S. (1997). Functional analysis of microphthalmia-associated transcription factor in pigment cell-specific transcription of the human tyrosinase family genes. *J. Biol. Chem., 272*, 503-509.

[93] Aksan, I. & Goding, C. R. (1998). Targeting the microphthalmia basic helix-loop-helix-leucine zipper transcription factor to a subset of E-box elements *in vitro* and *in vivo. Mol. Cell. Biol., 18*. 6930-6938.

[94] Galibert, M. D., Yavuzer, U., Dexter, T. J. & Goding, C. R., (1999). Pax3 and regulation of the melanocyte-specific tyrosinase-related protein-1 promoter. *J. Biol. Chem., 274*, 26894-26900.

[95] Bertolotto, C., Buscà, R., Abbe, P., Bille, K., Aberdam, E., Ortonne, J. P. & Ballotti, R. (1998). Different *cis*-acting elements are involved in the regulation of TRP1 and TRP2 promoter activities by cyclic AMP: pivotal role of M boxes (GTCATGTGCT) and of microphthalmia. *Mol. Cell. Biol., 18*, 694-702.

[96] Bentley, N. J., Eisen, T. & Goding, C. R. (1994). Melanocyte-specific expression of the human tyrosinase promoter: activation by the microphthalmia gene product and role of the initiator. *Mol. Cell. Biol., 14*, 7996-8006.

[97] Hemesath, T. J., Steingrímsson, E., McGill, G., Hansen, M. J., Vaught, J., Hodgkinson, C. A., Arnheiter, H., Copeland, N. G., Jenkins, N. A. & Fisher, D. E. (1994). microphthalmia, a critical factor in melanocyte development, defines a discrete transcription factor family. *Genes Dev., 8*, 2770-2780.

[98] Lin, C. B., Babiarz, L., Liebel, F., Roydon, P. E., Kizoulis, M., Gendimenico, G. J., Fisher, D. E. & Seiberg, M. (2002). Modulation of microphthalmia-associated transcription factor gene expression alters skin pigmentation., *J. Invest. Dermatol., 119*, 1330-1340.

[99] Yasumoto, K., Yokoyama, K., Shibata, K., Tomita, Y. & Shibahara, S. (1994). Microphthalmia-associated transcription factor as a regulator for melanocyte-specific transcription of the human tyrosinase gene. *Mol. Cell. Biol., 14*, 8058-8070.

[100] Moore, K. J. (1995). Insight into the microphthalmia gene. *Trends Genet., 11*, 442-448.

[101] Widlund, H. R. & Fisher, D. E. (2003). Microphthalamia-associated transcription factor: A critical regulator of pigment cell development and survival. *Oncogene, 22*, 3035-3041.

[102] Yamaguchi, Y., Brenner, M. & Hearing, V. J. (2007). The regulation of skin pigmentation. *J. Biol. Chem., 282*, 27557-27561.

[103] Kim, Y. J. & Uyama, H. (2005). Tyrosinase inhibitors from natural and synthetic sources: structure, inhibition mechanism and perspective for the future. *Cell Mol. Life Sci., 62*, 1707-1723.

[104] Wan, P., Hu, Y., & He, L. (2011). Regulation of melanocyte pivotal transcription factor MITF by some other transcription factors. *Mol. Cell Biochem., 354*, 241-246.

[105] Passeron, T., Valencia, J. C., Bertolotto, C., Hoashi, T., Le, P. E., Takahashi, K., Ballotti, R. & Hearing, V. J. (2007). SOX9 is a key player in ultraviolet B-induced melanocyte differentiation and pigmentation. *Proc. Natl. Acad. Sci. USA., 104*, 13984-13989.

[106] Jiao, Z., Mollaaghababa, R., Pavan, W. J., Antonellis, A., Green, E. D. & Hornyak, T. J. (2004). Direct interaction of Sox10 with the promoter of murine dopachrome

tautomerase (DCT) and synergistic activation of DCT expression with MITF. *Pigment Cell Melanoma Res., 17*, 352-362.

[107] Ludwig, A., Rehberg, S. & Wegner, M. (2004). Melanocyte-specific expression of dopachrome tautomerase is dependent on synergistic gene activation by the Sox10 and MITF transcription factors. *FEBS Lett., 556*, 236-244.

[108] Watanabe, A., Takeda, K., Ploplis, B. & Tachibana, M. (1998). Epistatic relationship between Waardenburg syndrome genes MITF and PAX3. *Nat Genet., 18*, 283-286.

[109] Bondurand, N., Pingault, V., Goerich, D. E., Lemort, N., Sock, E., Le, C. C., Wegner, M. & Goossens, M. (2000). Interaction among SOX10, PAX3 and MITF, three genes altered in Waardenburg syndrome. *Hum. Mol. Genet., 9*, 1907-1917.

[110] Hearing, V. J. (2000). The melanosome: the perfect model for cellular responses to the environment. *Pigment Cell Melanoma Res., 13*, 23-34.

[111] Thomas, A. J. & Erickson, C. A. (2009). FOXD3 regulates the lineage switch between neural crest-derived glial cells and pigment cells by repressing MITF through a non-canonical mechanism. *Development, 136*, 1849-1858.

[112] Curran, K., Lister, J. A., Kunkel, G. R., Prendergast, A., Parichy, D. M. & Raible, D. W. (2010). Interplay between Foxd3 and Mitf regulates cell fate plasticity in the zebrafish neural crest. *Dev. Biol., 344*, 107-118.

[113] Hemesath, T. J., Price, E. R., Takemoto, C., Badalian, T. & Fisher D. E. (1998). MAP kinase links the transcription factor Microphthalmia to c-Kit signalling in melanocytes. *Nature., 391*, 298-301.

[114] Solano, F., Briganti, S., Picardo, M. & Ghanem, G. (2006). Hypopigmenting agents: an updated review on biological, chemical and clinical aspects. *Pigment Cell Melanoma Res., 19*, 550-571.

[115] Saha, B., Singh, S. K., Sarkar, C., Bera, R., Ratha, J., Tobin, D. J. & Bhadra, R. (2006). Activation of the Mitf promoter by lipid-stimulated activation of p38-stress signalling to CREB. *Pigment Cell Melanoma Res., 19*, 595-605.

[116] Kim, D. S., Park, S. H., Kwon, S. B., Na, J. I., Huh, C. H., & Park, K. C. (2007). Additive effects of heat and p38 MAPK inhibitor treatment on melanin synthesis. *Arch. Pharm. Res., 30*, 581-586.

[117] Singh, S. K., Sarkar, C., Mallick, S., Saha, B., Bera, R., & Bhadra, R. (2005). Human placental lipid induces melanogenesis through p38 MAPK in B16F10 mouse melanoma. *Pigment Cell Melanoma Res., 18*, 113-121.

[118] Bellei, B., Maresca, V., Flori, E., Pitisci, A., Larue, L. & Picardo, M. (2010). p38 regulates pigmentation via proteasomal degradation of tyrosinase. *J. Biol. Chem., 285*, 7288-7299

[119] Oka, M., Nagai, H., Ando, H., Matsumura, M., Araki, K., Ogawa, W., Miki, T., Sakaue, M., Tsukamoto, K., Konishi, H., Kikkawa, U. & Ichihashi, M. (2000). Regulation of melanogenesis through phosphatidylinositol 3-kinase-Akt pathway in human G361 melanoma cells. *J. Invest. Dermatol., 115*, 699-703.

[120] Kim, D. S., Park, S. H., Kwon, S. B., Park, E. S., Huh, C. H., Youn, S. W. & Park, K. C. (2006). Sphingosylphosphorylcholine-induced ERK activation inhibits melanin synthesis in human melanocytes. *Pigment Cell Res., 19,* 146-153.

[121] Kim, D. S., Hwang, E. S., Lee, J. E., Kim, S. Y., Kwon, S.B. & Park, K.C. (2003). Sphingosine-1-phosphate decreases melanin synthesis via sustained ERK activation and subsequent MITF degradation. *J. Cell Sci., 116,* 1699-1706.

[122] Kim, D. S., Kim, S. Y., Chung, J. H., Kim, K. H., Eun, H. C. & Park, K. C. (2002). Delayed ERK activation by ceramide reduces melanin synthesis in human melanocytes. *Cell. Signal., 14,* 779-785.

[123] Yang, G., Li, Y., Nishimura, E. K., Xin, H., Zhou, A., Guo, Y., Dong, L., Denning, M. F., Nickoloff, B.J. & Cui, R. (2008). Inhibition of PAX3 by TGF-β modulates melanocyte viability. *Mol. Cell. Biol., 32,* 554-563.

[124] Englaro, W., Bertolotto, C., Buscà, R., Brunet, A., Pagès, G., Ortonne, J. P. & Ballotti, R. (1998). Inhibition of the mitogen-activated protein kinase pathway triggers B16 melanoma cell differentiation. *J. Biol. Chem., 273,* 9966-9970.

[125] Kim, D. S., Park, S. H. & Park, K. C. (2004). Transforming growth factor-β1 decreases melanin synthesis via delayed extracellular signal-regulated kinase activation. *Int. J. Biochem., 36,* 1482-1491.

[126] Hida, T., Wakamatsu, K., Sviderskaya, E. V., Donkin, A. J., Montoliu, L., Lynn Lamoreux, M., Yu, B., Millhauser, G. L., Ito, S., Barsh, G. S., Jimbow, K. & Bennett, D. C. (2009). Agouti protein, mahogunin, and attractin in pheomelanogenesis and melanoblast-like alteration of melanocytes: a cAMP-independent pathway. *Pigment Cell Melanoma Res., 22,* 623-634.

[127] Slominski, A. & Wortsman, J. (2000). Neuroendocrinology of the skin., *Endocr. Rev., 21,* 457-487.

[128] Zbytek, B., Wortsman, J. & Slominski, A. (2006). Characterization of a ultraviolet B-induced corticotropin-releasing hormone-proopiomelanocortin system in human melanocytes. *Mol. Endocrinol., 20*, 2539-2547.

[129] Nylander, K., Bourdon, J. C., Bray, S. E., Gibbs, N. K., Kay, R., Hart, I. & Hall, P. A. (2000). Transcriptional activation of tyrosinase and TRP-1 by p53 links UV irradiation to the protective tanning response. *J. Pathol.,190,* 39-46.

[130] Cui, R., Widlund, H. R., Feige, E., Lin, J.Y., Wilensky, D.L., Igras, V.E., D'Orazio, J., Fung, C.Y., Schanbacher, C.F., Granter, S.R. & Fisher, D.E. (2007). Central role of p53 in the suntan response and pathologic hyperpigmentation. *Cell, 128,* 853-864.

[131] Kichina, J., Green, A. & Rauth, S. (1996). Tumor suppressor p53 down-regulates tissue-specific expression of tyrosinase gene in human melanoma cell lines. *Pigment Cell Melanoma Res., 9,* 85-91.

[132] Khlgatian, M. K., Hadshiew, I. M., Asawanonda, P., Yaar, M., Eller, M. S., Fujita, M., Norris, D. A. & Gilchrest, B. A. (2002). Tyrosinase gene expression is regulated by p53. *J. Invest. Dermatol., 118,* 126-132.

[133] Tadokoro, T., Rouzaud, F., Itami, S., Hearing, V. J. & Yoshikawa, K. (2003). The inhibitory effect of androgen and sex-hormone-binding globulin on the intracellular cAMP level and tyrosinase activity of normal human melanocytes. *Pigment Cell Melanoma Res., 16,* 190-197.

[134] Schallreuter, K. U., Hasse, S., Rokos, H., Chavan, B., Shalbaf, M., Spencer, J. D. & Wood, J. M. (2009). Cholesterol regulates melanogenesis in human epidermal melanocytes and melanoma cells. *Exp. Dermatol., 18,* 680-688.

[135] Glinka, A., Wu, W., Delius, H., Monaghan, A, P., Blumenstock, C. & Niehrs, C. (1998). Dickkopf-1 is a member of a new family of secreted proteins and functions in head induction. *Nature, 391,* 357-362.

[136] Yamaguchi, Y., Itami, S., Watabe, H., Yasumoto, K., Abdel-Malek, Z. A., Kubo, T., Rouzaud, F., Tanemura, A., Yoshikawa, K. & Hearing, V.J. (2004). Mesenchymal-

epithelial interactions in the skin: increased expression of dickkopf1 by palmoplantar fibroblasts inhibits melanocyte growth and differentiation. *J. Cell Biol., 165,* 275-285.

[137] Yamaguchi, Y., Passeron, T., Hoashi, T., Watabe, H., Rouzaud, F., Yasumoto, K., Hara, T., Tohyama, C., Katayama, I., Miki, T. & Hearing, V.J. (2008). Dickkopf 1 (DKK1) regulates skin pigmentation and thickness by affecting Wnt/b-catenin signaling in keratinocytes. *Faseb J., 22,* 1009-1020.

[138] Urabe, K. N., J.; Hori, Y., Nordlund, J. J., Boissy, R. E., Hearing, V. J., King, R. A., Oetting, W. S. & Ortonne, J. P. (1998). Mixed epidermal and dermal hypermelanoses. *The Pigmentary System: Physiology and Pathophysiology.* 909-913.

[139] Virador, V., Matsunaga, N., Matsunaga, J., Valencia, J., Oldham, R. J., Kameyama, K., Peck, G. L., Ferrans, V. J., Vieira, W. D., Abdel-Malek, Z. A. & Hearing, V. J. (2001). Production of melanocyte-specific antibodies to human melanosomal proteins: Expression patterns in normal human skin and in cutaneous pigmented lesions. *Pigment Cell Melanoma Res., 14,* 289-297.

[140] Cullen, M. K., Norlund, J. J., Boissy, R. E., Hearing, V. J., Norlund, J. J., Boissy, R.E., Hearing, V.J., King, R.A. & Ortonne, J.P. (1998). Genetic epidermal syndromes: disorders characterized by lentigines. *The Pigmentary System: Physiology and Pathophysiology* 760-766.

[141] Tomita, Y. & Suzuki, T. (2004). Genetics of pigmentary disorders. *Am. J. Med. Genet. C., 131C,* 75-81.

[142] Boissy, R. E. & Nordlund, J. J. (1997). Molecular basis of congenital hypopigmentary disorders in humans: a review. *Pigment Cell Melanoma Res., 10,* 12-24.

[143] Wei, M. L. (2006). Hermansky-Pudlak syndrome: a disease of protein trafficking and organelle function. *Pigment Cell Melanoma Res., 19,* 19-42.

[144] Spritz, R. A., Chiang, P, W., Oiso, N. & Alkhateeb, A. (2003). Human and mouse disorders of pigmentation. *Curr. Opin. Genet. Dev., 13,* 284-289.

[145] Ménasché, G., Ho, C. H., Sanal, O., Feldmann, J., Tezcan, I., Ersoy, F., Houdusse, A., Fischer, A. & de Saint Basile, G. (2003). Griscelli syndrome restricted to hypopigmentation results from a melanophilin defect (GS3) or a MYO5AF-exon deletion (GS1). *J. Clin. Invest., 112,* 450-456.

[146] Huizing, M., Helip-Wooley, A., Westbroek, W., Gunay-Aygun, M., & Gahi, W. A. (2008). Disorders of lysosome-related organelle biogenesis: clinical and molecular genetics. *Annu. Rev. Genomics Hum. Genet., 9,* 359-386.

[147] Van Gele, M., Dynoodt, P. & Lambert, J. (2009). Griscelli syndrome: a model system to study vesicular trafficking. *Pigment Cell Melanoma Res., 22,* 268-282.

[148] Steingrímsson, E., Copeland, N. G. & Jenkins, N. A. (2004). Melanocytes and the microphthalmia transcription factor network. *Annu. Rev. Genet. 38,* 365-411.

[149] Takeda, K., & Shibahara, S. (2007). Transcriptional Regulation of Melanocyte Function. *The Pigmentary System: Physiology and Pathophysiology (2nd).* 242-260. Blackwell Publishing Ltd.

[150] Gillbro, J. M. & Olsson, M. J. (2011). The melanogenesis and mechanisms of skin-lightening agents- existing and new approaches. *Int. J. Cosmet. Sci., 33,* 210-221.

[151] Smit, N., Vicanova, J. & Pavel, S. (2009). The hunt for natural skin whitening agents. *Int. J. Mol. Sci., 10,* 5326-5349.

[152] Chiang, H. M., Lin, J. W., Hsiao, P. L., Tsai, S. Y., & Wen, K. C. (2011). Hydrolysates of citrus plants stimulate melanogenesis protecting against UV-induced dermal damage. *Phytother. Res., 25,* 569-576.

[153] Ando, H., Matsui, M. S., & Ichihashi, M. (2010). Quasi-drugs developed in Japan for the prevention or treatment of hyperpigmentary disorders. *Int. J. Mol. Sci., 11,* 2566-2575.

[154] Parvez, S., Kang, M., Chung, H. S. & Bae, H. (2007). Naturally occurring tyrosinase inhibitors: mechanism and applications in skin health, cosmetics and agriculture industries. *Phytother. Res., 21,* 805-816.

[155] Briganti, S., Camera, E. & Picardo, M. (2003). Chemical and instrumental approaches to treat hyperpigmentation. *Pigment Cell Melanoma Res., 16,* 101-110.

[156] Ando, H., Ichihashi, M. & Hearing, V. J. (2009). Role of the ubiquitin proteasome system in regulating skin pigmentation. *Int. J. Mol. Sci., 10,* 4428-4434.

[157] Nakayama, T., Sato, T., Fukui, Y., Yonekura-Sakakibara, K., Hayashi, H., Tanaka, Y., Kusumi, T. & Nishino, T. (2001). Specificity analysis and mechanism of aurone synthesis catalyzed by aureusidin synthase, a polyphenol oxidase homolog responsible for flower coloration. *FEBS Lett., 499,* 107-111.

[158] Jin, Y. Z., Li, G. H., Ahn, S. Y., Row, K. H. & Kim, E. K. (2006). Extraction and purification of depigmenting agents from Chinese plants. *Chem. Res. Chin. Univ., 22,* 162-167.

[159] Wang, K. H., Lin, R. D., Hsu, F. L., Huang, Y. H., Chang, H. C., Huang, C. Y. & Lee, M, H. (2006). Cosmetic applications of selected traditional Chinese herbal medicines. *J. Ethnopharmacol., 106,* 353-359.

[160] Liu, S. H., Chu, I. M. & Pan, I. H. (2008). Effects of hydroxybenzyl alcohols on melanogenesis in melanocyte-keratinocyte co-culture and monolayer culture of melanocytes. *J. Enzym. Inhib. Med. Chem., 23,* 526-534.

[161] Zhong, S., Wu, Y., Soo-Mi, A., Zhao, J., Wang, K., Yang, S., Jae-Ho, Y. & Zhu, X. (2006). Depigmentation of melanocytes by the treatment of extracts from traditional Chinese herbs: a cell culture assay. *Biol. Pharm. Bull., 29,* 1947-1951.

[162] Greatens, A., Hakozaki, T., Koshoffer, A., Epstein, H., Schwemberger, S., Babcock, G., Bissett, D., Takiwaki, H., Arase, S., Wickett, R. R. & Boissy, R. E. (2005). Effective inhibition of melanosome transfer to keratinocytes by lectins and niacinamide is reversible. *Exp. Dermatol., 14,* 498-508.

[163] Yamakoshi, J., Otsuka, F., Sano, A., Tokutake, S., Saito, M., Kikuchi, M. & Kubota, Y. (2003). Lightening effect on ultraviolet-induced pigmentation of guinea pig skin by oral administration of a proanthocyanidin-rich extract from grape seeds. *Pigment Cell Melanoma Res., 16,* 629-638.

[164] Yoshimura, M., Watanabe, Y., Kasai, K., Yamakoshi, J. & Koga, T. (2005). Inhibitory effect of an ellagic acid-rich pomegranate extract on tyrosinase activity and ultraviolet-induced pigmentation. *Biosci. Biotechnol. Biochem., 69,* 2368-2373.

[165] Duval, C., Smit, N. P., Kolb, A. M., Régnier, M., Pavel, S. & Schmidt, R. (2002). Keratinocytes control the pheo/eumelanin ratio in cultured normal human melanocytes. *Pigment Cell Melanoma Res., 15,* 440-446.

[166] Choi, T. Y., Kim, J. H., Ko, D. H., Kim, C. H., Hwang, J. S., Ahn, S., Kim, S. Y., Kim, C. D., Lee, J. H. & Yoon, T. J. (2007). Zebrafish as a new model for phenotype-based

screening of melanogenic regulatory compounds. *Pigment Cell Melanoma Res., 20,* 120-127.

[167] Tsujishita, Y., Asaoka, Y. & Nishizuka, Y. (1994). Regulation of phospholipase A2 in human leukemia cell lines: Its implication for intracellular signaling. *Proc. Natl. Acad. Sci. USA, 91,* 6274-6278.

[168] Chawla, A., Repa, J. J., Evans, R. M. & Mangelsdorf, D. J. (2001). Nuclear receptors and lipid physiology: Opening the X-files. *Science, 294,* 1866-1870.

[169] Clarke, S. D. (2004). The multi-dimensional regulation of gene expression by fatty acids: Polyunsaturated fats as nutrient sensors. *Curr. Opin. Lipidology, 15,* 13-18.

[170] Ando, H., Wen Z. M., Kim, H. Y., Valencia, J. C., Costin G. E., Watabe, H., Yasumoto, K., Niki, Y., Kondoh, H., Ichihashi, M. & Hearing V. J. (2006). Intracellular composition of fatty acid affects the processing and function of tyrosinase through the ubiquitin-proteasome pathway. *Biochem. J., 394,* 43-50.

[171] Ando, H., Funasaka, Y., Oka, M., Ohashi, A., Furumura, M., Matsunaga, J., Matsunaga, N., Hearing, V. J. & Ichihashi, M. (1999). Possible involvement of proteolytic degradation of tyrosinase in the regulatory effect of fatty acids on melanogenesis. *J. Lipid Res., 40,* 1312-1316.

[172] Dahlmann, B., Rutschmann, M., Kuehn, L. & Reinauer, H. (1985). Activation of the multicatalytic proteinase from rat skeletal muscle by fatty acids or sodium dodecyl sulphate. *Biochem J., 228,* 171-177.

[173] Santulli, R. J., Derian, C. K., Darrow, A. L., Tomko, K. A., Eckardt, A. J., Seiberg, M., Scarborough, R. M. & Andrade-Gordon, P. (1995). Evidence for the presence of a protease-activated receptor distinct from the thrombin receptor in human keratinocytes. *Proc. Natl. Acad. Sci. USA. 92,* 9151-9155.

[174] Sharlow, E. R., Paine, C.S., Babiarz, L., Eisinger, M., Shapiro, S. & Seiberg, M. (2000). The protease-activated receptor-2 upregulates keratinocyte phagocytosis. *J. Cell Sci., 113,* 3093-3101.

[175] Paine, C., Sharlow, E., Liebel, F., Eisinger, M., Shapiro, S. & Seiberg, M. (2001). An alternative approach to depigmentation by soybean extracts via inhibition of the PAR-2 pathway. *J. Invest. Dermatol., 116,* 587-595.

[176] Scott, G., Leopardi, S., Parker, L., Babiarz, L., Seiberg, M. & Han, R. (2003). The proteinase-activated receptor-2 mediates phagocytosis in a Rho-dependent manner in human keratinocytes. *J. Invest. Dermatol., 121,* 529-541.

[177] Saeki, Y., Kanamaru, A., Matsumoto, A. & Tada, A. (2003). The inhibitory effects of centaureidin on the outgrowth of dendrites, melanosome transfer and melanogenesis in normal human melanogenesis. *Pigment Cell Melanoma Res., 16,* 593.

[178] Ito, Y., Kanamaru, A. & Tada, A. (2006). Centaureidin promotes dendrite retraction of melanocytes by activating Rho. *Biochim. Biophys. Acta-Gen. Subj., 1760,* 487-494.

[179] Ito, Y., Kanamaru, A. & Tada, A. (2006). Effects of methylophiopogonanone B on melanosome transfer and dendrite retraction. *J. Dermatol. Sci., 42,* 68-70.

[180] Hakozaki, T., Minwalla, L., Zhuang, J., Chhoa, M., Matsubara, A., Miyamoto, K., Greatens, A., Hillebrand, G. G., Bissett, D. L. & Boissy, R. E. (2002). The effect of niacinamide on reducing cutaneous pigmentation and suppression of melanosome transfer. *Br. J. Dermatol., 147,* 20-31.

[181] Yoon, T. J., Lei, T. C., Yamaguchi, Y., Batzer, J., Wolber, R. & Hearing, V. J. (2003). Reconstituted 3-dimensional human skin of various ethnic origins as an in vitro model for studies of pigmentation. *Anal. Biochem., 318,* 260-269.

[182] Lei, T. C., Virador, V. M., Vieira, W. D. & Hearing, V. J. (2002). A melanocyte-keratinocyte coculture model to assess regulators of pigmentation in vitro. *Anal. Biochem., 305,* 260-268.

[183] Brenner, M. & Hearing, V. J. (2008). Modifying skin pigmentation-approaches through intrinsic biochemistry and exogenous agents. *Drug Discov. Today Dis. Mech., 5,* 189-199.

[184] Imokawa, G., Kobayashi, T., Miyagishi, M., Higashi, K. & Yada, Y. (1997). The role of endothelin-1 in epidermal hyperpigmentation and signaling mechanisms of mitogenesis and melanogenesis. *Pigment Cell Melanoma Res., 10,* 218-228.

[185] Hachiya, A., Kobayashi, A., Yoshida, Y., Kitahara, T., Takema, Y. & Imokawa, G. (2004). Biphasic expression of two paracrine melanogenic cytokines, stem cell factor and endothelin-1, in ultraviolet B-induced human melanogenesis. *Am. J. Pathol., 165,* 2099-2109.

[186] Hirobe, T. & Ootaka, H. (2007). Interleukin-1alpha stimulates the differentiation of melanocytes but inhibits the proliferation of melanoblasts from neonatal mouse epidermis. *Zool. Sci., 24,* 959-970.

[187] Hachiya, A., Kobayashi, T., Takema, Y. & Imokawa, G. (2002). Biochemical characterization of endothelin-converting enzyme-1alpha in cultured skin-derived cells and its postulated role in the stimulation of melanogenesis in human epidermis. *J. Biol. Chem., 277,* 5395-5403.

[188] Kawaguchi, Y., Mori, N. & Nakayama, A. (2001). Kit(+) melanocytes seem to contribute to melanocyte proliferation after UV exposure as precursor cells. *J. Invest. Dermatol., 116,* 920-925.

[189] Maeda, K. & Naganuma, M. (1997). Melanocyte-stimulating properties of secretory phospholipase A2, *Photochem. Photobiol., 65,* 145-149.

[190] Pentland, A. P. & Mahoney, M. G. (1990). Keratinocyte prostaglandin synthesis is enhanced by IL-1. *J. Invest. Dermatol., 94,* 43-46.

[191] Hachiya, A., Kobayashi, A., Ohuchi, A., Kitahara, T. & Takema, Y. (2001). The inhibitory effect of an extract of *Sanguisorba officinalis* L. on ultraviolet B-induced pigmentation *via* the suppression of endothelin-converting enzyme-1alpha. *Biol. Pharm. Bull., 24,* 688-692.

[192] Kobayashi, A., Hachiya, A., Ohuchi, A., Kitahara, T. & Takema, Y. (2002). Inhibitory mechanism of an extract of *Althaea officinalis* L. on endothelin-1-induced melanocyte activation. *Biol. Pharm. Bull., 25,* 229-234.

[193] Shimoda, H., Tanaka, J., Shan, S. J. & Maoka, T. (2010). Anti-pigmentary activity of fucoxanthin and its influence on skin mRNA expression of melanogenic molecules. *J. Pharm. Pharmacol., 62,* 1137-1145.

[194] Hasegawa, T., Takano, F., Takata, T., Niiyama, M. & Ohta, T. (2008). Bioactive monoterpene glycosides conjugated with gallic acid from the leaves of *Eucalyptus globulus*. *Phytochemistry, 69,* 747-753.

[195] Kawabata, T., Cui, M. Y., Hasegawa, T., Takano, F. & Ohta, T. (2011). Anti-inflammatory and anti-melanogenic steroidal saponin glycosides from Fenugreek (Trigonella foenum-graecum L.) seeds. *Planta Med., 77,* 705-710.

[196] Takashi, K. (2000). Development of new skin whitening agents. Whitening effect of Guava leaves extract. *Fragrance J, 28,* 86-90.

[197] Öhman, H. & Vahlquist, A. (1994). *In vivo* studies concerning a pH gradient in human stratum corneum and upper epidermis. *Acta Derm.-Venereol., 74,* 375-379.

[198] Sondell, B., Thornell, L.E. & Egelrud, T. (1995). Evidence that stratum corneum chymotryptic enzyme is transported to the stratum corneum extracellular space *via* lamellar bodies. *J. Invest. Dermatol., 104,* 819-823.

[199] Ekholm, I. E., Brattsand, M. & Egelrud, T. (2000). Stratum corneum tryptic enzyme in normal epidermis: a missing link in the desquamation process? *J. Invest. Dermatol., 114,* 56-63.

[200] Horikoshi, T., Arany, I., Rajaraman, S., Chen, S. H., Brysk, H., Lei, G., Tyring, S. K. & Brysk, M. M. (1998). Isoforms of cathepsin D and human epidermal differentiation. *Biochimie, 80,* 605-612.

[201] Zhu, W. & Zhang, R. (2006). Cosmetic Science and Technology Series. *In Cosmetic Formulation of Skin Care Products: Skin Lightening Agents. New York.* 205-218.

[202] Bowe, W. P. & Shalita, A. R. (2008). Effective over-the-counter acne treatments. *Semin. Cutan. Med. Surg., 27,* 170-176.

[203] Badreshia-Bansal, S. & Draelos, Z. D. (2007). Insight into skin lightening cosmeceuticals for women of color. *J. Drugs Dermatol., 6,* 32-39.

[204] Smith, W. P. (1999). The effects of topical (+) lactic Acid and ascorbic Acid on skin whitening. *Int. J. Cosmet Sci, 21,* 33-40.

[205] Yamamoto, Y., Uede, K., Yonei, N., Kishioka, A., Ohtani, T. & Furukawa, F. (2006). Effects of alpha-hydroxy acids on the human skin of Japanese subjects: the rationale for chemical peeling. *J. Dermatol., 33,* 16-22.

[206] Bellemère, G., Stamatas, G. N., Bruère, V., Bertin, C., Issachar, N. & Oddos, T. (2009). Antiaging action of retinol: from molecular to clinical. *Skin Pharmacol. Physiol., 22,* 200-209.

[207] Amer, M. & Metwalli, M. (2000). Topical liquiritin improves melasma. *Int. J. Dermatol., 39,* 299-301.

[208] Zhu, W. & Gao, J. (2008). The use of botanical extracts as topical skin-lightening agents for the improvement of skin pigmentation disorders. *J. Investig. Dermatol. Symp. Proc., 13,* 20-24.

[209] Riley, P. A. (1969). Hydroxyanisole depigmentation: *in-vitro* studies. *J. Pathol., 97,* 193-206.

[210] Naish-Byfield, S., Cooksey, C. J., Latter, A. M., Johnson, C. I. & Riley, P. A. (1991). *In vitro* assessment of the structure-activity relationship of tyrosinase-dependent cytotoxicity of a series of substitutedphenols. *Melanoma Res., 4,* 273-287.

[211] Smit, N. P., Peters, K., Menko, W., Westerhof, W., Pavel, S. & Riley, P. A. (1992). Cytotoxicity of a selected series of substituted phenols towards cultured melanoma cells. *Melanoma Res., 2,* 295-304.

[212] Sugai, T. (1992). Clinical effects of arbutin in patients with chloasma. *Skin Res. (Hifu), 34,* 522-529.

[213] Polnikorn, N. (2010). Treatment of refractory melasma with the MedLite C6 Q-switched Nd: YAG laser and alpha arbutin: a prospective study. *J Cosmet Laser Ther, 12,* 126-131.

[214] Boissy, R. E., Visscher, M. & DeLong, M. A. (2005). DeoxyArbutin: a novel reversible tyrosinase inhibitor with effective *in vivo* skin lightening potency. *Exp. Dermatol., 14,* 601-608.

[215] Chawla, S., deLong, M. A., Visscher, M. O., Wickett, R. R., Manga, P. & Boissy, R. E. (2008). Mechanism of tyrosinase inhibition by deoxyArbutin and its second-generation derivatives. *Br. J. Dermato., 159,* 1267-1274.

[216] Mishima, Y., Ohyama, Y., Shibata, T., Seto, H. & Hatae, S. (1994). Inhibitory action of kojic acid on melanogenesis and its therapeutic effect for various human hyper-pigmentation disorders. *Skin Res. (Hifu), 36,* 134-150.

[217] Takizawa, T., Mitsumori, K., Tamura, T., Nasu, M., Ueda, M., Imai, T. & Hirose, M. (2003). Hepatocellular tumor induction in heterozygous p53-deficient CBA mice by a 26-week dietary administration of kojic acid. *Toxicol. Sci., 73,* 287-293.

[218] Higa, Y., Kawabe, M., Nabae, K., Toda, Y., Kitamoto, S., Hara, T., Tanaka, N., Kariya, K. & Takahashi, M. (2007). Kojic acid -absence of tumor-initiating activity in rat liver, and of carcinogenic and photo-genotoxic potential in mouse skin. *J. Toxicol. Sci., 32,* 143-159.

[219] Kumano, Y., Sakamoto, T., Egawa, M., Iwai, I., Tanaka, M. & Yamamoto, I. (1998). *In vitro* and *in vivo* prolonged biological activities of novel vitamin C derivative, 2-O-alpha-D-glucopyranosyl-L-ascorbic acid (AA-2G), in cosmetic fields. *J. Nutr. Sci. Vitaminol., 44,* 345-359.

[220] Kameyama, K., Sakai, C., Kondoh, S., Yonemoto, K., Nishiyama, S., Tagawa, M., Murata, T., Ohnuma, T., Quigley, J., Dorsky, A., Bucks, D. & Blanock, K. (1996). Inhibitory effect of magnesium L-ascorbyl-2-phosphate (VC-PMG) on melanogenesis *in vitro* and *in vivo*. *J. Am. Acad. Dermatol, 34,* 29-33.

[221] Miyai, E., Yamamoto, I., Akiyama, J. & Yanagida, M. (1996). Inhibitory effect of ascorbic acid 2-O-α-glucoside on the pigmentation of skin by exposure to ultraviolet light. *Nishinihon J. Dermatol., 58,* 439-443.

[222] Katagiri, T., Okubo, T., Oyobikawa, M., Futaki, K., Shaku, M., Kawai, M. & Takenouchi, M. (2001). Inhibitory action of 4-n-butylresorcinol (Rucinol®) on melanogenesis and its skin whitening effects. *J. Cosmet. Chem. Jpn., 35,* 42-49.

[223] Shimogaki, H., Tanaka, Y., Tamai, H. & Masuda, M. (2000). *In vitro* and *in vivo* evaluation of ellagic acid on melanogenesis inhibition. *Int. J. Cosmet. Sci., 22,* 291-303.

[224] Kamide, R., Arase, S., Takiwaki, H., Watanabe, S., Watanabe, Y. & Kageyama, S. (1995). Clinical effects of XSC-29 formulation on UV-induced pigmentation. *Nishinihon J. Dermatol., 57,* 136-142.

[225] Ichihashi, M., Kobayashi, A., Okuda, M. & Imokawa, G. (1999). Effect of chamomilla extracts application on UV-induced pigmentation. *Skin Research (Hifu), 41,* 475-480.

[226] Kawashima, M., Okuda, M., Kobayashi, A. & Imokawa, G. (1999). Inhibitory effect of chamomilla extracts on UV-induced pigmentation. *Nishinihon J. Dermatol., 61,* 682-685.

[227] Nakamura, K., Yoshida, M., Uchiwa, H., Kawa, Y. & Mizoguchi, M. (2003). Down-regulation of melanin synthesis by a biphenyl derivative and its mechanism. *Pigment Cell Res., 16,* 494-500.

[228] Takeda, K., Yokota, T., Ikemoto, T., Kakishima, H. & Matsuo, T. (2006). Inhibitory effect of a formulation containing 0.5% Magnolignan® (5, 5'-dipropyl-biphenyl-2, 2'-diol) on UV-induced skin pigmentation. *Nishinihon J. Dermatol., 68,* 288-292.

[229] Takeda, K., Arase, S., Sagawa, Y., Shikata, Y., Okada, H., Watanabe, S., Yokota, T., Ikemoto, T., Kakishima, H. & Matsuo, T. (2006). Clinical evaluation of the topical application of Magnolignan® (5, 5'-dipropyl-biphenyl-2, 2'-diol) for hyperpigmentation on the face. *Nishinihon J. Dermatol., 68,* 293-298.

[230] Grimes, P. E. (1995). Melasma. Etiologic and therapeutic considerations. *Arch Dermatol., 131,* 1453-1457.

[231] Nguyen, Q. H. & Bui, T. P. (1995). Azelaic acid: pharmacokinetic and pharmacodynamic properties and its therapeutic role in hyperpigmentary disorders and acne. *Int. J. Dermatol., 34,* 75-84.

[232] Breathnach, A. S. (1996). Melanin hyperpigmentation of skin: melasma, topical treatment with azelaic acid, and other therapies. *Cutis, 57,* 36-45.

[233] Lowe, N. J., Rizk, D., Grimes, P., Billips, M. & Pincus, S. (1998). Azelaic acid 20% cream in the treatment of facial hyperpigmentation in darker-skinned patients. *Clin. Ther., 20,* 945-959.

[234] Verallo-Rowell, V. M., Verallo, V., Graupe, K., Lopez-Villafuerte, L. & Garcia-Lopez, M. (1989). Double-blind comparison of azelaic acid and hydroquinone in the treatment of melasma. *Acta Derm. Venereol. Suppl. (Stockh), 143,* 58-61.

[235] Chang, W. C., Shi, G. Y., Chow, Y. H., Chang, L. C., Hau, J. S., Lin, M. T., Jen, C. J., Wing, L. Y. & Wu, H. L. (1993). Human plasmin induces a receptor-mediated arachidonate release coupled with G proteins in endothelial cells. *Am. J. Physiol., 264,* C271-C281.

[236] Wang, N., Zhang, L., Miles, L. & Hoover-Plow, J. (2004). Plasminogen regulates pro-opiomelanocortin processing. *J. Thromb. Haemost., 2,* 785-796.

[237] Maeda, K. & Naganuma, M. (1998). Topical trans-4-aminomethylcyclohexane carboxylic acid prevents ultraviolet radiation-induced pigmentation. *J. Photochem. Photobiol. B-Biol., 47,* 136-141.

[238] Furukawa, F., Kanehara, S., Harano, F., Shinohara, S., Kamimura, J., Kawabata, S., Igarashi, S., Kawamura, M., Yamamoto, Y. & Miyachi, Y. (2008). Effects of adenosine 5'-monophosphate on epidermal turnover. *Arch. Dermatol. Res., 300,* 485-493.

[239] Kawashima, M., Mizuno, A. & Murata, Y. (2008). Improvement of hyperpigmentation based on accelerated epidermal turnover: Clinical effects of disodium adenosine monophosphate in patients with melasma. *Jpn. J. Clin. Dermatol., 62,* 250-257.

[240] Jimbow, K. (1991). N-acetyl-4-S-cysteaminylphenol as a new type of depigmenting agent for the melanoderma of patients with melasma. *Arch Dermatol., 127,* 1528-1534.

[241] Clinical trial group for linoleic acid-containing gel. (1998). Clinical trial for liver spots using a linoleic acid-containing gel. *Nishinihon J. Dermatol.,60,* 537-542.

[242] Ando, H., Ryu, A., Hashimoto, A., Oka, M. & Ichihashi, M. (1998). Linoleic acid and alpha-linolenic acid lightens ultraviolet-induced hyperpigmentation of the skin. *Arch. Dermatol. Res., 290,* 375-381.

[243] Shigeta, Y., Imanaka, H., Ando, H., Ryu, A., Oku, N., Baba, N. & Makino, T. (2004). Skin whitening effect of linoleic acid is enhanced by liposomal formulations. *Biol. Pharm. Bull., 27,* 591-594.

[244] Thibault, P. K., Wlodarczyk, J. & Wenck, A. (1998). A double-blind randomized clinical trial on the effectiveness of a daily glycolic acid 5% formulation in the treatment of photoaging. *Dermatol. Surg., 24,* 573-578.

[245] Javaheri, S. M., Handa, S., Kaur, I. & Kumar, B. (2001). Safety and efficacy of glycolic acid facial peel in Indian women with melasma. *Int. J. Dermatol., 40,* 354-357.

[246] Sharquie, K. E., Al-Tikreety, M. M. & Al-Mashhadani, S. A. (2005). Lactic acid as a new therapeutic peeling agent in melasma. *Dermatol. Surg., 31,* 149-154.

[247] Stiller, M. J., Bartolone, J., Stern, R., Smith, S., Kollias, N., Gillies, R. & Drake, L. A. (1996). Topical 8% glycolic acid and 8% L-lactic acid creams for the treatment of photodamaged skin. A double-blind vehicle-controlled clinical trial. *Arch Dermatol, 132,* 631-636.

[248] Ahn, H. H. & Kim, I. H. (2006). Whitening effect of salicylic acid peels in Asian patients. *Dermatol. Surg., 32,* 372-375.

[249] Kubo, I., Kinst-Hori, I. & Yokokawa, Y. (1994). Tyrosinase inhibitors from Anacardium occidentale fruits. *J. Nat. Prod., 57,* 545-551.

[250] Chen, Y. R., Y-Y, R., Lin, T. Y., Huang, C. P., Tang, W. C., Chen, S. T. & Lin, S. B. (2009). Identification of an Alkylhydroquinone from Rhus succedanea as an Inhibitor of Tyrosinase and Melanogenesis. *J. Agric. Food Chem., 57,* 2200-2205.

[251] Kubo, I. & Kinst-Hori, I. (1999). 2-Hydroxy-4-methoxybenzaldehyde: a potent tyrosinase inhibitor from African medicinal plants. *Planta Med., 65,* 19-22.

[252] Kim, Y. J., No, J. K., Lee, J. S., Kim, M. S. & Chung, H. Y. (2006). Antimelanogenic activity of 3,4-dihydroxyacetophenone: inhibition of tyrosinase and MITF. *Biosci. Biotechnol. Biochem., 70,* 532-534.

[253] Lim, J. Y., Ishiguro, K. & Kubo, I. (1999). Tyrosinase inhibitory *p*-coumaric acid from ginseng leaves. *Phytother. Res., 13,* 371-375.

[254] An, S. M., Lee, S. I., Choi, S. W., Moon, S. W. & Boo, Y. C. (2008). *p*-Coumaric acid, a constituent of Sasa quelpaertensis Nakai, inhibits cellular melanogenesis stimulated by alpha-melanocyte stimulating hormone. *Br. J. Dermatol., 159,* 292-299.

[255] Mapunya, M. B., Hussein, A. A., Rodriguez, B. & Lall, N. (2011). Tyrosinase activity of *Greyia flanaganii* (Bolus) constituents. *Phytomedicine, 18,* 1006-1012.

[256] No, J. K., Kim, M. S., Kim, Y. J., Bae, S. J., Choi, J. S. & Chung, H. Y. (2004). Inhibition of tyrosinase by protocatechuic aldehyde. *Am. J. Chin. Med., 32,* 97-103.

[257] Kang, H. S., Choi, J. H., Cho, W. K., Park, J. C. & Choi, J. S. (2004). A sphingolipid and tyrosinase inhibitors from the fruiting body of Phellinus linteus. *Arch. Pharm. Res., 27,* 742-750.

[258] Miyazawa, M., Oshima, T., Koshio, K., Itsuzaki, Y. & Anzai, J. (2003). Tyrosinase inhibitor from black rice bran. *J. Agric Food Chem., 51,* 6953-6956.

[259] Kang, H. S., Kim, H. R., Byun, D. S., Son, B. W., Nam, T. J. & Choi, J. S. (2004). Tyrosinase inhibitors isolated from the edible brown alga *Ecklonia stolonifera*. *Arch. Pharm. Res., 27,* 1226-1232.

[260] Heo, S. J., Ko, S. C., Cha, S. H., Kang, D. H., Park, H. S., Choi, Y. U., Kim, D., Jung, W. K. & Jeon, Y. J. (2009). Effect of phlorotannins isolated from *Ecklonia cava* on melanogenesis and their protective effect against photo-oxidative stress induced by UV-B radiation, *Toxicol. In. Vitro., 23,* 1123-1130.

[261] Yoon, N. Y., Eom, T. K., Kim, M. M. & Kim, S. K. (2009). Inhibitory effect of phlorotannins isolated from *Ecklonia cava* on mushroom tyrosinase activity and melanin formation in mouse B16F10 melanoma cells, *J. Agric. Food Chem., 57,* 4124-4129.

[262] Ngoc, T. M., Lee, I., Ha do, T., Kim, H., Min, B. & Bae, K. (2009). Tyrosinase-inhibitory constituents from the twigs of *Cinnamomum cassia*. *J. Nat. Prod., 72,* 1205-1208.

[263] Lee, S. H., Choi, S. Y., Kim, H., Hwang, J. S., Lee, B. G., Gao, J. J. & Kim, S. Y. (2002). Mulberroside F isolated from the leaves of *Morus alba* inhibits melanin biosynthesis. *Biol. Pharm. Bull., 25,* 1045-1048.

[264] Shimizu, K., Kondo, R. & Sakai, K. (2000). Inhibition of tyrosinase by flavonoids, stilbenes and related 4-substituted resorcinols: structure-activity investigations. *Planta. Med., 66,* 11-15.

[265] Cho, Y., Kim, K. H., Shim, J. S. & Hwang, J. K. (2008). Inhibitory effects of macelignan isolated from *Myristica fragrans* HOUTT. on melanin biosynthesis. *Biol. Pharm. Bull., 31,* 986-989.

[266] Masuda, M., Murata, K., Fukuhama, A., Naruto, S., Fujita, T., Uwaya, A., Isami, F. & Matsuda, H. (2009). Inhibitory effects of constituents of *Morinda citrifolia* seeds on elastase and tyrosinase. *J. Nat. Med., 63,* 267-273.

[267] Iwai, K., Kishimoto, N., Kakino, Y., Mochida, K. & Fujita, T. (2004). *In vitro* antioxidative effects and tyrosinase inhibitory activities of seven hydroxycinnamoyl derivatives in green coffee beans. *J. Agric. Food Chem., 52,* 4893-4898.

[268] Lee, H. S. (2002). Tyrosinase inhibitors of *Pulsatilla cernua* root-derived materials. *J. Agric. Food Chem., 50,* 1400-1403.

[269] Wang, H., Chou, Y. T., Hong, Z. L., Chen, H. A., Chang, Y. C., Yang, W. L., Chang, H. C., Mai, C.T., & Chen, C. Y. (2011). Bioconstituents from stems of *Synsepalum dulcificum* Daniell (Sapotaceae) inhibit human melanoma proliferation, reduce mushroom tyrosinase activity and have antioxidant properties. *Journal of the Taiwan Institute of Chemical Engineers, 42,* 204-211.

[270] Cho, M., Ryu, M., Jeong, Y., Chung, Y. H., Kim, D. E., Cho, H. S., Han, J. S., Chang M. Y., Lee, C. K., Jin, M., Kim, H. J. & Oh, S. (2009). Cardamonin suppresses melanogenesis by inhibition of Wnt/beta-catenin signaling, *Biochem. Biophys. Res. Commun., 390,* 500-505.

[271] Yoon, J. H., Shim, J. S., Cho, Y., Baek, N. I., Lee, C. W., Kim, H. S., & Hwang, J. K. (2007). Depigmentation of melanocytes by isopanduratin A and 4-hydroxypanduratin A isolated from *Kaempferia pandurat*a ROXB. *Biol. Pharm. Bull., 30,* 2141-2145.

[272] Shirota, S., Miyazaki, K., Aiyama, R., Ichioka, M. & Yokokura, T. (1994). Tyrosinase inhibitors from crude drugs. *Biol. Pharm. Bull., 17,* 266-269.

[273] Kim, J. H., Sapers, G. M. & Choi, S. W. (1998). Identification of tyrosinase inhibitor from *Galla rhois*. *Food. Sci. Biotechnol, 7*. 56-59.

[274] Chen, L. G., Chang, W. L., Lee, C. J., Lee, L. T., Shih, C. M. & Wang, C. C. (2009). Melanogenesis inhibition by gallotannins from Chinese galls in B16 mouse melanoma cells. *Biol. Pharm. Bull., 32*. 1447-1452.

[275] Kubo, I., Kinst-Hori, I., Nihei, K., Soria, F., Takasaki, M., Calderon, J. S. & Cespedes, C. L. (2003). Tyrosinase inhibitors from galls of *Rhus javanica* leaves and their effects on insects. *Z. Naturforsch., 58,* 719-725.

[276] Park, J. S., Park, H. Y., Rho, H. S., Ahn, S., Kim, D. H. & Chang, I. S. (2008). Statistically designed enzymatic hydrolysis for optimized production of icariside II as a novel melanogenesis inhibitor. *J. Microbiol. Biotechnol., 18*. 110-117.

[277] Koo, J. H., Kim, H. T., Yoon, H. Y., Kwon, K. B., Choi, I. W., Jung, S. H., Kim, H. U., Park, B. H. & Park, J. W. (2008). Effect of xanthohumol on melanogenesis in B16 melanoma cells. *Exp. Mol. Med., 40,* 313-319.

[278] Okunji, C., Komarnytsky, S., Fear, G., Poulev, A., Ribnicky, D. M., Awachie, P. I., Ito, Y. & Raskin, I. (2007). Preparative isolation and identification of tyrosinase inhibitors from the seeds of *Garcinia kola* by high-speed counter-current chromatography. *J. Chromatogr. A., 1151,* 45-50.

[279] Masuda, T., Yamashita, D., Takeda, Y. & Yonemori, S. (2005). Screening for tyrosinase inhibitors among extracts of seashore plants and identification of potent inhibitors from *Garcinia subelliptica*. *Biosci. Biotechnol. Biochem., 69,* 197-201.

[280] Kubo, I., Kinst-Hori, I., Chaudhuri, S. K., Kubo, Y., Sanchez, Y. & Ogura, T. (2000). Flavonoids from *Heterotheca inuloides*: tyrosinase inhibitory activity and structural criteria. *Bioorg. Med. Chem., 8,* 1749-1755.

[281] Choi, M. Y., Song, H. S., Hur, H. S. & Sim, S. S. (2008). Whitening activity of luteolin related to the inhibition of cAMP pathway in alpha-MSH-stimulated B16 melanoma cells. *Arch. Pharm. Res., 31,* 1166-1171.

[282] Roh, J. S., Han, J. Y., Kim, J. H. & Hwang, J. K. (2004). Inhibitory effects of active compounds isolated from safflower (*Carthamus tinctorius* L.) seeds for melanogenesis. *Biol. Pharm. Bull., 27,* 1976-1978.

[283] Fujita, H., Motokawa, T., Katagiri, T., Yokota, S., Yamamoto, A., Himeno, M. & Tanaka, Y. (2009). Inulavosin, a melanogenesis inhibitor, leads to mistargeting of tyrosinase to lysosomes and accelerates its degradation. *J. Invest. Dermatol., 129,* 1489-1499.

[284] Nakashima, S., Matsuda, H., Oda, Y., Nakamura, S., Xu, F. & Yoshikawa, M. (2010). Melanogenesis inhibitors from the desert plant *Anastatica hierochuntica* in B16 melanoma cells. *Bioorg. Med. Chem., 18,* 2337-2345.

[285] Choo, S. J., Ryoo, I. J., Kim, Y. H., Xu, G. H., Kim, W. G., Kim, K. H., Moon, S. J., Son, E. D., Bae, K. & Yoo, I. D. (2009). Silymarin inhibits melanin synthesis in melanocyte cells. *J. Pharm. Pharmacol., 61,* 663-667.

[286] Chiari, M. E., Vera, D. M., Palacios, S. M. & Carpinella, M. C. (2011). Tyrosinase inhibitory activity of a 6-isoprenoid-substituted flavanone isolated from *Dalea elegans*. *Bioorg. Med. Chem., 19,* 3474-3482.

[287] Son, J. K., Park, J. S., Kim, J. A., Kim, Y., Chung, S. R. & Lee, S. H. (2003). Prenylated flavonoids from the roots of *Sophora flavescens* with tyrosinase inhibitory activity. *Planta. Med., 69,* 559-561.

[288] Ryu, Y. B., Westwood, I. M., Kang, N. S., Kim, H. Y., Kim, J. H., Moon, Y. H., & Park, K. H. (2008). Kurarinol, tyrosinase inhibitor isolated from the root of *Sophora flavescens*, *Phytomedicine, 15,* 612-618.

[289] Kim, S. J., Son, K. H., Chang, H. W., Kang, S. S. & Kim, H. P. (2003). Tyrosinase inhibitory prenylated flavonoids from *Sophora flavescens*. *Biol. Pharm. Bull., 26,* 1348-1350.

[290] Ha, T. J., Yang, M. S., Jang, D. S., Choi, S. U. & Park, K. H. (2001). Inhibitory activity of flavanone derivatives isolated from *Sophora flavescens* for melanogenesis. *Bull. Korean. Chem. Soc., 22,* 97-99.

[291] Hyun, S. K., Lee, W. H., Jeong da, M., Kim, Y. & Choi, J. S. (2008). Inhibitory effects of kurarinol, kuraridinol, and trifolirhizin from *Sophora flavescens* on tyrosinase and melanin synthesis. *Biol. Pharm. Bull., 31,* 154-158.

[292] Lo, Y. H., Lin, R. D., Lin, Y. P., Liu, Y. L. & Lee, M. H. (2009). Active constituents from *Sophora japonica* exhibiting cellular tyrosinase inhibition in human epidermal melanocytes. *J. Ethnopharmacol., 124,* 625-629.

[293] Baek, S., Kim, J., Kim, D., Lee, C. & Chung, D. K. (2008). Inhibitory effect of dalbergioidin isolated from the trunk of *Lespedeza cyrtobotrya* on melanin biosynthesis. *J. Microbiol. Biotechnol., 18,* 874-879.

[294] Kim, J. H., Baek, S. H., Kim, D. H., Choi, T. Y., Yoon, T. J., Hwang, J. S., Kim, M. R., Kwon, H. J. & Lee, C. H. (2008). Downregulation of melanin synthesis by haginin A and its application to *in vivo* lightening model. *J. Invest. Dermatol., 128,* 1227-1235.

[295] Kim, H. J., Seo, S. H., Lee, B. G. & Lee, Y. S. (2005). Identification of tyrosinase inhibitors from *Glycyrrhiza uralensis*. *Planta. Med., 71,* 785-787.

[296] Fu, B., Li, H., Wang, X., Lee, F. S. & Cui, S. (2005). Isolation and identification of flavonoids in licorice and a study of their inhibitory effects on tyrosinase. *J. Agric. Food Chem., 53,* 7408-7414.

[297] Kim, J. H., Kim, M. R., Lee, E. S. & Lee, C. H. (2009). Inhibitory effects of calycosin isolated from the root of *Astragalus membranaceus* on melanin biosynthesis. *Biol. Pharm. Bull., 32,* 264-268.

[298] Lee, M. H., Lin, Y. P., Hsu, F. L., Zhan, G. R. & Yen, K. Y. (2006) Bioactive constituents of *Spatholobus suberectus* in regulating tyrosinase-related proteins and mRNA in HEMn cells. *Phytochemistry, 67,* 1262-1270.

[299] Ko, R. K., Kim, G.O., Hyun, C. G., Jung, D. S. & Lee, N.H. (2011). Compounds with tyrosinase inhibition, elastase inhibition and DPPH radical scavenging activities from the branches of *Distylium racemosum* Sieb. et Zucc. *Phytother. Res.*

[300] Karioti, A., Protopappa, A., Megoulas, N. & Skaltsa, H. (2007). Identification of tyrosinase inhibitors from *Marrubium velutinum* and *Marrubium cylleneum*. *Bioorg. Med Chem., 15,* 2708-2714.

[301] Kubo, I. & Kinst-Hori, I. (1999). Flavonols from saffron flower: tyrosinase inhibitory activity and inhibition mechanism. *J. Agric. Food Chem., 47,* 4121-4125.

[302] Oozeki, H., Tajima, R. & Nihei, K. (2008). Molecular design of potent tyrosinase inhibitors having the bibenzyl skeleton. *Bioorg. Med. Chem. Lett., 18,* 5252-5254.

[303] Kim, D. H., Kim, J. H., Baek, S. H., Seo, J. H., Kho, Y. H., Oh, T. K. & Lee, C. H. (2004). Enhancement of tyrosinase inhibition of the extract of *Veratrum patulum* using cellulase. *Biotechnol. Bioeng., 87,* 849-854.

[304] Yagi, A., Kanbara, T. & Morinobu, N. (1987). Inhibition of mushroom-tyrosinase by *aloe* extract. *Planta Med., 53,* 515-517.

[305] Wang, Z., Li, X., Yang, Z., He, X., Tu, J. & Zhang, T. (2008). Effects of aloesin on melanogenesis in pigmented skin equivalents. *Int. J. Cosmet. Sci., 30,* 121-130.

[306] Zheng, Z. P., Cheng, K. W., To, J. T., Li, H. & Wang, M. (2008). Isolation of tyrosinase inhibitors from *Artocarpus heterophyllus* and use of its extract as antibrowning agent. *Mol. Nutr. Food Res., 52,* 1530-1538.

[307] Likhitwitayawuid, K., Sritularak, B. & De-Eknamkul, W. (2000). Tyrosinase inhibitors from *Artocarpus gomezianus*. *Planta Med., 66,* 275-277.

[308] Arung, E. T., Shimizu, K., Tanaka, H. & Kondo, R. (2010). 3-Prenyl luteolin, a new prenylated flavone with melanin biosynthesis inhibitory activity from wood of *Artocarpus heterophyllus*. *Fitoterapia, 81,* 640-643.

[309] Baek, Y. S., Ryu, Y. B., Curtis-Long, M. J., Ha, T. J., Rengasamy, R., Yang, M. S. & Park, K. H. (2009). Tyrosinase inhibitory effects of 1,3-diphenylpropanes from *Broussonetia kazinoki*. *Bioorg. Med. Chem., 17,* 35-41.

[310] Shimizu, K., Yasutake, S. & Kondo, R. (2003). A new stilbene with tyrosinase inhibitory activity from *Chlorophora excelsa*. *Chem. Pharm. Bull. (Tokyo), 51,* 318-319.

[311] Zheng, Z. P., Zhu, Q., Fan, C. L., Tan, H. Y. & Wang, M. (2011). Phenolic tyrosinase inhibitors from the stems of *Cudrania cochinchinensis*. *Food Funct., 2,* 259-264.

[312] Zhang, X., Hu, X., Hou, A. & Wang, H. (2009). Inhibitory effect of 2,4,2',4'-tetrahydroxy-3-(3-methyl-2-butenyl)-chalcone on tyrosinase activity and melanin biosynthesis. *Biol. Pharm. Bull., 32,* 86-90.

[313] Shin, N. H., Ryu, S. Y., Choi, E. J., Kang, S. H., Chang, I. M., Min, K. R. & Kim, Y. (1998). Oxyresveratrol as the potent inhibitor on dopa oxidase activity of mushroom tyrosinase. *Biochem. Biophys. Res. Commun.,243,* 801-803.

[314] Jeong, S. H., Ryu, Y. B., Curtis-Long, M. J., Ryu, H. W., Baek, Y. S., Kang, J. E., Lee, W. S. & Park, K. H. (2009). Tyrosinase inhibitory polyphenols from roots of *Morus lhou*. *J. Agric. Food Chem., 57,* 1195-1203.

[315] Nattapong, S. & Omboon, L. (2008). A new source of whitening agent from a Thai Mulberry plant and its betulinic acid quantitation. *Nat. Prod. Res., 22,* 727-734.

[316] Hanamura, T., Uchida, E. & Aoki, H. (2008). Skin-lightening effect of a polyphenol extract from Acerola (*Malpighia emarginata* DC.) fruit on UV-induced pigmentation. *Biosci. Biotechnol. Biochem., 72,* 3211-3218.

[317] Ding, H. Y., Lin, H. C. & Chang, T. S. (2009). Tyrosinase inhibitors isolated from the roots of *Paeonia suffruticosa*. *J. Cosmet. Sci., 60,* 347-352.

[318] Cheng, K. T., Hsu, F. L., Chen, S. H., Hsieh, P. K., Huang, H. S., Lee, C. K. & Lee, M. H. (2007). New constituent from *Podocarpus macrophyllus* var. *macrophyllus* shows anti-tyrosinase effect and regulates tyrosinase-related proteins and mRNA in human epidermal melanocytes. *Chem. Pharm. Bull. (Tokyo), 55,* 757-761.

[319] Leu, Y. L., Hwang, T. L., Hu, J. W. & Fang, J. Y. (2008). Anthraquinones from *Polygonum cuspidatum* as tyrosinase inhibitors for dermal use. *Phytother. Res., 22,* 552-556.

[320] Miyazawa, M. & Tamura, N. (2007). Inhibitory compound of tyrosinase activity from the sprout of *Polygonum hydropiper* L. (Benitade). *Biol. Pharm. Bull., 30,* 595-597.

[321] Fujii, T. & Saito, M. (2009). Inhibitory effect of quercetin isolated from rose hip (*Rosa canina* L.) against melanogenesis by mouse melanoma cells. *Biosci. Biotechnol. Biochem., 73,* 1989-1993.

[322] Sasaki, K. & Yoshizaki, F. (2002). Nobiletin as a tyrosinase inhibitor from the peel of *Citrus* fruit. *Biol. Pharm. Bull., 25,* 806-808.

[323] Magid, A. A., Voutquenne-Nazabadioko, L., Bontemps, G., Litaudon, M. & Lavaud, C. (2008). Tyrosinase inhibitors and sesquiterpene diglycosides from *Guioa villosa*. *Planta Med., 74,* 55-60.

[324] Momtaz, S., Mapunya, B. M., Houghton, P. J., Edgerly, C., Hussein, A., Naidoo, S. & Lall, N. (2008). Tyrosinase inhibition by extracts and constituents of *Sideroxylon*

inerme L. stem bark, used in South Africa for skin lightening. *J. Ethnopharmacol., 119,* 507-512.

[325] Azhar, U. Haq., Malik, A., Khan, M. T., Anwar, U. H., Khan, S. B., Ahmad, A. & Choudhary, M. I. (2006). Tyrosinase inhibitory lignans from the methanol extract of the roots of *Vitex negundo* Linn. and their structure-activity relationship. *Phytomedicine, 13,* 255-260.

[326] Ohguchi, K., Tanaka, T., Iliya, I., Ito, T., Iinuma, M., Matsumoto, K., Akao, Y. & Nozawa, Y. (2003). Gnetol as a potent tyrosinase inhibitor from genus *Gnetum. Biosci. Biotechnol. Biochem., 67,* 663-665.

[327] No, J. K., Soung, D. Y., Kim, Y. J., Shim, K. H., Jun, Y. S., Rhee, S. H., Yokozawa, T. & Chung, H. Y. (1999). Inhibition of tyrosinase by green tea components. *Life Sci., 65,* PL241-246.

[328] Choi, S. W., Lee, S. K., Kim, E. O., Oh, J. H., Yoon, K. S., Parris, N., Hicks, K. B. & Moreau, R. A. (2007). Antioxidant and antimelanogenic activities of polyamine conjugates from corn bran and related hydroxycinnamic acids. *J. Agric. Food Chem., 55,* 3920-3925.

[329] Park, J. S., Kim, D. H., Lee, J. K., Lee, J. Y., Kim, D. H., Kim, H. K., Lee, H. J. & Kim, H. C. (2010). Natural ortho-dihydroxyisoflavone derivatives from aged Korean fermented soybean paste as potent tyrosinase and melanin formation inhibitors. *Bioorg. Med. Chem. Lett., 20,* 1162-1164.

[330] Kim, D. C., Rho, S. H., Shin, J. C., Park, H. H. & Kim, D. (2011). Inhibition of melanogenesis by 5,7-dihydroxyflavone (chrysin) via blocking adenylyl cyclase activity. *Biochem. Biophys. Res. Commun., 411,* 121-125.

[331] Sung, J. H., Park, S. H., Seo, D. H., Lee, J. H., Hong, S. W. & Hong, S. S. (2009). Antioxidative and skin-whitening effect of an aqueous extract of *Salicornia herbacea. Biosci. Biotechnol. Biochem., 73,* 552-556.

[332] Cho, Y. H., Kim, J. H., Park, S. M., Lee, B. C., Pyo, H. B. & Park, H. D. (2006). New cosmetic agents for skin whitening from *Angelica dahurica. J. Cosmet Sci., 57,* 11-21.

[333] Kubo, I., Yokokawa, Y. & Kinst-Hori, I. (1988). Tyrosinase inhibitors from cumin. *J. Agric. Food Chem., 46,* 5338-5341.

[334] Lee, K. K. & Choi, J. D. (1999). The effects of *Areca catechu* L extract on anti-inflammation and anti-melanogenesis. *Int. J. Cosmet. Sci., 21,* 275-284.

[335] Behera, B. C., Adawadkar, B. & Makhija, U. (2006). Tyrosinase-inhibitory activity in some species of the lichen family Graphidaceae. *J. Herb Pharmacother., 6,* 55-69.

[336] Luo, L. H., Kim, H. J., Nguyen, D. H., Lee, H. B., Lee, N. H. & Kim, E. K. (2009). Depigmentation of melanocytes by (2Z,8Z)-matricaria acid methyl ester isolated from *Erigeron breviscapus. Biol. Pharm Bull., 32,* 1091-1094.

[337] Chang, Y. H., Kim, C., Jung, M., Lim, Y. H., Lee, S. & Kang, S. (2007). Inhibition of melanogenesis by selina-4(14),7(11)-dien-8-one isolated from *Atractylodis Rhizoma* Alba. *Biol. Pharm. Bull., 30,* 719-723.

[338] Choi, H., Ahn, S., Lee, B. G., Chang, I. & Hwang, J. S. (2005). Inhibition of skin pigmentation by an extract of *Lepidium apetalum* and its possible implication in IL-6 mediated signaling. *Pigment Cell Res., 18,* 439-446.

[339] Wu, B., He, S., Wu, X. D. & Pan, Y. J. (2008). New tyrosinase inhibitory sesquiterpenes from *Chloranthus henryi. Chem. Biodivers., 5,* 1298-1303.

[340] Wu, B., Chen, J., Qu, H. & Cheng, Y. (2008). Complex sesquiterpenoids with tyrosinase inhibitory activity from the leaves of *Chloranthus tianmushanensis*. *J. Nat. Prod., 71*. 877-880.

[341] Khan, M. T., Khan, S. B. & Ather, A. (2006). Tyrosinase inhibitory cycloartane type triterpenoids from the methanol extract of the whole plant of *Amberboa ramosa* Jafri and their structure-activity relationship. *Bioorg Med. Chem., 14*, 938-943.

[342] Choi, J. Y., Choi, E. H., Jung, H. W., Oh, J. S., Lee, W. H., Lee, J. G., Son, J. K., Kim, Y. & Lee, S. H. (2008). Melanogenesis inhibitory compounds from *Saussureae Radix*. *Arch. Pharm. Res., 31,* 294-299.

[343] Issa, R. A., Afifi, F. U. & Amro, B. I. (2008). Studying the anti-tyrosinase effect of *Arbutus andrachne* L. extracts. *Int. J. Cosmet. Sci., 30,* 271-276.

[344] Masamoto, Y., Ando, H., Murata, Y., Shimoishi, Y., Tada, M. & Takahata, K. (2003). Mushroom tyrosinase inhibitory activity of esculetin isolated from seeds of *Euphorbia lathyris* L. *Biosci. Biotechnol. Biochem., 67,* 631-634.

[345] Sabudak, T., Tareq Hassan Khan, M., Iqbal Choudhary, M. & Oksuz, S. (2006). Potent tyrosinase inhibitors from *Trifolium balansae*. *Nat. Prod. Res., 20,* 665-670.

[346] Baurin, N., Arnoult, E., Scior, T., Do, Q. T. & Bernard, P. (2002). Preliminary screening of some tropical plants for anti-tyrosinase activity. *J. Ethnopharmacol., 82,* 155-158.

[347] Li, C. Y., Lee, E. J. & Wu, T. S. (2004). Antityrosinase principles and constituents of the petals of *Crocus sativus*. *J. Nat. Prod., 67,* 437-440.

[348] Lee, S. E., Kim, M. O., Lee, S. G., Ahn, Y. J. & Lee, H. S. (2000). Inhibitory effects of *Cinnamomum cassia* bark-derived materials on mushroom tyrosinase. *Food Sci. Biotechnol., 9,* 330-333.

[349] Wang, H. M., Chen, C. Y. & Wen, Z. H. (2011). Identifying melanogenesis inhibitors from *Cinnamomum subavenium* with *in vitro* and *in vivo* screening systems by targeting the human tyrosinase. *Exp. Dermatol., 20,* 242-248.

[350] Wang, H. M., Chen, C. Y., Chen, C. Y., Ho, M. L., Chou, Y. T., Chang, H. C., Lee, C. H., Wang, C. Z. & Chu, I. M. (2010). (-)-N-Formylanonaine from *Michelia alba* as a human tyrosinase inhibitor and antioxidant. *Bioorg. Med. Chem., 18,* 5241-5247.

[351] Jang, S. G., Jeon, K. S., Lee, E. H., Kong, W. S. & Cho, J. Y. (2009). Isolation of 1',3'-dilinolenoyl'-2'-linoleoylglycerol with tyrosinase inhibitory activity from *Flammulina velutipes*. *J. Microbiol. Biotechnol., 19,* 681-684.

[352] Chang, L. W., Juang, L. J., Wang, B. S., Wang, M. Y., Tai, H. M., Hung, W. J., Chen, Y. J. & Huang, M. H. (2011). Antioxidant and antityrosinase activity of mulberry (*Morus alba* L.) twigs and root bark. *Food Chem. Toxicol., 49,* 785-790.

[353] Kubo, I. & Kinst-Hori, I. (1999). Tyrosinase inhibitory activity of the olive oil flavor compounds. *J. Agric. Food Chem., 47,* 4574-4578.

[354] Wu, L. C., Chang L. H., Chen, S. H., Fan, N. C. & Ho, J. A. (2009). Antioxidant activity and melanogenesis inhibitory effect of the acetonic extract of *Osmanthus fragrans*: a potential natural and functional food flavor additive. LWT- *Food Sci. Technol., 42,* 1513-1519.

[355] Behera, B. C., Verma, N., Sonone, A. & Makhija, U. (2007). Tissue culture of some lichens and screening of their antioxidant, antityrosinase and antibacterial properties. *Phytother. Res., 21,* 1159-1170.

[356] Kumar, C. M., Sathisha, U. V., Dharmesh, S., Rao, A. G. & Singh, S. A. (2011). Interaction of sesamol (3,4-methylenedioxyphenol) with tyrosinase and its effect on melanin synthesis. *Biochimie., 93,* 562-569.

[357] Sharma, V. K., Choi, J., Sharma, N., Choi, M. & Seo, S. Y. (2004). *In vitro* anti-tyrosinase activity of 5-(hydroxymethyl)-2-furfural isolated from *Dictyophora indusiata. Phytother. Res., 18,* 841-844.

[358] Kim, K. S., Kim, J. A., Eom, S. Y., Lee, S. H., Min, K. R. & Kim, Y. (2006). Inhibitory effect of piperlonguminine on melanin production in melanoma B16 cell line by downregulation of tyrosinase expression. *Pigment Cell Res., 19,* 90-98.

[359] Masuda, T., Odaka, Y., Ogawa, N., Nakamoto, K. & Kuninaga, H. (2008). Identification of geranic acid, a tyrosinase inhibitor in lemongrass (*Cymbopogon citratus*). *J. Agric. Food Chem., 56,* 597-601.

[360] Silveira, J. E., Pereda Mdel, C., Eberlin, S., Dieamant, G. C. & Di Stasi, L. C. (2008). Effects of *Coccoloba uvifera* L. on UV-stimulated melanocytes. *Photodermatol. Photoimmunol. Photomed., 24,* 308-313.

[361] Chien, C. C., Tsai, M. L., Chen, C. C., Chang, S. J. & Tseng, C. H. (2008). Effects on tyrosinase activity by the extracts of *Ganoderma lucidum* and related mushrooms. *Mycopathologia., 166,* 117-120.

[362] Jang, J. Y., Lee, J. H., Kang, B. W., Chung, K. T., Choi, Y. H. & Choi, B. T. (2009). Dichloromethane fraction of *Cimicifuga heracleifolia* decreases the level of melanin synthesis by activating the ERK or AKT signaling pathway in B16F10 cells. *Exp. Dermatol., 18,* 232-237.

[363] Itoh, K., Hirata, N., Masuda, M., Naruto, S., Murata, K., Wakabayashi, K. & Matsuda, H. (2009). Inhibitory effects of *Citrus hassaku* extract and its flavanone glycosides on melanogenesis. *Biol. Pharm. Bull., 32,* 410-415.

[364] Rangkadilok, N., Sitthimonchai, S., Worasuttayangkurn, L., Mahidol, C., Ruchirawat, M. & Satayavivad, J. (2007). Evaluation of free radical scavenging and antityrosinase activities of standardized longan fruit extract. *Food Chem. Toxicol., 45,* 328-336.

[365] Oh, E. Y., Jang, J. Y., Choi, Y. H., Choi, Y. W. & Choi, B. T. (2010). Inhibitory effects of 1-O-methyl-fructofuranose from *Schisandra chinensis* fruit on melanogenesis in B16F0 melanoma cells. *J .Ethnopharmacol., 132,* 219-224.

[366] Husni, A., Jeon, J. S., Um, B. H., Han, N. S. & Chung, D. (2011). Tyrosinase inhibition by water and ethanol extracts of a far eastern sea cucumber, *Stichopus japonicus. J. Sci. Food Agric., 91,* 1541-1547.

[367] Villareal, M. O., Han, J., Yamada, P., Shigemori, H. & Isoda, H. (2010). Hirseins inhibit melanogenesis by regulating the gene expressions of Mitf and melanogenesis enzymes. *Exp. Dermatol., 19,* 450-457.

[368] Goetghebeur, M. & Kermasha, S. (1996). Inhibition of polyphenol oxidase by copper-metallothionein from *Aspergillus niger. Phytochemistry, 42,* 935-940.

[369] Piao, X. L., Baek, S. H., Park, M. K. & Park, J. H. (2004). Tyrosinase-inhibitory furanocoumarin from *Angelica dahurica. Biol. Pharm. Bull., 27,* 1144-1146.

[370] Panich, U., Kongtaphan, K., Onkoksoong, T., Jaemsak, K., Phadungrakwittaya, R., Thaworn, A., Akarasereenont, P., & Wongkajornsilp, A. (2010). Modulation of antioxidant defense by *Alpinia galanga* and *Curcuma aromatica* extracts correlates with their inhibition of UVA-induced melanogenesis. *Cell Biol. Toxicol., 26,* 103-116.

[371] Jang, J. Y., Lee, J. H., Jeong, S. Y., Chung, K. T., Choi, Y. H. & Choi, B. T. (2009). Partially purified *Curcuma longa* inhibits alpha-melanocyte-stimulating hormone-stimulated melanogenesis through extracellular signal-regulated kinase or Akt activation-mediated signalling in B16F10 cells. *Exp. Dermatol., 18,* 689-694.

[372] Jeon, H. J., Noda, M., Maruyama, M., Matoba, Y., Kumagai, T. & Sugiyama, M. (2006). Identification and kinetic study of tyrosinase inhibitors found in sake lees. *J. Agric. Food Chem., 54,* 9827-9833.

[373] Wang, B. S., Chang L.W., Wu H. C., Huang S. L., Chu H. L. & Huang M. H. (2011). Antioxidant and antityrosinase activity of aqueous extracts of green asparagus. *Food Chem., 127,* 141-146.

[374] Pinon, A., Limami, Y., Micallef, L., Cook-Moreau, J., Liagre, B., Delage, C., Duval, R. E. & Simon, A. (2011). A novel form of melanoma apoptosis resistance: melanogenesis up-regulation in apoptotic B16-F0 cells delays ursolic acid-triggered cell death. *Exp. Cell Res., 317,* 1669-1676.

[375] Ye, Y., Chu, J. H., Wang, H., Xu, H., Chou, G. X., Leung, A. K., Fong, W. F. & Yu, Z. L. (2010). Involvement of p38 MAPK signaling pathway in the anti-melanogenic effect of San-bai-tang, a Chinese herbal formula, in B16 cells. *J. Ethnopharmacol., 132,* 533-535.

[376] Minwalla, L., Zhao, Y., Cornelius, J., Babcock, G. F., Wickett, R. R., Le Poole, I. C. & Boissy, R. E. (2001). Inhibition of melanosome transfer from melanocytes to keratinocytes by lectins and neoglycoproteins in an *in vitro* model system., *Pigment Cell Res., 14,* 185-194.

[377] Brenner, M. & Hearing, V. J. (2008). Modifying skin pigmentation–approaches through intrinsic biochemistry and exogenous agents. *Drug Discov. Today Dis. Mech., 5,* 189-199.

[378] Akihisa, T., Noto, T., Takahashi, A., Fujita, Y., Banno, N., Tokuda, H., Koike, K., Suzuki, T., Yasukawa, K. & Kimura, Y. (2009). Melanogenesis inhibitory, anti-inflammatory, and chemopreventive effects of limonoids from the seeds of *Azadirachta indicia* A. Juss. (neem). *J. Oleo. Sci., 58,* 581-594.

[379] Yokota, T., Nishio, H., Kubota, Y. & Mizoguchi, M. (1998). The inhibitory effect of glabridin from licorice extracts on melanogenesis and inflammation. *Pigment Cell Res., 11,* 355-361.

[380] Kim, Y. J., Kang, K. S. & Yokozawa, T. (2008). The anti-melanogenic effect of pycnogenol by its anti-oxidative actions. *Food Chem. Toxicol., 46,* 2466-2471.

[381] Heo, S. J., Ko, S. C., Cha, S. H., Kang, D. H., Park, H. S., Choi, Y. U., Kim, D., Jung, W. K. & Jeon, Y. J. (2009). Effect of phlorotannins isolated from *Ecklonia cava* on melanogenesis and their protective effect against photo-oxidative stress induced by UV-B radiation. *Toxicol. Vitro, 23,* 1123-1130.

[382] Heo, S. J., Ko, S. C., Kang, S. M., Cha, S. H., Lee, S. H., Kang, D. H., Jung, W. K., Affan, A., Oh, C. & Jeon, Y. J. (2010). Inhibitory effect of diphlorethohydroxycarmalol on melanogenesis and its protective effect against UV-B radiation-induced cell damage. *Food Chem. Toxicol., 48,* 1355-1361.

[383] Huang, H. C., Chiu, S. H. & Chang, T. M. (2011). Inhibitory Effect of [6]-Gingerol on Melanogenesis in B16F10 Melanoma Cells and a Possible Mechanism of Action. *Biosci. Biotechnol. Biochem., 75,* 1067-1072.

[384] Hamed, S. H., Sriwiriyanont, P., de Long, M. A., Visscher, M. O., Wickett, R. R. & Boissy, R. E. (2006). Comparative efficacy and safety of deoxyarbutin, a new tyrosinase-inhibiting agent. *J. Cosmet. Sci., 57,* 291-308.

[385] Miyamoto, K., Takiwaki, H., Hillebrand, G. G. & Arase, S. (2002). Utilization of a high-resolution digital imaging system for the objective and quantitative assessment of hyperpigmented spots on the face. *Skin Res. Technol., 8,* 73-77.

[386] Kasai, K., Yoshimura, M., Koga, T., Arii, M. & Kawasaki, S. (2006). Effects of oral administration of ellagic acid-rich pomegranate extract on ultraviolet-induced pigmentation in the human skin. *J. Nutr. Sci. Vitaminol. (Tokyo), 52,* 383-388.

[387] Ertam, I., Mutlu, B., Unal, I., Alper, S., Kivcak, B. & Ozer, O. (2008). Efficiency of ellagic acid and arbutin in melasma: a randomized, prospective, open-label study. *J. Dermatol., 35,* 570-574.

[388] Mafune, E., Morimoto, Y. & Iizuka, Y. (2008). Tranexamic acid and melasma. *Farumashia., 44,* 437-442.

Index

D

E

F

G

H

I

N

O

P

Q

R

T

U

V

W

X

Y

Z